Praise for Taking Charge of ADHD

"Dr. Barkley is a foremost researcher who has devoted his career to teaching and helping those with ADHD. This book brings together in one place everything that parents need to cope with daily challenges and make important decisions about their child's care. Dr. Barkley's knowledge, brilliance, and dedication shine through on every page like a beacon of hope."

—Edward M. Hallowell, MD, coauthor of *Driven to Distraction*

"An invaluable, comprehensive resource. The book arms you with the most current scientific facts, including a clear explanation of executive functions and their role in ADHD. Dr. Barkley has a gift for providing practical, easy-to-understand guidance that empowers you to become an effective advocate for your child."

—Chris A. Zeigler Dendy, MS, parent and author of *Teaching Teens with ADD, ADHD & Executive Function Deficits*

"Dr. Barkley helps parents make order out of chaos and problem-solve more effectively. That's what I love about this book! *Taking Charge* treats parents respectfully and intelligently. You'll go back repeatedly—maybe even every day—to the sections on becoming an executive parent and managing life with ADHD."

—Mary Fowler, parent and author of *Maybe You Know My Kid*

"This is not just another book. This is a great book....Although aimed at parents, it has something for everyone involved with ADHD kids: teachers, psychologists, doctors, and family. I am not going to lend this book to parents (although I will show it to them) because they need to buy it so they have it on hand to read and reread."

—*Pediatric News* (review by J. Clyde Ralph, MD)

"An excellent and readable book that will empower parents of children with ADHD."

—*NAMI Advocate*

"As a starting point for parents, or for smaller libraries that can only afford one title, Barkley's book is the first choice."

—*Library Journal*

"I am always looking for the best book, the right book or the latest book. Let me tell you about one: Russell A. Barkley, PhD's, *Taking Charge of ADHD.*"

—*Psychiatric Times* (review by Ellen R. Fischbein, MD)

"This book features pioneering research that provides new insight into preventing ADHD from becoming a major obstacle in a child's (and parent's) life....Parents will appreciate having this book on hand, and teachers will want a copy to show parents who are ready for a resource."

—*Intervention in School and Clinic*

"If any professional knows about ADHD, it is Russell Barkley....All in all, this is a splendid book."

—*Child and Family Behavior Therapy*

Taking Charge of ADHD

Selected works from Russell A. Barkley

For more information, visit the author's website: *www.russellbarkley.org*

For General Readers

Taking Charge of Adult ADHD
Russell A. Barkley with Christine M. Benton

Your Defiant Child, Second Edition: Eight Steps to Better Behavior
Russell A. Barkley and Christine M. Benton

Your Defiant Teen: 10 Steps to Resolve Conflict and Rebuild Your Relationship
Russell A. Barkley and Arthur L. Robin with Christine M. Benton

For Professionals

ADHD and the Nature of Self-Control
Russell A. Barkley

ADHD in Adults: What the Science Says
Russell A. Barkley, Kevin R. Murphy, and Mariellen Fischer

Attention-Deficit Hyperactivity Disorder, Third Edition:
A Clinical Workbook
Russell A. Barkley and Kevin R. Murphy

Attention-Deficit Hyperactivity Disorder, Third Edition:
A Handbook for Diagnosis and Treatment
Russell A. Barkley

Barkley Deficits in Executive Functioning Scale—
Children and Adolescents (BDEFS-CA)
Russell A. Barkley

Barkley Functional Impairment Scale—
Children and Adolescents (BFIS-CA)
Russell A. Barkley

Executive Functions:
What They Are, How They Work, and Why They Evolved
Russell A. Barkley

Taking Charge *of* ADHD

THIRD EDITION

The Complete, Authoritative Guide for Parents

RUSSELL A. BARKLEY, PhD

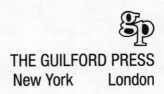

THE GUILFORD PRESS
New York London

A Division of Guilford Publications, Inc.
370 Seventh Avenue, Suite 1200, New York, NY 10001
www.guilford.com

The information in this volume is not intended as a substitute for consultation with healthcare professionals. Each individual's health concerns should be evaluated by a qualified professional.

Printed in the United States of America

This book is printed on acid-free paper.

Last digit is print number: 9 8 7 6 5 4

Library of Congress Cataloging-in-Publication Data

Barkley, Russell A., 1949–
Taking charge of ADHD : the complete, authoritative guide for parents / Russell A. Barkley. — Third edition.
pages cm
Includes bibliographical references and index.
ISBN 978-1-4625-0851-8 (hardcover : alk. paper) — ISBN 978-1-4625-0789-4 (pbk. : alk. paper)
1. Attention-deficit hyperactivity disorder—Popular works. 2. Child rearing—Popular works. I. Title.
RJ506.H9B373 2013
618.92′8589—dc23

2012050510

To Sandra F. Thomas and Mary Fowler,
two extraordinary parents who started a movement
and awakened a nation to the suffering of children
with attention-deficit/hyperactivity disorder

Contents

Preface xi

Introduction: A Guiding Philosophy for Parents of Children with ADHD 1

Part I
Understanding ADHD

1 What Is Attention-Deficit/Hyperactivity Disorder? 19

2 "What's Really Wrong with My Child?": Poor Self-Control 53

3 What Causes ADHD? 71

4 What to Expect: The Nature of the Disorder 100

5 The Family Context of a Child with ADHD 120

Part II
Taking Charge:
How to Be a Successful Executive Parent

6 Deciding to Have Your Child Evaluated for ADHD 131

7 Preparing for the Evaluation 139

8 Coping with the Diagnosis of ADHD 152

9 Fourteen Guiding Principles for Raising a Child with ADHD 158

10 Just for Parents: How to Take Care of Yourself 169

Part III

Managing Life with ADHD: How to Cope at Home and at School

11 Eight Steps to Better Behavior 181

12 Taking Charge at Home: The Art of Problem Solving 210

13 How to Help Your Child with Peer Problems 216

14 Getting through Adolescence 226
with Arthur L. Robin, PhD

15 Off to School on the Right Foot: Managing Your Child's Education 246
with Linda J. Pfiffner, PhD

16 Enhancing Education at School and at Home: Methods for Success from Kindergarten through Grade 12 263
with Linda J. Pfiffner, PhD

17 Keeping School Performance in Perspective 284

Part IV

Medications for ADHD

18 The Approved Effective Medicines: Stimulants and Nonstimulants 293

19 Other Medicines: Antidepressants and Antihypertensives 319

Support Services for Parents 327

Suggested Reading and Videos 329

References 343

Index 351

About the Author 363

Purchasers may download and print select practical tools from this book at *www.guilford.com/p/barkley.*

Preface

It is quite normal for children to be more active, more exuberant, less attentive, and more impulsive than adults. It is hardly surprising that children have more problems than adults in following through on directions and consistently finishing their work. So when parents complain that their child has difficulty paying attention, controlling his activity, or resisting impulses, others may be quick to dismiss these problems simply as normal behavior and to reassure parents that they are natural qualities of children and there is no need for alarm. If a child's behavior problems seem a little excessive, even for a child, it is probably the case that he is simply a little immature and will likely outgrow these problems.

Usually this is true—but there are times when it is not. In some cases a child's attention span is so short, activity level so high, and impulse control so limited that her behavior in these areas is clearly extreme for her age. Most people have known such a child—one who is having trouble completing schoolwork, who may not be getting along well with the neighborhood children, whose inability to follow through and complete assigned chores without parental supervision is causing conflict at home.

Behavior problems in these areas that have become so severe as to impair a child's adjustment are not likely to be outgrown, and they can hardly be considered normal. If you have such a child, it is not only misguided but potentially harmful to your child's psychological and social well-being to downplay the problems or simply to give your child time to mature a little more. Doing so could also cause future problems for you and other family members who must deal with this child every day.

Children whose problems with attention, overactivity, and lack of inhibition reach a certain level have a developmental disability known as *attention-deficit/hyperactivity disorder,* or *ADHD*. This book is about ADHD. It is intended for parents who are raising a child with ADHD and for others who wish to know more about the disorder and its management. The main goal is to empower parents to take charge of the care of these often demanding children in a way that ensures the health of the entire family, collectively and individually.

Numerous books on this subject directed to parents have already been published. Most are pretty good, and there are a few I recommend to the families we see at our clinic. Why, then, did I want to write another? The answer is that the books available just don't go far enough in educating parents about what is currently known about ADHD and, more important, about what can be done to help those with the disorder. Most books for parents successfully convey what has been gained from years of clinical experience in treating children with ADHD and their families, but they fail to integrate the most current scientific breakthroughs. The growth in research on ADHD over the last 20 years alone, since the original edition of this book was published, has been nothing short of astounding. Yet in most other books on this subject, the conclusions and recommendations come only from the clinical experience of the author—and have often been wrong. For instance, in the last 10 years, advances in the molecular genetics of ADHD have progressed at a rapid pace and continue to do so today. At least seven genes for the disorder have been reliably identified, and researchers expect that a number of others will be found in the next few years. The entire human genome has been scanned for ADHD risk genes, and at least 25–40 locations appear to be relevant to the disorder. Brain imaging research has also shown us the regions implicated in ADHD and even linked some of the activities in these areas to some of the risk genes for the disorder. The pace of research is rapid and the results are piling up quickly.

These findings have important implications for parents. They continue to underscore the conclusion of the previous editions of this book that ADHD is a largely biologically caused disorder that has a substantial genetic/hereditary basis. Those findings also point to possible future breakthroughs in diagnosis and treatment over the next decade because they imply that genetic testing for the disorder eventually may be possible. And so may be the development of much safer, more effective medications for the management of the disorder. Parents need to be aware of these sorts of developments so that they can better understand the disorder and respond to scientifically illiterate critics who continue to insist that ADHD arises from poor parenting, diet, or excessive TV viewing.

For instance, for several decades, most clinical professionals operated according to the fallacious notions that ADHD was caused by poor parenting; that children would eventually outgrow it by adolescence; that stimulant medications would be effective only with children (not with older adolescents and adults) and should be used only on school days; and that children with ADHD would benefit from a diet free of certain food additives and sugar—all despite the absence of any set of findings in the scientific literature to support such claims. More recently, some authors have claimed that the disorder results from too much playing of video games, too much TV viewing, or the increased pace of modern culture. We now understand that many children with ADHD have inherited a genetic form of the disorder, that many do not outgrow their problems by adolescence, that medication can be taken year-round by adolescents and adults as well as children, and that altering sugar in diets does little to benefit most people with ADHD. And we also know that ADHD does not arise from video games, TV, or the fast pace of modern life. How far we have come in just 40 years of research! In fact exciting changes, some profound, have taken place over the last 10 years and continue to do so as of this writing. These changes pertain not only to a better understanding of the causes of ADHD, but also to a richer scientific understanding of the nature of ADHD that has been radically changing the way we look at this disorder.

Within the last decade scientific studies have shown, for example, that ADHD probably is not primarily a disorder of paying attention but one of *self-regulation*: how our sense of self develops so that we can manage ourselves within the larger realm of social behavior. Thus, even the name *ADHD* may now be incorrect, though it will continue to be used for the time being for various legal reasons. To label it a disorder of attention trivializes the disorder, since it grossly understates the substantial and dramatic problems these children face in trying to meet the challenges of their daily lives and the increasing demands of their families, schools, and society to regulate themselves as they mature. Calling the disorder an attention deficit is also not able to account for the myriad ways that it diminishes individuals' capacity to meet their responsibilities toward self and others. For instance, my own studies and later those of others have shown that children and adults with ADHD have a disturbed ability to manage themselves relative to time itself. They do not use their sense of time to guide their behavior as well as others, and therefore cannot manage themselves relative to time, deadlines, and the future generally as well as others are able to do. This includes intervals of time as short as 10–20 seconds. Time escapes them, and they are never as able to deal with it as effectively as others of their age group do.

In spite of how debilitating ADHD can be, it is not surprising that many remain skeptical about the seriousness of the disorder. All of us occasionally have trouble paying attention, and children do especially. Conquering impulsivity and restlessness, some people claim, is just a matter of buckling down. Or is it? Teachers, relatives, neighbors, and others may try to convince you that it is. They don't understand what you do: that there is something fundamentally and significantly wrong with your child's conduct. Many stories on TV and in the print media have claimed that the disorder is a myth perpetrated in order to label merely adventuresome children, especially boys—the Tom Sawyers and Huck Finns of modern life—with a psychiatric diagnosis. Fringe religious groups have challenged the very existence of the disorder and scathingly criticize the use of medication for its management. A thorough understanding of the scientific literature clearly reveals the fallacies in these ideas, yet parents may continue to be bombarded periodically with these or other scientifically unfounded claims about ADHD. All of these misconceptions will be dealt with in this book, in the chapters that address the nature of the disorder and its causes as we now understand them.

In contrast to these relatively popular but indefensible views, the phenomenon we call ADHD is, I have come to believe, a disturbance in a child's ability to inhibit immediate reactions to the moment so as to use self-control with regard to time and the future. That is, those with ADHD ultimately suffer from an inability to use a sense of time and of the past and future to guide their behavior. What is not developing properly in your child is the capacity to shift from focusing on the here and now to focusing on what is likely to come next in life and the future more generally. When all a child focuses on is the moment, acting impulsively makes sense. The child simply wants to do what is fun or interesting at the moment and escape from what is not reinforcing at the time, maximizing immediate gratification as much as possible. From the child's perspective, it is always "now." But this can be disastrous when the child is expected to be developing a focus on what lies ahead and what needs to be done to meet the future effectively. That capacity is crucial to our ability as human beings to be organized, planful, and goal-directed, and it is directly dependent on how much control we have over our impulses. It frees us from being controlled by the moment and allows us to be influenced by the future. This view of ADHD significantly dignifies the condition and its consequent problems. It explains why those with ADHD are not always able to act as others act, and it provides us with the basis for respecting them, deepening our understanding of how ADHD impairs a person's daily life. This book has much more to say on this point and what it means for understanding ADHD. Indeed, the chief reason I wrote it originally was to develop this idea for parents, and my principal goal in revising it is to bring this view up to date. I believe this view comes much closer to conveying the scientific reality of ADHD than other viewpoints have done.

I also felt compelled to write this book because I saw a need to teach parents to be *scientific* in their attempts to get information or seek help from professionals. To be scientific is to be both inquisitive and skeptical, to pursue and yet challenge your sources of information for their rationale. So another goal of this book is to give you as a parent the tools you need to stay well informed and to question *everything* you hear and read—including the information in this book. This need for an optimistic and inquisitive form of skepticism is even more necessary now than it was for the original edition of this book. That is because we are now experiencing a veritable information explosion in modern culture, due largely to the increasingly widespread availability of the personal computer and in particular the development and widespread availability of the Internet. Every household with a computer and an Internet connection or a smart phone can now connect to the information highway. Unfortunately, what gets on that highway is frequently not the most accurate information on a subject. Because it is not peer-reviewed or critiqued, the information that awaits you there is often a thinly veiled sales pitch for some product, herbal remedy, or political point of view. And it is not just the websites related to ADHD that can be misinforming, but the blogs and chat rooms as well. Here everyone with harebrained ideas can hold forth on these opinions, with no credentials in this area of research and no scientific information to back them up. My visits to those blogs or chat rooms have convinced me that the vast majority of information exchanged on them is largely unscientific opinion and is largely wrong. So, whether at your local library, bookstore, or online, never let your skepticism down.

But don't stop inquiring either. You need all the information you can get about ADHD to raise your child. Arming yourself with the facts as they are uncovered is the first step toward becoming an "executive parent," one who retains the ultimate decision-making authority over the child's care by others, whether physicians, psychologists, nurses, social workers, or educators. These professionals are merely your advisers in their areas of specialization. No one—and I mean *no one*—knows your child as well as you do. An underlying tenet of this book is that *you* are in charge of your child's professional and educational care. Each of the following chapters has been written with the goal of *empowering you* to take that responsibility, to relieve you of the distressing feeling that you are losing control of your child's care—and perhaps, in the process, your child. In short, this book will teach you *how* to make decisions and even *when* they should be made. But it cannot and should not make your decisions about your child for you. Neither should any other book or person.

The lessons offered in this volume have emerged from my clinical work and research with several thousand families of children with ADHD over the last 35 years. They have also evolved from my own continuing journey of attempted self-improvement as a person, a father, a husband, a scientist, a teacher, a supervisor, and a clinical professional. It was no single case that resulted in the conclusions in this book. No one book shaped my ideas. No great flash of insight occurred. Instead, I had an ever-growing sense of the importance of certain principles as I worked with each new family, read each new book on the subject, and taught each new student. Unlike the techniques of management I have taught to parents, or the facts I have provided them about the disorder and the treatments currently available, these principles cut across a wide variety of situations, families, and problem areas. They can form a bedrock attitude for any actions you may take on behalf of your child with ADHD.

The information and advice contained in this book are similar to what I would say to a parent whose child I had evaluated. These recommendations have been drawn from extensive scientific research and represent the equivalent of approximately 20–25 sessions of counseling or therapy. Still, you will not find everything you need in this one book. It is impossible to encapsulate here the thousands of scientific articles on the subject. And even though ADHD is among the most well studied of all childhood psychological disorders, as clinical scientists there is much that my colleagues and I still do not know. ADHD remains misunderstood and controversial in the minds of the general public as well as the educational establishment.

This volume attempts to cut through myths and misinformation about ADHD by relying on what is currently understood to be accurate and scientifically verifiable. For particular issues about which no information is available or about which the information is not certain, I have said so. Our research continues. Also, every case of ADHD is unique. I must leave it to you to tailor information and advice to the circumstances of your own child's case and your own family's unique context. Where you still have questions about how to handle certain problems with your child, I strongly suggest that you seek out the professionals in your community who are most informed about ADHD to see if they can be of help.

What you will find in this book is much of what you need to know about ADHD and about the special changes you will have to make in your life and your child's life to raise your child to a well-adjusted adulthood. Throughout, this information is presented with the goal of teaching you executive parenthood, scientific inquiry, and principle-centered action. Although the ideas expressed here have been influenced by many people over my 35 years of clinical work, the opinions expressed here are strictly my own, or those of my coauthors in those chapters so designated.

I once more wish to thank my wife, Pat, and our sons, Ken and Steve, for their support of my writing in general and this project in particular. As Milton says, "They also serve who only stand and wait," and this is surely true of the members of an author's family.

Again, I wish to express my deepest gratitude to Kitty Moore, Seymour Weingarten, and Bob Matloff of The Guilford Press for their support of the idea for this book and their nurturance of the manuscript to its final, published stage, both for the original edition and now for this revised one. Among the many members of the Guilford "family," substantial credit must go to Christine M. Benton for her tremendous investment in the editing and organization of the book through all of its editions and her constant encouragement of me to say what I wanted and needed to say in the most effective way. The book reads and lives as it does mostly because of her.

Finally, I continue to thank all of those parents of children with ADHD who have shared their lives with me in seeking assistance for their children. Much of what you will learn from this book they have taught me. I can only hope that I have continued to learn their lessons well enough to benefit you and your child.

Taking Charge of ADHD

Introduction

A GUIDING PHILOSOPHY FOR PARENTS OF CHILDREN WITH ADHD

"Help me. I'm losing my child."

More than 20 years ago, in 1990, I was part of the herculean effort by parents and professionals to gain access to special education services for children with ADHD. In the midst of my preoccupation with a battle waged on federal and state levels, I received one of life's profound lessons—a lesson that shed much light on the monumental task this book encourages you to undertake on behalf of your child's academic success.

The best clinicians say that they may learn as much from some of their clients as their clients do from them, if only they will listen and be guided and moved by what they hear. This particular lesson was taught to me one very busy morning in my practice at our ADHD clinic several years ago, and the wise mother who offered it probably has no idea how her family's dilemma affected me or how many subsequent families she may have helped through the change she inspired in my own professional practices. This was an experience that shook me mentally to the core. The wonderment of it lasted several days, and the lesson from it has stayed with me ever since.

The morning I was to meet this mother and her 8-year-old child, whom I'll call Steve, was hectic even before our scheduled 9:00 A.M. appointment. I am sure I must have entered the clinic with a flurry of activity, charts and papers about me, probably apologizing for running late. As I quickly scanned the chart for the demographic form and its information that we obtain routinely by mail before the appointment, I was fully expecting the usual complaints from the mother about how terribly her child and

---

Portions of this chapter are adapted from the speech "Help Me, I'm Losing My Child" that I gave as keynote speaker at the national convention of Children and Adults with Attention-Deficit/Hyperactivity Disorder (CHADD) in Chicago on October 15, 1992. The complete transcript is available on tape from CHADD, (301) 306-7070; *www.chadd.org.*

their family were doing. When I ask my typical first question—either “What are you most concerned about with your child?” or “What brings you to our clinic today?”—it is a rare parent who does not immediately respond with myriad school-related problems; second to this is often an equally long list of all of the child’s negative and unruly behaviors at home. So conditioned are we clinicians to hear this response that we virtually hallucinate hearing this litany before parents speak it. I had, in fact, already headed my paper with “School Problems” and “Home Problems” in such anticipation.

This mother’s response was so astonishing to me, so unpredictable, that I was stunned into silence. I am sure my mouth must have hung open in surprise. For she did not say what I knew to expect: “My child is failing at school,” “My child is about to be suspended,” or “My child won’t listen to anything I say.” No, quite the contrary: what she said was “Help me. I’m losing my child.”

In shock, I must have said, “Pardon me?” She simply said it again. “Help me. I’m losing my child.” What on earth could she mean?, I thought to myself. What new species of parent was this? “I see,” I said, nodding with a knowing, sympathetic glance. “You are in the midst of a custody battle with your ex-husband.”

A clinician who is caught off-guard once can gloss over the fact quickly by moving on with the interview, but to be stunned twice by unexpected responses left me off-balance and utterly bewildered. My only response to her “No” while trying to regain my composure was “I’m sorry, I don’t think I understand what you mean.” Clearly this was true. There was no place on my notepad for such a response.

Tears came to her eyes then, further adding to my own clumsiness and discomfort, and she proceeded to explain. “It has been going on for some time,” she said, “at least a few years. I can’t pinpoint when it started, but I sense it is happening as surely as a mother can know her own child. I am losing him; Steve is drifting away from me, and I may never get him back. That would be the worst thing in the world for me.”

I had no clinical hunches to guide me, so I softly asked her to go on.

“He is my first child,” she said, “and we were always very close until this all began to happen several years ago. Now I think he hates me. I know he doesn’t want to spend time with me.”

“Why do you say that?” I asked.

“Because when I come into a room, he becomes cool toward me, very clipped when I speak with him, and sometimes even sarcastic,” she replied. “If I suggest we do things together, which he used to love to do, he says ‘No’ and seems to find any excuse to avoid me. When I try to talk with him, he doesn’t look at me the way he used to do, but turns away and tries to quickly end the conversation. He is also spending more time away from home, at friends’ houses, and doesn’t bring his friends around here the way he used to do. He always seemed proud that I was his mom, until this began to happen. Now he doesn’t even acknowledge that I exist unless he absolutely has to, and certainly doesn’t introduce his new friends to me the way he used to do.”

“Go on,” I said, still not fully comprehending the problem or the exact nature of her grief. She then explained in detail how her relationship with her son seemed lost, ruined, and possibly even irreparable. This is what she had lost or was in the process of losing: her bond with her first child, the natural reciprocal love between parent and offspring, the foundation on which all of the rest of successful and fulfilling parenting truly depends. Oh, you can certainly raise a child without this bond—in some technical, logistical, or pragmatic sense, but not in the real sense, not in that emotional or spiritual sense of having fully brought up a child.

I have never known a parent to cut so quickly to the root issue in her life, the very crux of her own—and probably her son's—unhappiness. The loss she was describing is so deeply embedded in family life that it is rarely articulated even when it is happening. It is a loss that may be exceeded only by the real loss of a child through death. The relationship she was losing is the dynamic that truly drives all parent–child interactions and all actions by parents on behalf of their families. It has been said about death that when we lose our parents we lose our past, but to lose a child is to lose the future. How true for this mother who sensed the loss of her bond with her child! She could not see what meaningful future lay before her without the love and friendship of her child, whom she had once known so deeply.

She spoke so clearly of this change in her relationship with her child that I could not help examining, in parallel, my own relationship to my two sons. Was I losing them, as she was? What a fool I seemed to myself in the presence of this woman's profound wisdom about her life—our lives. How blind I was not to have seen in countless cases before her, in the unhappiness I had encountered in families who had come to our clinic, that this had really been the significant issue in their lives all along!

You may be reading this book because you too feel you are losing your child. Your child has been diagnosed as having ADHD, and you have been doing your best to help the child and the rest of your family to adjust. But it just isn't working.

Or perhaps you have not reached this stage; you know something is wrong with your child and are beginning to seek professional help. So far, however, you have more questions than answers.

Wherever you and your family stand, you are not alone. Current figures put the number of children with ADHD at over 2.5 million of school age, conservatively estimated. Talk to a parent of any one of them and you're likely to hear a familiar story:

Something is clearly wrong with your child's behavior. He* is losing precious parts of his childhood, and you feel frustrated and confused about what is causing this to happen and what to do about it. Your child is not at peace within the dynamics of your family. There is much daily conflict over chores, homework, relations with siblings, and behavior at school or in the neighborhood. Your child has few if any friends. The phone calls from classmates, the knocks at the door by neighborhood children, the adventures such playmates share in growing up together, and the invitations to

*Note that throughout this book, I alternate between using masculine and feminine pronouns to describe a child with ADHD.

birthday parties and sleep-overs that are daily events in most young lives are either missing or rare in your child's life. Success at school and excitement about learning—grades, certificates of achievement and citizenship, compliments from teachers—are not where they should be for your child's ability and talent, and you know it.

Valuable years and experiences of childhood are being tarnished by something you cannot see but know is there. Whatever this problem may be, it handicaps the very fabric of your child's daily interaction with others. And more painful than all of this is that you sense—as only a parent can—that your child is not at peace with himself. He is gradually becoming aware that he is not what he wants to be, cannot control as well as others what he knows he should do, cannot make himself into the child he somehow knows you wish he could be. He discourages you, dissatisfies others, and disappoints himself, and at some primitive level of awareness he has come to know it. Perhaps you see a familiar sequence played out almost daily: the low self-esteem, the dragging through the door after school with a downcast look, the efforts to escape discussions about schoolwork, the lies to himself and others about how bad things really are, the promises to try harder next time that never quite materialize, and (for some children) the wish to be dead. You hurt; your child hurts.

What is wrong? Your child looks physically normal. Nothing outward suggests a problem. Your child is not mentally delayed. Most likely she walks, talks, hears, and sees normally and has at least normal intellect or better. Yet with each passing year she seems increasingly less able than other children to inhibit her behavior, manage herself, and meet the challenges the future is throwing at her. You know that if you do not do something to help soon, she is destined to lead a troubled life of underachievement as surely as today rises out of the past and the future out of today. Your desire for a normal, peaceful, loving family life with this child; your hopes for her educational and occupational success; your striving to give her a life perhaps better than you had yourself; your wish to have her stand on your shoulders to reach further ahead in life—now all these seem in jeopardy because of something you cannot quite see or understand. You are at times perplexed, puzzled, angry, sad, anxious, fearful, guilty, and helpless in the face of what afflicts your child. You seek answers and guidance.

Instinctively, you may have sensed that what you face with this child is in some way a disability of self-control or will. What constitutes our will? What makes us do what we know we should do, behave toward others as we know we ought to do, and complete the work that we know how to do and that must be done? More generally, what makes us self-disciplined and persistent so we can turn away from immediate gratification and meet the challenges of today to prepare for the future like others of our age? Whatever it is within us that permits us to act with self-control, to adhere to our morals and values, to "walk our talk," and to act with a sense of the future is not developing so well in your child. Perhaps that is what has brought you to this book. Perhaps your child has ADHD. This book can help you find out. It can also advise you on how to cope effectively if your child has the disorder.

The Challenge of Raising a Child with ADHD

Raising a child with ADHD can be incredibly challenging for any parent. These children are very inattentive, impulsive or uninhibited, overactive, and demanding. Their problems can place a burden on your role as a parent that you never thought possible when you first considered having a child. These problems may even have caused you to rethink the wisdom of that decision.

In areas where any reasonable and competent parent *wishes* to be involved in child rearing, parents of a child with ADHD *must* become involved—doubly involved. They must search out schools, teachers, professionals, and other community resources. They will find themselves having to supervise, monitor, teach, organize, plan, structure, reward, punish, guide, buffer, protect, and nurture their child far more than is demanded of a typical parent. They also will have to meet more often with other adults involved in the child's daily life: school staff, pediatricians, and mental health professionals. Then there is all the intervention with neighbors, Scout leaders, coaches, and others in the community necessitated by the greater behavior problems the child is likely to have when dealing with these outsiders.

To make matters more difficult, the increased need of a child with ADHD for parental guidance, protection, advocacy, love, and nurturance can be hidden behind a facade of excessive, demanding, and at times obnoxious behavior. Margaret Flacy from Dallas, mother of two boys (now young adults) with ADHD, put it beautifully when she wrote to me: "early in my career as a teacher [when] I was bemoaning my inability to cope with a particularly difficult child . . . who in hindsight was probably as [severely affected by] ADHD as they come . . . a wonderful and wise retired teacher took my hand and said, 'Margaret, the children who need love the most will always ask for it in the most unloving ways.' "

Many parents with whom I have had the privilege to work find that the challenge of raising a child with ADHD elevates parenting to a new, higher plane. Bringing up a child with ADHD may be the hardest thing you ever have to do. Some parents succumb to the stress such a child can place on them, winding up with a child or a family in constant crisis or, worse, with a family that breaks apart over time. But if you rise to the challenge, raising a child with ADHD can provide a tremendous opportunity for self-improvement, fulfillment as a parent, and even heroism in that role. You can watch your direct investment of time and energy pay off in the happiness and well-being of your child—not always, but often enough to make it richly fulfilling for many parents. To know that you are truly needed by such a child can bring a deeper purpose to your life than many other things can do.

The words of Margaret Flacy's mentor became the keystones for the rearing of Flacy's own sons and all the children she taught over 30 years. They also illustrate the importance of centering your child-rearing philosophy on certain proven principles. If you view your parental responsibility as resting on a tripod, the first leg is the principle-centered approach. Add executive parenthood and scientific thinking, and your strategy for raising a well-adjusted child will have a firm and balanced base.

Becoming a Principle-Centered Parent

For more than three decades I have counseled parents on the methods that seem most effective in managing children with ADHD. For the first 5 years of developing my clinical practice, that is all I did. Then, from both my practice and research, a feeling began to emerge that some larger, deeper principles were at work. As these became clearer, I wrote them down. They became some of the first things taught in my parent-training classes on child management, and I passed them on to my junior colleagues and to others through my many workshops for professionals. The list eventually grew to the 14 principles presented in Chapter 9. They are useful because, simply, when you see the "why," you are more likely to do the "how." That is, you are more likely to use the special management aids your child with ADHD needs—and to apply them creatively—when you know why you're using them and why they work.

Being principle-centered also keeps you on a straight course through a twisting, turning journey. It establishes a pattern whereby you act not on impulses, but on rules—from a sense of the future and what is right, not from the transitory feelings of the moment. It frees your behavior from control by the immediate actions of your child and the visceral negative emotions these actions may elicit, and it directs your behavior according to your ideals. Being principle-centered allows you to disengage from the downward spiraling of hostilities with your child (or others) and to act from a plan and sense of what is right. In short, it enables you to hold yourself to higher standards of parenting than others may follow.

Being principle-centered in your interactions with your child is both liberating and encumbering. It means you have far more control over the outcome of the interaction than your child does, because you have the freedom to act to change what happens. It means you cannot blame your child entirely for the conflicts or hostilities between you, that you cannot blame professionals or others who counsel you if things go wrong between you and your child, and that you cannot divert the responsibility for your actions with your child to your past or to others who raised and taught you. Principle-centered parenting means owning the responsibility of your self-determined actions. It makes you immensely free yet awesomely accountable.

As I continued my study of ADHD and my own journey of self-improvement, I came to realize that another set of principles, which I now think of as first-order principles, applies to *all* parents. Dr. Stephen R. Covey has spelled them out far more clearly and forcefully than I could in *The Seven Habits of Highly Effective People,* a book I highly recommend, but here I have rewritten them to apply to raising a child with ADHD:

1. *"Be proactive."* Far too often we *react* to our children's behavior, often on impulse, without regard for the consequences and with no plan for what we are trying to achieve. In those instances we are being acted on and not consciously choosing to act. Seeing a situation from a reactive frame of mind can sometimes make it seem hopeless—your destiny with your child is being controlled by the child or other outside agents. Negative interactions with your child simply wash over you unpredictably, knocking you off-balance like waves when you stand backward (and unprepared) in the surf. You feel helpless, and your relationship with your child can become hostile, negative, discouraging, stressful, or dysfunctional. But it is not *what your child does* or does to you that creates these problems for you, but *your responses.* Take responsibility for your own behavior as a parent and for the interactions and relationship with your child. Take the initiative to change what you do not like in the way you act toward your child, and accept the responsibility to make this relationship happen the way you would like it to be. You have the ability to subordinate your impulses to your values, Dr. Covey says. You have the freedom to choose your actions with your child. Develop that sense of choice, practice it, and exercise it.

2. *"Begin with the end in mind."* When faced with a problem, try to envision how you want it to turn out. You can apply this principle on a small scale, such as envisioning how you wish the evening's homework session to turn out before you begin, or on a larger scale, such as how you would like your child to reflect on your having helped him complete an important goal, like graduating from high school. Even more broadly, you can try an exercise Dr. Covey recommends. Picture your own funeral service. Your child with ADHD has been asked to say a few words about you during the service. What would you want him to say you were like as a parent? Beginning with the end in mind helps focus our mind more clearly on what matters most and see what we must do to make situations turn out the way we would like.

You cannot have a plan without a goal, a map without a destination, or a set of strategies to use with your child without knowing what outcome you desire. For instance, at a time when you might be prepared to get your child to work with you on putting together a science project or just doing daily homework, envision how you want this homework time to conclude. Probably, you not only want to see the work done but also want the time to end peaceably, with your relationship with your child intact and possibly enriched by this experience. Having it end with smiles or even some laughter would be great. You will notice how these images guide you in your decisions about and reactions to your child. You are choosing to act to keep the interaction positive, upbeat, instructive, guiding, and even humorous. And so it is likely to be. Your relationship with your child and the manner in which smaller interactions turn out by design or by default are entirely up to you. I find that this principle is most needed in situations of potential conflict. Before acting, see the end in your mind and clarify the goal; the steps toward your goal will emerge from this process.

3. *"Put first things first."* What is important in your relationship with your child? What matters most in your role as a parent to this child? What are the major hurdles

and responsibilities you must assist your child in overcoming or fulfilling? I have often counseled parents of children with ADHD to distinguish the "battles" from the "wars"—that is, to separate the trivial and unimportant things they must get done with their children (for example, making a bed before school) from the far more important goals to be accomplished (for example, being prepared for school and leaving home in a peaceful, loving atmosphere). Too often the parents of these children find themselves caught in struggles over trivial matters. Children with ADHD can do so many things wrong that parents could confront them on their transgressions throughout much of the day. But is this the kind of relationship you want with your child? Parents of children with ADHD must develop a sense of priorities.

Learn to distinguish among the four categories of work and responsibilities with your child: (a) urgent and important, (b) urgent and not important, (c) important but not urgent, and (d) not important and not urgent. As parents we are likely to accomplish category *a* and unlikely to waste much time on *d*. The hard part is distinguishing *b* from *c*. Racing around and arguing with your child to meet deadlines for less important activities (sports, clubs, music lessons, etc.) can often take precedence over more important but nonurgent things. For instance, you may well get your child to a piano lesson on time but destroy your relationship with that child in the process.

On Sunday evening as you contemplate the busy week ahead, think about what is important for you and your child and concentrate on doing these things first. Insert them into your calendar first, so they don't get swept away by the onrush of the seemingly urgent but relatively unimportant things that you will have to attend to that week (such as returning calls to others, doing housework, preparing meals on time, getting children to bed on time, etc.). And it is not just your activities with and for your child with ADHD that require sorting out by this method. Think about your own work and obligations apart from this child. Have you overcommitted yourself to committee work, volunteer activities, babysitting for others' children, or the like? Do you need to learn to say "No" to others who call and ask you to help with things about which you do not feel strongly?

4. *"Think win/win."* Throughout your daily life with your child with ADHD, especially as the teenage years approach, you will have to ask your child to do schoolwork and chores, keep social commitments, and adhere to household rules. Each of these requests constitutes a negotiation. As Dr. Covey says, when you enter into a negotiation with anyone, think win/win. That is, approach the interaction with the idea that whenever possible you want both you and your child to get what you want. Don't concentrate only on what you want the child to do; you must try to understand how difficult it may be for her to do as you ask. Do you ever find yourself simply spewing forth commands for obedience all day long? It's certainly easy to do, but is it the kind of relationship you want with your child? Begin with the end in mind and ask yourself how you wish to be remembered: as a tyrant or as a respectful negotiator?

Say you typically have your daughter clean up her room once a week, usually on Saturday. As you approach the designated cleanup time, think about what might make this chore a winning situation for your child, not just for you. Would she enjoy some extra time playing her favorite video game, the chance to rent a DVD for the evening, the opportunity to play a game with you, or the chance to earn some extra money for the week? Choose any reward you think will be appealing and make it part of the verbal contract you make with your daughter on Saturday morning: "If you clean up your room by noon, we can spend the afternoon at the beach," for example.

5. *"Seek first to understand, then to be understood."* Dr. Covey uses the metaphor of an emotional bank account to convince us of the importance of this principle. It refers to the amount of trust that has been built up in a relationship with someone—in this case, your child with ADHD. By being honest, kind, courteous, and keeping your promises, you make deposits into this account. Avoiding discourtesy, disrespect, dishonesty, overreaction, threats, insults or putdowns, and betrayals of trust increases your balance with your child. Then, when it is most important that your child seek you out and follow your advice, he is likely to do so; when you most need him to understand and help you, he will be there for you.

Remember that your love for your child with ADHD is a bedrock of emotional support that he can count on because he is your child and belongs to your family. Be sure he knows that it has no strings attached—that your love is not dependent on how well he behaved that day, how well he did in school, how many friends he has, or how terrific he is at sports or other recreational pursuits.

Dr. Covey describes six types of deposits you can make into this account, but the first is the most important: (a) Understand your child's point of view and make what is important to him important to you. Be a good listener—reflect what you think he has said in your own words and see the situation from his point of view. (b) Attend to the little things, the small kindnesses and courtesies. (c) Keep your commitments to your child. (d) Make your expectations clear and explicit at the beginning of any task or negotiation with your child. (e) Show personal integrity; do not be two-faced or dishonest; make your behavior conform to your words. (f) Apologize sincerely to your child when you make a withdrawal from that account; that is, admit when you are wrong, have been unkind or disrespectful, have embarrassed or humiliated your child, or have failed to make the other five deposits. Only when you have really tried to see things from your child's point of view should you seek to make yourself understood.

6. *"Synergize."* Work with your child in creative cooperation and strive to combine all of the foregoing principles into your interactions with your child. The combination, as Dr. Covey says, unleashes the greatest power within people, freeing us to act imaginatively with others. This means being open to whatever outcomes this creative cooperation with your child may bring forth. If you truly strive not to have everything go your way but to incorporate the other five principles into your parenting of your child with ADHD, the course and outcome of your relationship will not be entirely predictable. They will flow and change as your child grows, and you must be open to that change. Some parents will be frightened by this uncertainty, but if you come to relish the adventure, you will be prepared for whatever may come, secure in the strength

of your relationship and your trust in each other. Value the differences between your child and others, be open to new ways of solving difficulties you may face together, and remember that there is no one "right" way to raise your child. There may, in fact, be several excellent ways to work together in facing the challenges life holds for you both.

7. *"Renewal."* This principle supports all the others. It recognizes that you are the most important resource that you and your child with ADHD have and that you must care for yourself to renew that resource. As Dr. Covey says, just as machinery requires downtime, effective people need rejuvenation. Dr. Covey identifies four dimensions of our lives that require renewal: physical, mental, social/emotional, and spiritual. Renewing the physical dimension of your life may mean proper nutrition, exercise, and stress management. Mental maintenance may mean reading and broadening your knowledge, continuing education, engaging in creative pursuits, visualizing and planning your goals, or writing. Socially and emotionally, you may want to be of service to others, show empathy, act synergistically with others, create a closer relationship with your spouse or partner, and draw on your inner security that comes from habits one through six. Caring for the spiritual dimension may mean continuing to clarify your values and commitments, studying your relationship to your world, and thinking about your morals and your life's purposes.

Too often parents of children with ADHD dedicate so much of their time and energy exclusively to their children that they exhaust themselves. Such martyrdom may seem heroic and altruistic at first glance, but is actually foolish and destructive in the long run. Failing to take time to renew yourself leaves you increasingly less to give to your child. Industrial machinery that is never shut down may be tremendously productive in the short run but will have a brief life, says Dr. Covey. The best gift you can give your child with ADHD is your gift of self-renewal.

If you find that you are not using many of these seven effective habits, you are hardly alone—nor are you a bad parent or a horrible person. All of us get tired, stressed, angry, and shortsighted at times, and this interferes with our ability to keep these principles in mind and to act accordingly. It is the striving toward self-improvement that matters most, and all of us can succeed at committing ourselves to that course even though we fall short of it occasionally.

Becoming an Executive Parent

Many parents of children with ADHD have told me of the shame and humiliation they have experienced at the hands of educators and professionals involved with their children. Some have described feeling lost or misunderstood or being treated like children themselves during school planning meetings. They felt that their views and opinions were dismissed as biased or naive. Their overall impression was that those involved simply wanted to reach some quick conclusion—to do what was cheap and expedient for the school system or a professional, and not what was best for a child. The outcome of such meetings is often disillusionment, dissatisfaction, and distrust in the parent–school relationship, as well as a sense of loss of control over a child's fate. In encounters with physicians and mental health specialists, parents of a child with ADHD have been dismissed as hysterical, easily stressed, or naive, especially if the child was well behaved during the appointment. Or the professionals have launched the child on a treatment program without asking about the parents' concerns and without explaining the program's rationale, goals, or side effects.

"The last time we had a school meeting there were six people there—his teacher, a psychologist, a social worker, someone called an LD specialist, his counselor, and the principal. I couldn't understand most of what they said. What can I do next time to avoid feeling intimidated and make sure my son gets the help he needs?"

Meetings with *your* advisers—which is how you should view the educators and professionals involved with your child—do not have to go that way. Maintaining an attitude of executive parenting gives you the self-confidence of knowing that *you* are ultimately in charge of this meeting and of what happens to your child.

You are the *case manager* of your child's life, and you must be a proactive executive prepared to take charge—and to keep it longer than most parents must. As you watch other parents increasingly relinquish responsibility and control to their maturing children, your child's deficits in self-control and willpower guarantee that you will have to retain much of the management and control of her behavior. You are the child's advocate with others in the community who control the resources you will need. You are the child's buffer from excessive criticism and rejection.

No doubt you already know all this, but your encounters with those who are supposed to work for you and your child may have left you feeling disenfranchised and disenchanted. Being an executive parent is the way to take back that power. No matter how much help they offer, you cannot rely on professionals to take on this role for you. There are, of course, many competent and compassionate professionals available for consulting. But professionals come and go, and even when they stay put, they have other things on their agenda.

Only you are in a position to make your child a top priority. Others can provide medication, special education, counseling, tutoring, and coaching in sports, among other special services. But you are always the pivotal person who coordinates these activities and who ultimately determines when and how much of these services your child requires and can stand at one time. You can change or terminate your child's involvement whenever you believe it is not in your child's best interests to continue with those services. Yes, you should listen and actively evaluate information given to you, but any professional who bullies or browbeats you into submitting your child to activities or services just because the professional has more advanced degrees or higher education than you have should be replaced.

This theme of being an executive parent to your child with ADHD echoes throughout this book. Explicitly reminding yourself of your role as decision maker will encourage you to act more like an executive: to solicit advice and information, to ask questions of others when they are unclear, to make your feelings about your child's care in each system (the school system, the health care system, etc.) known, to help flesh out the variety of options before you, to select among them, and to give your consent to the best of these choices. Use the information in this book to empower yourself as an executive parent who takes every step with your child's best interest in mind.

The benefits can be extraordinary. Just thinking in the executive mode provides you with an inner sense of control over your fate and that of your child. It removes the sense of helplessness or second-class status that can come from allowing others to usurp your role. All of this makes you a far more effective decision maker as a parent of a child with ADHD. As a side benefit, it will also bring with it a deeper sense of respect from the professionals and specialists with whom you must deal, and of pride and respect for yourself as you strengthen your role as a parent.

Becoming a Scientific Parent

Buttressing your work as an executive parent is an approach I call *scientific parenting.* Scientists admit their uncertainty about something and then seek as much information as they can on that subject. They question everything. They remain open to new information, but also are generally skeptical toward claims not supported by facts. Finally, they experiment with new ways of doing things and revise their plans based on the results. These steps can be just as useful in being a parent of a child with ADHD as they are in discovering a cure for cancer.

Admit Uncertainty

To be a scientific parent, therefore, means to start out admitting that you (and I as well as any other professional) do not know everything there is to know about raising your child with ADHD. When you face a new problem with your child, remember that it is when you are most certain about something that you are most likely to be wrong. Many parents become so wedded to an idea about the cause or treatment of their child's ADHD that they are blinded to other potentially useful information.

Seek Knowledge

Admitting that you don't know something naturally leads to the second thing that good scientists do: seek knowledge. So should you. Be voracious about it. You need to learn as much as you can about ADHD and the treatments that may help your child. You cannot be an executive or a scientific parent without the facts. Before scientists study a problem, they conduct a search of the available literature on the topic. Even if they don't find the answer to their questions, they can discover what mistakes others have made and thus avoid repeating them. But they are also likely to find information that points them in a better direction than they might have taken originally. You must do the same. Read! Listen! Seek! Question! Find out as much as you can, reasonably, about your child's disorder. You have started this process just by reading this book. Like a scientist, the more you know about ADHD as a parent, the less likely you are to fall prey to the past mistakes of others and the better prepared you will be to discover the right direction to take with your child.

Evaluate Information Critically

A good scientist remains open to new ideas but challenges those ideas, subjecting them to experiments before accepting them as part of the body of scientific findings on the topic. So whatever you discover, be open-minded about it and entertain the value of the information to your research, but question everything. Be prepared to abandon any theory or hypothesis that does not stand up to critical scrutiny.

Be an especially critical consumer of new information on ADHD. Do not accept everything you hear or read. Be open to an idea, but challenge it, test it, criticize it. Ask others what they think about it. If the new information can stand up to this kind of logical inspection, maybe it is true and can be of help to you in understanding and raising your child with ADHD. But always ask for the evidence that supports a new idea, especially if it disagrees with information you already have.

Call national parent support groups like Children and Adults with Attention-Deficit/Hyperactivity Disorder (CHADD) or the Attention Deficit Disorders Association (ADDA)—addresses and phone numbers are at the back of this book—to see what they know about this new concept. Talk with local professionals about their opinions on the subject. Ask the people promoting a new treatment for any copies of published research articles that support their claims. This can keep you from leaping into an unproven treatment that may be a waste of your time and money or may even be detrimental to your child.

If you are among the many families with home Internet access, you might consider going online to get more information about ADHD, but be very cautious about what you find. A search, such as using Google, is likely to produce a list of millions of "hits" and hundreds of websites, many of them commercially oriented while others are just propaganda from extremist groups. This means that, along with information and advice, these sites have products to sell or positions to promote. In my experience, the information offered is not especially accurate, can be heavily biased, and typically progresses into sales pitches for proprietary products, many of which represent unproven "alternative" therapies. The best, most informative, and most helpful sites I have seen were created by professional organizations or nonprofit groups that are devoted to advocating for children with ADHD and have nothing to sell. I have listed these sites at the back of this book.

Also be particularly critical of opinions expressed about ADHD. In the time since the original edition of this book was published, the popular media and various special interest groups have made false and misleading claims about the legitimacy of ADHD as a disorder, about the rate of diagnosis, about its causes, and about the medications used to treat it. Despite the fact that these claims lack the support of scientific fact, they have become widespread and are passed along as if backed by valid research. Objective, fact-based discussions of these issues are presented throughout this revised edition, particularly in Chapters 1–4, 8, and 18.

One point that will be made frequently throughout this book is that truth is an assembled entity. It comes from no single source, text, or person, but emerges as we acquire more and more information about a subject.

Experiment and Revise

The logical next step is experimentation. This means trying new ways of parenting or managing your child's behavior, including some of the methods recommended later in this book, when the old ways just don't seem to be working. Use the results of your experiments to revise your thinking about the problem and to chart the course for your next experiment on the problem. Indeed, experimenting and revising are never-ending processes for parents of a child with ADHD.

When an experiment fails, do not be discouraged. Use what you have learned to try solving the problem a different way. This time, what you do might just help your child. Above all, keep trying. Never conclude that the failure of a particular plan means you are a bad parent. As you go back to the drawing board, reassure yourself that you are doing the best you can as this child's executive parent to develop plans that may help.

What You'll Find in This Book

The ultimate purpose of this volume is, therefore, to empower you, to help you become a scientific, principle-centered, executive parent who is as effective as possible in meeting the many challenges involved in raising any child with this disorder. In the following chapters you'll find the most up-to-date information available, as well as guidelines for finding the ever-emerging new resources that can keep you informed as our knowledge of the subject evolves. You'll find advice for taking care of your child, preserving your family, and protecting your own health and welfare in the process. Throughout the book I'll remind you of those fundamental truths that thousands of parents have helped me to see—the principles that can keep you on a steady course in your daily effort to raise a happy, healthy child and keep you from veering off into a downward spiral of knee-jerk reactions, frustration, and resentment.

The book is divided into four major sections. Part I will tell you what the latest research has revealed: what ADHD is, what causes it (and, just as important, what doesn't cause it), and what all of this tells us about how to treat it. Integral to this discussion is my theory that ADHD is more than just a deficiency in attention and impulse control. Rather, I believe it is a fundamental deficiency in self-regulation generally and executive functioning specifically—the ability to look toward the future and to control one's behavior based on that foresight. You'll also learn in this section about what features and problems you can expect to encounter as a child with ADHD grows and how ADHD in children typically affects their families. With this knowledge in hand, you should be well equipped to pursue your responsibilities as a scientific parent.

Part II prepares you to become an effective executive parent, beginning with your child's evaluation for ADHD by a professional. Knowing what to expect and what resources may be at your disposal will help you take charge of your child's destiny from the start. Here you will also find my 14 principles for managing children with ADHD. Use these to supplement the more general habits of effective parenting discussed here, and you will have a solid framework for meeting a wealth of everyday challenges that ADHD in the family can present. Because all smart executives take care of themselves as well as their job responsibilities, Part II also attends to *your* needs, telling you how to cope with the natural emotional reactions to your child's diagnosis of ADHD and how to renew yourself throughout your years in this demanding role.

In Part III, you will find full descriptions of the most effective methods for managing ADHD symptoms and associated problems with your child, whether a preschooler or an adolescent. Here are dozens of proven techniques designed to acknowledge and work with your child's disabilities rather than to deny and struggle futilely against them. Maximally applied, these methods can restore harmony to your home; help your child fit in with peers, improve achievement at school, and enhance the all-important self-esteem that goes with these things; and generally improve behavior to set your child on the road to well-adjusted adulthood. I cannot and will not promise miracles, but you will undoubtedly be surprised by how much you and your child can accomplish together with perseverance—and understanding.

Finally, Part IV provides current information on the medications that are often recommended for helping to manage the symptoms of ADHD.

Part I

Understanding ADHD

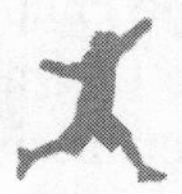

1 What Is Attention-Deficit/ Hyperactivity Disorder?

Attention-deficit/hyperactivity disorder, or ADHD, is a developmental disorder of self-control. It consists of obvious problems with attention span, impulse control, and activity level. But, as you will discover here, it is much more. The disorder is also reflected in impairment in will or the capacity to control the child's own behavior relative to the passage of time, that is, to keep future goals and consequences in mind. It is not, as other books will tell you, just a matter of being inattentive and overactive. It is not just a temporary state that will be outgrown in most cases, a trying but normal phase of childhood. It is not caused by parental failure to properly discipline or raise the child, and it is not a sign of some sort of inherent "badness" or moral failing in the child.

ADHD is real: a real disorder, a real problem, and often a real obstacle. It can be heartbreaking and nerve-wracking when not treated properly.

"Why Don't They Do Something about That Kid?"

It's easy to see why many people find it hard to view ADHD as a disability like blindness, deafness, cerebral palsy, or other physical disabilities. Children with ADHD look normal. There is no outward sign that something is physically wrong within their central nervous system or brain. Yet research clearly shows that it is an imperfection in the brain that causes the constant motion, the poor impulse control, the distractibility, and the other behavior that people find so intolerable in a child who has ADHD.

By now you may be familiar with the way others react to ADHD behavior. At first many adults attempt to overlook the child's interruptions, blurted remarks, and violation of rules. With repeated encounters, however, they try to exert more control over the child. When the child fails to respond, the vast majority of adults decide that the child is being willfully and intentionally disruptive. Ultimately most will come to one conclusion, albeit a false one: the child's problems result from how the child is being raised: The child needs more discipline, more structure, more limit setting, and less coddling. The child's parents are considered to be ignorant, careless, permissive, uninvolved, unloving, or, in contemporary parlance, "dysfunctional."

"So, why don't they do something about that kid?"

Of course the parents often *are* doing something. But when they explain that the child has been diagnosed as having ADHD, judgmental outsiders may react with skepticism. They see the label as simply an excuse by the parents to avoid the responsibility of child rearing and an attempt to make the child yet one more type of helpless victim unaccountable for his actions. This hypocritical response—viewing the child's behavior so negatively, while at the same time labeling the child as "just normal"—leaves outsiders free to continue blaming the parents.

Even the less critical reaction of considering ADHD behavior a stage to be outgrown is not so benign in the long run. Many adults, including some professionals, counsel the parents not to worry. "Just hang in there" or "keep them busy," they advise, "and by adolescence these children will have outgrown it." This is certainly true in some milder forms of ADHD: in perhaps one-sixth to one-third of cases diagnosed in childhood, the behaviors are likely to be within the broadly normal range by adulthood, though still relatively frequent. If your preschool child has more serious problems with ADHD symptoms, however, such advice is small comfort. Being advised to "hang in there" for 7–10 years is hardly consoling. Worse, it is often grossly mistaken or harmful advice. The life of a child whose ADHD is left unrecognized and untreated for years is likely to be filled with failure and underachievement. Up to 30–50% of these children may be retained in a grade in school at least once. As many as 35% fail to complete high school. For half of such children, social relationships are seriously impaired, and for 60% or more of them seriously defiant behavior leads to misunderstanding and resentment by siblings, frequent scolding and punishment, and a greater potential for delinquency and substance abuse later on. Failure by the adults in a child's life to recognize and treat ADHD can leave that child with an unremitting sense of failure in many domains of major life activities.

"Isn't ADHD overdiagnosed? Aren't most children inattentive, active, and impulsive?"

No and yes. ADHD is *underdiagnosed* in most populations, with 40–60% of such children in any given community in the United States not being diagnosed or treated. But most children do show occasional signs of inattention, overactivity, or impulsiveness. What distinguishes children with ADHD from other children is the far greater frequency and severity with which these behaviors are demonstrated and the far greater impairment children with ADHD are likely to experience in many domains of life.

Imagine the toll on society when, conservatively estimated, 5–8%, or 2.5–4 million school-age children, have ADHD. This means that at least one or even two children with ADHD are in every classroom throughout the United States. It also means that ADHD is one of the most common childhood disorders of which professionals are aware. Finally, it means that all of us know someone with the disorder, whether we can identify it by name or not.

The costs of ADHD to society are staggering, not only in lost productivity and underemployment in adults, but also in reeducation. And what of the costs to society in individuals being undereducated, more accident-prone, and more likely to engage in antisocial behavior, crime, and substance abuse? More than 20% of children with ADHD have set serious fires in their communities, more than 30% have engaged in theft, more than 40% drift into early tobacco and alcohol use, and more than 25% are expelled from high school because of serious misconduct. Recently the effects of ADHD on driving have also been studied. Within their first 5–10 years of independent driving, adolescents and young adults with a diagnosis of ADHD have nearly four to five times as many citations for speeding, two to three times as many auto accidents, have accidents that are two to three times more expensive in damages or likelihood of causing bodily injuries, and have three times as many total traffic citations as young drivers without ADHD. Health economists have also calculated that the cost to society of a teenager's not graduating from high school will be between $370,000 and $450,000 in lost wages, taxes, and other contributions to society as well as in the need for additional social or medical services. Other economists have also shown that raising a child with ADHD results in more than twice the expense in medical bills of families of typical children, and this does not include the extra costs related to actually treating the child's ADHD. It results mostly from the child's greater use of emergency room services and other outpatient medical services. All of this is to say that ADHD is not an economically neutral or benign disorder but a costly one to the family, to the community, and to society more generally.

Recognition of these consequences has spawned a huge effort to understand ADHD. More than 10,000 scientific papers and more than 100 textbooks have been devoted to the subject, with again as many books written for parents and teachers. Countless newspaper stories have addressed ADHD over the course of the 230 years that medical science has recognized the disorder as a serious problem. Many local parents' support associations have sprung up, most notably Children and Adults with Attention-Deficit/Hyperactivity Disorder (CHADD), which has grown into a national organization of more than 50,000 members. At least five professional organizations include a number of scientific presentations on the subject in their convention programs each year, and one was created in the last decade that is devoted entirely to professionals who specialize in ADHD (American Professional Society for ADHD and Related Disorders). (See "Support Services for Parents" at the back of the book for more information on these resources.) All this is hardly what you would expect if the disorder were not "real," as some critics continue to claim.

Fact versus Fiction

As mentioned in the Introduction, various unsubstantiated claims about the legitimacy of the disorder we call ADHD make the media rounds periodically. Trying to sort through these, in addition to facing the skepticism of friends, family, and teachers, can make it difficult for parents to accept a diagnosis of ADHD and move forward into productive treatment of their child. It may be reassuring to know that more than a decade has passed since a consortium of almost 100 scientists from around the world, many of whom have dedicated a significant portion of their careers to the scientific study of ADHD, signed a consensus statement in January 2002 attesting to the validity of ADHD and its adverse impact on the lives of those diagnosed. The full text can be found on my website *(www.russellbarkley.org)* or in *Clinical Child and Family Psychology Review* (vol. 5, no. 2, pages 89–111) for those who are interested. More than 100 European professionals signed this document as well in a version published in Germany a few years later. In addition, here is what we know to date:

Fiction: ADHD is not real, because there is no evidence that it is associated with or is the result of a clear-cut disease or gross brain damage.

Fact: Many legitimate disorders exist without any evident underlying disease or pathology. ADHD is among them.

Disorders for which there is no evidence of brain damage or disease include the vast majority of cases of mental retardation (various brain-scanning methods reveal no obvious disease or damage in children with Down syndrome, for example), childhood autism, reading disabilities, language disorders, bipolar disorders, major depression, and psychosis, as well as medical disorders involving early-stage Alzheimer's disease, the initial onset of multiple sclerosis, and many of the epilepsies. Many disorders arise due to problems in the way the brain has developed or the way it is functioning at the level of nerve cells. Some of these are genetic disorders, in which the condition arises from an error in development rather than from a destructive process or an invading micro-organism. The fact that we do not yet know the precise causes of many of these disorders at the level of the molecules in the brain does not mean they are not legitimate. A disorder, as explained under "What Is ADHD?" later in this chapter, is defined as a "harmful dysfunction," not by the existence of obvious pathological causes.

As for ADHD, the evidence is now unquestionable that we are dealing in most cases with either a delay in or subtle brain injuries sustained during early brain development or abnormal brain functioning that originates in genetics in more than two-thirds of all cases and in pregnancy, birth, or early childhood injuries in the remainder. Chapter 3 explains in more depth what we know about the genetic origins of ADHD. In cases of hereditary origin, many studies using brain-imaging techniques have found the brain to be 3–10% smaller than in other children of the same age, especially in the frontal area, and 2–3 years delayed in maturation. Certain parts of the brain are also found to be less aroused or active or to manifest abnormal forms of activity. Although most cases of ADHD appear to arise from such genetic effects and difficulties with brain development and functioning, ADHD can certainly arise from direct damage to or diseases of the brain as well. A mother's consumption of alcohol or tobacco during pregnancy can increase the risk that her child will develop ADHD 2.5 times over that of the normal population. ADHD is associated not only with fetal alcohol syndrome, but also with repeated infections of the mother during pregnancy that create a higher risk of the disorder in children. Prematurity of birth sufficient to warrant placement in a neonatal intensive care unit can be associated with small brain hemorrhages and thus a higher risk for ADHD in later development. And it is well known that children suffering significant trauma to the frontal part of their brain are likely to develop symptoms of ADHD as a consequence. All of this indicates to scientists that any process that disrupts the normal development or functioning of the frontal part of the brain and its connections to several other brain regions, such as the striatum, anterior cingulate, and cerebellum, is likely to result in ADHD. It just so happens that most cases are not due to such gross damage, but seem to arise from problems in the neural development of these critical brain regions or in their normal functioning. Someday soon we will understand the nature of those problems with greater precision. But for now, the lack of such a precise understanding does not mean that the disorder is not valid or real. If the demonstration of damage or disease were the critical test for diagnosis, then the vast majority of mental disorders, nearly all developmental disabilities, and many medical conditions would have to be considered invalid. Countless people suffering from very real problems would go untreated, and their problems would be unexplored.

Fiction: If ADHD were real, there would be a lab test to detect it.

Fact: There is no medical test for any currently known "real" mental disorder.

Just as we cannot give children with ADHD a test guaranteed to detect it, neither is there a sure-fire lab test for schizophrenia, bipolar disorder, alcoholism, Tourette syndrome, depression, anxiety disorders, or any of the other well-established mental disorders, or for many widespread medical disorders such as arthritis or the early stages of multiple sclerosis or Alzheimer's disease. Yet they are all very real in being harmful dysfunctions.

Fiction: ADHD must be an American fabrication, since it is diagnosed only in the United States.

Fact: Many studies conducted in numerous foreign countries show that all cultures and ethnic groups have children with ADHD. The worldwide prevalence has now been established to be 4.5–5.5% of children and 3.5–4.5% of adults.

For instance, Japan has identified up to 7% of children as having the disorder, China up to 6–8%, France up to 7%, and New Zealand up to 7%, just to name a few of the many countries that have been studied to date. All of this means that ADHD is a universal disorder found in every country studied so far. Other countries may not refer to ADHD by this term, they may not know as much about its causes or treatment, and (depending on the countries' level of development) they may not even recognize it yet as a legitimate disorder. But there is no question that ADHD is a legitimate disorder and is found worldwide.

Fiction: Because the rate of diagnosis of ADHD and the prescription of stimulants to treat it have risen markedly in the last decade or two, ADHD is now widely overdiagnosed.

Fact: As the National Institutes of Health (NIH) Consensus Development Conference on ADHD concluded in late 1998, the surgeon general in a report on children's mental health in the United States in 2002, the Centers for Disease Control and Prevention in the *National Health Interview Survey* in 2005, and NIMH again in the *National Comorbidity Survey Replication* in 2005 and 2010, it is *under*diagnosis and *under*treatment of ADHD (and other disorders) in children that remain the big problems in the United States today.

Several studies indicate that fewer than 60% of all children who have ADHD are diagnosed or treated properly for the disorder and that only half or fewer of these are treated with medication. The greatest problems for our children continue to be that a large percentage of those with legitimate disorders in need of treatment are not being referred, diagnosed, or treated properly and that services across the United States for children with ADHD are inconsistent, erratic, and often well below what is considered the standard of care for the disorder. Thus, proclamations that we are overdiagnosing or overmedicating ADHD or any other child mental disorder in the United States lack credible scientific evidence, as Judith Warner, columnist for the *New York Times,* showed in her 2011 book *We've Got Issues: Children and Parents in the Age of Medication.*

One possible reason for the rise in diagnosis and stimulant treatment of ADHD is that the prevalence of the disorder has actually increased. However, we do not have a lot of research that has measured the rates of children's mental disorders across multiple generations. The little research we do have indicates that ADHD has not been on the rise over the last two generations of children, but that a few other disorders may be, such as oppositional defiant disorder (ODD; see the case of Amy, below). Mainly what we have been witnessing is an increase in the recognition of the disorder by the general population, and therefore an increase in the number of children *being referred and diagnosed* with the disorder. Tremendous strides have been made to educate the American public about ADHD in the last 20 years. Thanks to a substantial upsurge in research on the disorder, to the various parent advocacy groups raising the level of public and political awareness about ADHD (such as CHADD and ADDA—see "Support Services for Parents" at the back of the book), to increased professional education on the disorder, and to the recognition of ADHD as a legitimate disability in the Individuals with Disabilities in Education Act and the Americans with Disabilities Act, more children (and adults) with this disorder are getting proper diagnosis and management. But again, we still have a long way to go.

The same scenario seems to have been occurring more recently in other countries, such as Australia, Great Britain, Italy, Spain, and Scandinavia, where greater efforts have been made to educate the public and professional communities about the disorder. The result has been a marked increase in the number of children being referred for professional help, diagnosed properly, and possibly being treated with ADHD medications, among other treatments. Therefore most of the increase in diagnosis in the United States is likely due to greater awareness of the disorder.

In conclusion, a number of facts suggest that we do not have widespread overdiagnosis or overmedication, despite the marked rise in both in the United States over the last 10–20 years. That is not to say that there may not be some locales within the United States where more children than expected are being diagnosed or where more medication than would be prudent is being prescribed. But these appear to be very local problems and not an epidemic.

A Question of Perspective

Intense interest in demystifying ADHD has instigated voluminous research. More than 300 articles per year are published in scientific journals on the disorder, and more than 3,000 have been published since 2006. As I will describe in detail in Chapter 2, the research done up through 1994 led me to develop a new view of ADHD in 1997—a view that has been reinforced by studies undertaken since the theory was first introduced. This view has been refined and expanded further in my 2012 book, *The Executive Functions: What They Are, How They Work, and Why They Evolved*. I see ADHD as a developmental disorder of the ability to self-regulate behavior with an eye toward the future. I believe the disorder stems from underactivity in specific areas of the brain that, as they mature, provide ever-greater means of behavioral inhibition, self-organization, self-regulation, foresight, and time management. Relatively hidden from view in a child's moment-to-moment behavior, the behavioral deformity this underactivity causes is pernicious, insidious, and disastrous in its impact on a person's ability to manage the critical day-to-day affairs through which human beings prepare for the future, both near and far.

The fact that its daily impact is subtle but its consequences for the child's adaptive functioning are severe has led to many changes in the labels and concepts applied to the disorder over the last century. It explains why clinical science, in its attempts to pin down the nature of the problem, has moved from vague, unfocused notions of attention disorders in 1775 (Melchior Adam Weikard in Germany, as discussed in Barkley & Peters, 2012) and 1798 (Alexander Crichton in Scotland) to defective moral control in 1902 (George Still in England) to sharper, more specific concepts of hyperactivity, inattention, and impulsivity in the 1960s to 1980s. This evolution of our knowledge from the very general to the very specific has made great leaps forward in our understanding of the abnormalities of children with ADHD, but it has caused us to lose our larger perspective on how those behaviors affect the social adaptation of these children over long periods of time.

In the 1990s, however, clinical science began stepping back from its microscope on the specific social interactions of children with ADHD and once again peered through its telescope at longer term social development and other outcomes, thanks in large part to the publication of studies of children with ADHD followed over 20 years to adulthood, such as my study with Dr. Mariellen Fischer at the Medical College of Wisconsin in Milwaukee and those of Drs. Mannuzza and Klein at New York University Medical School, Drs. Weiss and Hechtman at Montreal Children's Hospital, Dr. Hinshaw and colleagues at the University of California at Berkeley, and Dr. Christopher Gillberg and colleagues in Gothenberg, Sweden, among others (see the Barkley, Murphy, & Fischer, 2008, book). We now understand how these "atoms" of momentary ADHD behavior come to form "molecules" of daily life, how these daily "molecules" form the larger "compounds" of weekly and monthly social existence, and how these social "compounds" form the larger stages or structures of a life played out over many years and across many domains of major life activities. As a result, we see that ADHD is not just the hyperactivity or distractibility of the moment or the inability to get the day's work done, but a relative impairment in how behavior is organized and directed toward the tomorrows of life. This larger, longer view of ADHD as a disorder of executive functioning (future-directed behavior) and the self-regulation it provides has clarified why those with the disorder struggle in their adaptation to the demands of social life. It further shows why they so often fail to reach the goals and futures that they have tried to set for themselves or that others demand of them. If we remember that the behavior of those with ADHD is focused on the moment, and not on the "laters" of life, and that this results from a neurological basis, we won't judge their actions so harshly. No one would understand half of what we "normal" adults do if these actions were judged solely by their immediate consequences. Many of the actions we take have been planned with the future in mind. Likewise, we don't understand—and are quick to criticize—the behavior of those with ADHD because we are expecting them to act with self-restraint and foresight when they have always focused instead on the moment. We find it difficult to tolerate the way those with ADHD behave, the decisions they make, and their complaining about the negative consequences that befall them because *we,* who do not have the disorder, can foresee where it is all likely to be leading and use that mental vision to determine our current behavior while they cannot. Only now is clinical science coming to understand this very important feature of ADHD as being a disorder of future-directed behavior.

Have You Seen These Children?

The children described in the following cases may be quite familiar to you. They are real cases from my 30-plus years in clinical practice (though their names and identities have been changed to preserve confidentiality). Their stories will give you some idea of the circumstances children with ADHD commonly find themselves in today. As you read, you will probably be able to see how their lives might be different if their parents, teachers, and others really understood their deficits in executive functioning—their inability to look toward the future and to regulate their own behavior. You also should know, however, how far we have come. To provide some perspective on how much better the prospects are for these children today than in the past, I'll also describe how such children might have been treated during earlier decades.

"Does my child have ADHD?"

Amy: Constant Struggle

Amy is an attractive 7-year-old girl whose parents, Rose and Michael, are quite concerned about her. They tell me they have to repeat their commands to her a lot more than with her brothers or sisters, and they sometimes have to guide her physically through tasks, such as getting dressed and undressed or picking up her toys. She seems to pay little attention to her homework, chores, or what others are saying to her unless she is interested in the activity at hand. She has great difficulty sitting still through a meal or when the family watches TV together, and in staying in bed at bedtime. She runs rather than walks everywhere and often climbs up on furniture as she tears about the room.

Amy seems unable to let others finish what they are saying at family meals before she blurts out her ideas and then changes the subject altogether. Her incessant chatter has moved her siblings to nickname her "Motor Mouth."

When her parents tell her not to do something, Amy often becomes argumentative, angry, resentful, and belligerent. She says, "But I don't care; I want that," repeating her demands and throwing a temper tantrum. When told to pick up her toys, put her dirty clothes away, or get ready for her bath, she pouts or crosses her arms over her chest and says "No!" or just ignores here parents' instructions while she continues to play or just walks out of the room.

Amy's parents have noticed that she does not seem to think before she acts. She lunges into other children's play without considering what they are doing and whether she is welcome to join them. She takes over the activity, bossing others about, and gets frustrated and visibly upset when others do not obey her commands. Her emotions seem to get the best of her during many social activities. At parties she becomes excited, giddy, and loud, often being more elated than the birthday child. She becomes even more excited during games and can't wait until others take their turns. Once a game ends, she has great trouble settling down to a quieter activity, such as having birthday cake. She has even been known to start opening the presents for the birthday child.

Amy easily becomes envious of other children and has on occasion taken home someone's new toy that she doesn't have. She brags about her accomplishments, manufacturing many details. Her peers and their parents find her blunt comments rude and her play behavior both unfocused and selfish. Amy has been losing friends and now is not often invited to other children's homes. Neighborhood children have begun to call her "weird" and "hyper." Her parents are worried that she will soon wind up friendless and that she may develop a poor self-image or even depression.

Despite her devil-may-care attitude about most things, Amy depends excessively on her parents or teachers for help with her schoolwork, which she constantly protests with "I'm bored!" and "I hate this!" Amy's completion of schoolwork lags behind the ability that testing has shown her to have, and she is beginning to fall behind her classmates. She finds it hard to concentrate on what the teacher is saying. Instead she talks to her neighbors, doodles, or gets up and moves about, exploring the aquarium at the back of the room and making frequent trips to the trash can and pencil sharpener.

The school psychologist has tested Amy and found her to be of normal intelligence. Her early academic skills are all average or better; no learning disability is causing her poor school performance. She is likely, however, to have to repeat second grade.

When Amy was born, she was premature and weighed less than 5 pounds. She did not have any other problems, but was slow to put on weight. She was a bit late in learning to walk, but spoke her first words earlier than most children. Her parents do not remember any serious medical problems during her development. At age 4, Amy's preschool teacher reported that she was "wild," always running around the room, climbing on furniture and shelves, taking toys from the other children, throwing things, and fidgeting during group story time. All of the behavior problems she now displays were also noticed during kindergarten.

When I first met them, Amy's parents were at their wits' end. Cutting sugary foods out of Amy's diet had had little effect; more discipline had also produced little improvement. Rose now feels she has somehow failed as a parent and complains of excessive stress and fatigue when she has had to be with Amy for long periods of time; Michael reports numerous confrontations with Amy over her behavior problems. Both parents fear that their marriage is suffering and find themselves fantasizing about the peaceful pleasantness of the early days of their marriage, before children.

Amy's case illustrates the classic symptoms seen with ADHD: inattention and poor ability to stay on a task to completion, impulsiveness and the inability to think about what she does before she acts, and overactivity or frequent restlessness. As for most children with ADHD, Amy's problems began in her preschool years but were not diagnosed until years later. Professional help was not sought until her behavior problems created difficulties outside the family—in this case at school, which is also fairly common. Amy is also fairly typical of many children with ADHD because she shows a second pattern of behavior: oppositional, defiant, and hostile behavior toward others, especially her parents. This pattern is known as ODD. Between 35 and 85% of children with ADHD who are referred to clinics will have this problem (the lower figure is more characteristic of children seen in primary-care settings, the higher one of those seen in psychiatric or mental health clinics). It occurs 11 times more often in children with ADHD than in the general population.

Over two centuries ago, in the 1770s, Amy would likely not have been diagnosed with a psychological disorder. Yet if she had been seen by Dr. Weikard in Germany, the first physician to describe disorders of attention, her "symptoms" might well have been noted but blamed on her upbringing. Probably only those raising her would have considered her to be a real problem. With nothing known scientifically and little known clinically about such children, outsiders would have considered her just a social oddity—a judgment that would not have prevented them from dealing harshly with her. In lieu of the appropriate management methods (such as those discussed in Parts II and III of this book), both her parents and others would have been likely to discipline her often, reduce distractions around her, put her in isolation, or recommend strange herbs, sour milk, and horseback riding as part of her cure, as Dr. Weikard suggested. By early adolescence, she might well have been turned out into the street to fend for herself given the chronic problems she posed for her parents and family, a not uncommon end for troublesome children.

Had she been born about 125 years later in England, she might have been referred to Dr. George Still, a British physician who published a description of 24 children like Amy from his clinical practice. Her parents might have been told that she suffered from a defect of willpower, or *volitional inhibition*, as Still called it. He might have said that her actions illustrated a serious defect in the moral control of her behavior and might have concluded that its cause was neurological. Even so, little was known about how to treat such a problem, so the prognosis for Amy would have been rather bleak by comparison with today's standards of treatment. Most likely Amy still would not have been diagnosed with any disorder, but would have been viewed as ill-mannered, immoral, excessively passionate (emotional), or even an idiot or imbecile despite normal intellectual development, given that anyone with any sort of psychological problems was likely to be so classified in this age before the recognition of specific psychological disorders. In those days she might very well have faced a life of social rejection and ostracism and of limited educational achievement. Today, however, early intervention offers hope not only for managing ADHD symptoms, but also for possibly minimizing the impact of ODD over the course of a child's development.

Ricky: A Damaged Self-Image

Ricky is an 8-year-old second grader whose parents, Richard and Danielle, have tried "everything" to get Ricky to do better at school. He was retained in first grade, and they fear he may be retained again before getting to middle school. Ricky is a noisy, restless gadfly who flits about his home or classroom, doing many things at once but not staying on-task long enough to finish any of them. Most days, notes home from his teacher tell his parents he has been "off-task," aggressive, and disruptive of other children's work and play activities. For little apparent reason, just this year he has taken to shoving other children, taking things from them, bullying peers during recess, and sabotaging others' work when he is not being supervised directly.

His mother believes that his teacher relies too much on punishment and too little on the positive feedback, one-to-one attention and assistance, and nurturing that Ricky needs. For the first time, his parents are having difficulty getting him to school. He complains of vague bodily aches and pains that are clearly intended to keep him home. Recently he has mentioned hating himself and wishing he were dead and has begun referring to himself as "stupid."

Ricky's parents have always taken his differences from his older brother and sister in stride as part of Ricky's unique personality. He frequently responds well to their praise of him and is seen as a loving, affectionate child toward all family members. Yet this year his self-esteem has plummeted, he is easily irritated, and at times he is on the verge of tears when frustrated by the simplest things. His parents see him as really hurting inside, yet cannot seem to provide more than temporary relief for him. They have developed an adversarial relationship with his teacher, seeing her harsh discipline and lack of forgiveness as a major contributor to Ricky's downhill slide in self-image.

Ricky met all the typical developmental milestones at a normal age, though as an infant he was always in motion. His parents were forced to put a net over his crib to keep him from wandering around the house while others were asleep. When he was a little older, he was found riding his tricycle in the driveway at 4:00 A.M. one morning with only the garage light to guide him. Ricky seemed accident-prone as a toddler and has always been seen as "a talker," easily engaging even strangers in conversation. Ricky's grandmother often remarked on the similarity between Ricky and his father at the same age.

Ricky, unlike Amy, does not have ODD. Yet, as is true for some children with ADHD, Ricky's self-esteem has begun to decline as he chronically underperforms at school and increasingly gets into trouble with other children. The unyielding and unsympathetic view of Ricky's teacher seems to have contributed to this decline in self-image and certainly makes for a more conflict-filled school day. That this has led him to the point of being depressed is also not uncommon for children with ADHD who show early signs of low self-esteem, although his statements about harming himself at such a young age are extreme for most such children.

If Ricky had been a child in the 1920s to 1940s in the United States, he might have been labeled as having *restlessness syndrome* or *organic drivenness*, terms in use in scientific journals at the time. He might even have been diagnosed as having a *post-encephalitic behavior disorder* if he had survived a recent serious infection of the nervous system (encephalitis). Some children with Ricky's pattern of behavior were being referred to as having *brain-injured child syndrome* because injuries to the brain from either disease or trauma could cause children to act this way. Therefore, any child who behaved like this, even if there was no obvious history of a brain injury, was thought of as having this syndrome. Ricky might have been placed in a special classroom where very little extra stimulation was available except for the material related to the lesson being taught. The teachers might have worn rather dull-colored clothing and no jewelry, and the classroom might have been kept undecorated to minimize distractions, seen as the greatest problem for children with the brain-injured child syndrome. But these classrooms were rare and quite unusual for their time, and as a result were not available to most families with children like Ricky.

If Ricky had been treated at the Emma Pendleton Bradley home for children in Providence, Rhode Island, in 1936–1938, he might have been tried on a stimulant medication known as *D*-amphetamine, or Dexedrine (its trade name), being tested on teenagers with behavior problems by Dr. William Bradley. Note would have been made of the dramatic improvement in behavior and the ability to complete schoolwork that this medication produced. Most likely, however, Ricky would not have had access to this unusual treatment, nor would he have been diagnosed with any psychological disorder.

Ricky's parents might have been advised that he was just "all boy" and would be likely to outgrow the behaviors. When his problems persisted into adolescence, he would have been viewed as a troublemaker or social misfit and probably would have dropped out of school as soon as possible, to work either on a farm or in a factory at low wages. Onlookers likely would have judged him a young adult lacking in "character," for which his parents would undoubtedly have been blamed.

Sandy: Doing Well with Lots of Help

Sandy is a 15-year-old in 10th grade at a small private school for children with learning difficulties. Her parents, Frances and John, placed her there when she began failing in public school years ago, despite having above-average intelligence and no signs of a learning disorder. Her greatest problems have always been inability to concentrate on her schoolwork and to apply persistent effort to boring but necessary tasks. She can rarely complete her high school assignments without assistance, yet usually knows the answers or the correct steps to get the problem solved. What others seem to provide for Sandy are some external structure, guidance, and discipline. Although she is somewhat restless, her activity level has decreased considerably since she was a young child and is now limited primarily to moving her feet back and forth while she is seated, tapping her fingers or pencil while she works, and shifting her posture frequently.

Sandy's schoolwork is often poorly organized, and her notebook is an organizational disaster. She often comes to class without something critical to the class work, such as pencils, the course text, or her lab equipment. When her many errors in homework are pointed out to her, however, she can quickly say what is wrong with them. Her teachers and parents have tried using daily assignment notebooks and behavior rating cards to support her school performance, with limited and temporary success. In class she typically raises her hand and then blurts out an answer, frequently the wrong answer. Her teachers nevertheless enjoy her spontaneity and view her as a bit immature, scattered, and unfocused.

Sandy's problems have existed since at least kindergarten and probably longer.

Throughout her schooling, teachers have complained about her inattentive and impulsive style and her poor follow-through on her assignments. Yet she has always had friends, has been well liked and included in other children's activities, and has had no discipline problems. She has been tested three times by various psychologists and school learning specialists and found to be at the 75th percentile in intelligence and average or better in all academic skills. Her handwriting is often noted to be poor and sluggish, however, and her fine motor coordination has been mildly delayed compared to that of other children.

Although Sandy gets along well with her parents and siblings, they have all shown academic accomplishments well beyond hers. All of her siblings as well as both her parents are college-educated and see this as a necessity for Sandy as well. Sandy's self-esteem is somewhat low, and she is periodically demoralized by her difficulties. She fears that she will continue to disappoint her family and is highly frustrated over what she can do to improve.

Sandy represents that rare child with ADHD who has gotten into adolescence relatively unscathed by the impact of the disorder. I believe this is because it has had its chief impact on her schooling rather than on her social and family life, because she has had a number of understanding teachers along the way who have tried to help her, and because her parents have tried to protect and assist her as much as possible (including moving her into a private school when the need arose). Not to be overlooked, however, is Sandy's own pleasant disposition, which may have caused others to forgive her problems with time management, organization, and completion of schoolwork and which may have allowed her to rebound quickly from any social criticism received. The power of close friendships to help buffer someone like Sandy also cannot be overlooked. Finally, the fact that she is above average in intelligence may have assisted her in finding more socially appropriate ways to cope with difficulties she has faced in school. Much research exists to show that high intelligence predicts a better academic outcome in children with ADHD, just as it does in children without ADHD.

If Sandy had been in school between the 1950s and 1970s, she might have been diagnosed as having *minimal brain damage* or *minimal brain dysfunction*, terms used in the clinical professional journals at that time. These terms came into use because many felt the term *brain-injured child syndrome* was being misused. To appease these critics while still focusing professional attention on a problem in the brain as causing the disorder, the term *minimal brain dysfunction*, or MBD for short, was coined. In the 1960s, terms like *hyperactive child syndrome* or *hyperkinetic reaction of childhood* might have been used instead to describe children like Sandy, since they capture one obvious facet of the child's behavior problems—her incessant movement and restlessness. At about this time, the use of stimulant medication such as Dexedrine or the new drug Ritalin (methylphenidate) would have been increasingly common, though not as widespread as today. If Sandy had been taken for professional help, her parents might have been made to feel to blame for her problems, and she might have received a long-term course of play therapy or psychotherapy to explore what then were thought to be the deep-seated emotional problems giving rise to her "symptoms." Like Ricky, Sandy might have stayed in school only until her early adolescence, dropping out when it became simply too difficult or aversive for her to stay any longer. She might also have been more likely to drift into the 1960s counterculture, where her behavioral problems might have even been viewed positively, reflecting the "free-spirit" attitude of the times.

Brad: A Parent's Puzzle

Brad is a 12-year-old in the sixth grade who consistently begins the school year with excellent grades and acceptable classroom behavior and gradually declines over the fall and winter to C's and D's and disruptive classroom behavior. Several times he has come close to having to repeat a grade, but his teachers have always given him the benefit of the doubt because of his above-average intellect and academic achievement skills. At school Brad is restless and hyperactive, concentrates poorly on work, and talks excessively. He is careless in his schoolwork and disruptive at his desk. Consequently, he demands a lot of the teacher's time and attention and is sent to the office once every few weeks. He complains to his parents and teachers that schoolwork is boring, and he often questions its relevance to what he claims he wants to do as an adult, which is to be a police detective.

Brad's parents noticed that his activity level and attention span were different from those of other children when he was 3 or 4 years old. He was always racing around from one play activity to another and getting into everything that aroused his curiosity. His mischief included pouring dishwashing detergent into the ventilation grate on his father's new stereo amplifier and decorating the family's new sofa with chocolate syrup. He was also known to take apart anything mechanical just to see how it worked: clocks, small appliances, and many toys. He would lose pieces in the process, so that most things could never be returned to working order.

At age 5, Brad began to argue with his parents over being told to clean up his toys, take a bath, go to church, or stay out of his sister's room. As he grew older, Brad began teasing other children; they gradually stopped coming over to play or inviting him to their homes. Despite frequent reminders immediately before he began to play with someone not to tease and to control his notorious temper, it would not be long before Brad would come whining to his parents about what the other child was doing that "wasn't fair," or the other child would leave abruptly to go home without much of an explanation. At one point Brad's parents placed him in a summer camp for help with his social skills, but none of the improvements seen at camp carried over into his life at home or school.

Like Amy's difficulties, Brad's problems are relatively typical of children with ADHD. Unlike the other children described here, however, Brad's ADHD affects his schoolwork episodically rather than more continuously. Brad's unusual pattern may stem from his intelligence, which enables him to pick up new information at the beginning of the school year with little effort but does not suffice once the workload increases and long-term projects are assigned.

If Brad's parents had gone for professional help during the early 1980s, Brad would have been given a diagnosis similar to the term used today: *attention deficit disorder*, or *ADD*. The treatments typically offered were similar to what are now provided, including counseling his parents on behavior modification methods to use at home, making educational adjustments in his regular classes, drawing on special education services if they were available and warranted, and even trying medication treatment (most likely with a stimulant drug such as Ritalin). Brad's parents might even have been told to watch his diet more carefully to remove any substances that contained unusually high levels of additives, artificial flavorings or colorings, preservatives, or sugar.

All of the children you have just met have ADHD. Yes, they are all different—different in their ages, genders, families, and even many of their problems. And had they lived in different eras, they would either not have been diagnosed with any psychological disorder or would have been labeled as having something entirely different from the diagnosis we use today. Certainly their treatment by professionals would have differed substantially across the decades. Most, however, would not have been diagnosed or treated, and their lives would have been filled with underachievement, missed opportunities, even substance abuse and delinquent or criminal conduct. It is less clear that society's reactions to them would have changed as much. Even today, as described earlier in this chapter, people not familiar with ADHD are likely to react harshly to those with the disorder.

What Is ADHD?

To claim that ADHD is a real developmental disorder, scientists must show that (1) it arises early in child development; (2) it clearly distinguishes these children from normal children or those who do not have the disorder; (3) it is relatively pervasive or occurs across many different situations, though not necessarily all of them; (4) it affects a child's ability to function successfully in meeting the typical demands placed on children of that age in various major life activities; (5) it is relatively persistent over time or development; (6) it is not readily accounted for by purely environmental or social causes; (7) it is related to abnormalities in brain functioning or development, which is to say that there exists a failure or deficit in the natural functioning of a mental ability that occurs in all normal humans; and (8) it is associated with other biological factors that can affect brain functioning or development (that is, genetics, injuries, toxins, etc.). Addressing these scientific issues has not been easy, but abundant evidence is now available for all eight of these requirements from the thousands of studies on ADHD. As you will read throughout this book, the evidence that ADHD is a valid disorder is not only abundant but of a long-standing nature and has been considered to be such by clinical scientists for decades if not centuries. The evidence is highly compelling, and some of it is described throughout the next four chapters.

The children just described also illustrate how ADHD represents a significant impairment in the ability to inhibit behavior and consider the later consequences of one's actions. In its early history as a distinctly recognizable phenomenon (about 1775), this attention disorder would have been attributed to bad child-rearing practices by parents, as noted above. By 1902, ADHD would have been seen as a problem in how children develop a capacity to willfully inhibit their behavior, to contemplate the future consequences of their actions for themselves and others, and to adhere to rules of social conduct—not simply social etiquette, but fundamental morals of the time. Ironically, despite its rather judgmental tone concerning morality, the essence of this view was not wholly inaccurate and is being revisited in the view of ADHD that I present in this book. That is because one of the many problems that uninhibited behavior leads to is impairment in how likely children are to think about the longer term implications of their pending actions and how well rules, instructions, and a child's internal (the mind's) voice or "conscience" help that child control behavior so as to be more appropriate, effective, and supportive of their longer term adjustment and welfare.

Over the next few decades, clinical scientists drifted away from focusing on just the behavior that characterized the disorder and concentrated more heavily on its possible causes. Scientists began arguing that the disorder seemed to arise out of the brain and conveyed this by using labels related to brain dysfunction (such as *brain-injured child syndrome*). But when many children were found to have no obvious gross underlying brain damage, the term was softened somewhat to *minimal brain dysfunction,* which still implied that something in the brain was awry. Later, clinical research returned to seeking a better description of the behavioral problems until more and better research could be done on the conjectured neurological origin of the condition. This refocusing on behavior such as hyperactivity led to the disorder's being called *hyperkinesis* or *hyperactive child syndrome.* The concept was then widened in the 1970s to acknowledge that deficits in impulse control and sustained attention were equally problematic for those with ADHD. Research subsequently shifted away from studies of activity level to studies on the nature of attention, its different types, and which types might be involved in the disorder.

At this point the disorder was renamed *attention deficit disorder* (ADD, with or without hyperactivity). As clinical research advanced, it became clear that the hyperactivity and the impulsiveness seen in children diagnosed as having ADD with hyperactivity were highly related to each other, suggesting that they formed a single problem of poor inhibitory control. In addition, research increasingly showed that this problem was as important as the problems with attention in distinguishing ADHD from other childhood disorders. Consequently the term was amended slightly in 1987 to *attention-deficit/hyperactivity disorder,* its current name. Most of what I have to say in this book pertains to ADHD that includes hyperactivity, as the term suggests. Children who are primarily inattentive but who are not hyperactive or impulsive are now referred to as having ADHD—predominantly inattentive presentation. I will have more to say about these children later because it now appears that up to half of them may actually have a newly discovered and distinct disorder of attention that is quite different from that seen in ADHD, one that is called sluggish cognitive tempo (SCT) by researchers, or, more recently, concentration deficit disorder (CDD).

It is important to understand the thinking about ADHD that has prevailed among many scientists and clinical professionals over the last 25 years because it is the point of view you are most likely to encounter now if you seek professional help for your child. So we will take a closer look at it in the sections that follow. Keep in mind, however, that even this view can stand to be modified to bring it into line with the latest evidence about ADHD emerging from the behavioral sciences, neurosciences, and behavioral genetics.

Today most clinical professionals—physicians, psychologists, psychiatrists, and others—believe that ADHD consists of three primary problems in a person's ability to control behavior: difficulties with sustained attention and increased distractibility, impulse control or inhibition, and self-regulating activity level. Other professionals (myself included) recognize that those with ADHD have additional problems with self-awareness and self-monitoring; working memory (remembering what is to be done); contemplating the future consequences of their proposed actions, including planning, time management, remembering and following rules and instructions; self-regulating emotion and motivation; problem solving to overcome obstacles to their goals; and excessive variability in their responses to situations (particularly doing work). All of these symptoms are subsumed under the term *executive functioning,* which refers to those mental abilities people use for self-regulation. This, I believe, is the hallmark of ADHD. Some clinical scientists in other countries have also reached this opinion recently. Scientists continue to debate the extent of and the reason for this problem with executive functioning—whether it applies to all cases and whether it is due to problems with regulating brain activation or arousal or to some deeper problem with brain growth (development) and nerve cell connectivity and functioning. Nevertheless, at this time most researchers agree that inhibiting behavior specifically and certain aspects of executive functioning more generally are central problems for most of the children having the disorder.

Difficulty Sustaining Attention

Parents and teachers often describe their ADHD children in these ways:

"My child doesn't seem to listen."

"My child fails to finish assigned tasks."

"My daughter often loses things."

"My child can't concentrate and is easily distracted."

"My son can't seem to work independently of supervision."

"My daughter requires more redirection."

"He shifts from one uncompleted activity to another."

"She is often forgetful in her daily activities."

All of these refer to problems with paying attention and concentrating.

ADHD is thought to involve a significant difficulty with sustained attention, attention span, or persistence of effort. In short, people with ADHD have trouble sticking with things for as long as others. They struggle, sometimes mightily, to sustain their attention to activities that are longer than usual, especially those that are boring, repetitious, or tedious. Uninteresting school assignments, lengthy household chores, and long lectures are troublesome, as are reading lengthy uninteresting works, paying attention to explanations of uninteresting subjects, and finishing extended projects. Our research tells us that although children with ADHD have a shorter attention span for much of what they are asked to do, keeping their attention on something over long periods of time is the most difficult part of paying attention for these children.

Unfortunately, as children grow up, we expect them to be able to do these things even if they are boring or effortful. The older they become, the more they should be able to do necessary but uninteresting tasks with little or no assistance. Those with ADHD will lag behind others in this ability, perhaps by as much as 30% or more. That means that a 10-year-old child with ADHD, for instance, may have the attention span of a 7-year-old child without ADHD. This will require that others step in to help guide, supervise, and structure their work and behavior for them. So it is easy to see how conflicts arise frequently between children with ADHD and their parents and teachers.

More than a hundred studies have now measured the attention problems of children with ADHD, and in the vast majority of these studies the children with ADHD were found to spend less time paying attention to what they were asked to do than the children who did not have ADHD. For instance, as long ago as 1975 I documented such differences in my study of 36 boys, half diagnosed as hyperactive (they now would be described as having ADHD) and half as not hyperactive. I asked them to perform a variety of activities in a clinic playroom at the department of psychology at Bowling Green State University in Ohio. One activity the boys were required to do was to wait in a playroom for 6 minutes by themselves before I came to take them to do some other tasks. Toys were available for play. I had placed thin black lines on the floor to form a grid or checkerboard to measure their activity by counting how many lines they crossed as they walked (or ran!) about the room. Through a one-way mirror, I observed and recorded the number of different toys they played with and how much time they spent playing with each toy. The boys with ADHD, I discovered, played with three times as many toys as the other boys and spent 50% less time playing with each toy.

I then took the boys to another room and asked them to sit and watch a short movie about a make-believe creature. I told them that I would ask questions about the movie when I returned. While they were watching the movie, I found that the boys with ADHD spent nearly twice as much time looking away from it as the other boys did. The boys with ADHD also answered 25% fewer questions correctly about the content of the movie than did the other boys when I quizzed them afterward. These and other measures I took during this experiment clearly showed that the boys with ADHD paid less attention to what they were doing. Many other researchers have found similar results, using a variety of procedures.

Filtering Information Is Not a Problem

Interestingly, our research also shows that children with ADHD do not have trouble filtering information—distinguishing the important from the irrelevant in what they are asked to attend to. They seem to pay attention to the same things that children without ADHD would when asked to look at or listen to something. It's just that children with ADHD cannot sustain this effort for as long as other children. They look away from the task more frequently than others. They are also more readily drawn to more rewarding activities. So, children with ADHD are not really overwhelmed by information or stimulation, as scientists believed in the 1950s. Instead, they cannot persist in their effort and attention, and they find themselves being drawn away by anything that might be more stimulating or interesting.

Are Children with ADHD More Distractible Than Children without ADHD?

Scientists are now more certain that ADHD involves being more distractible than other children. It is not that they perceive distractors better than others. Instead these children react more than others to events around them that are irrelevant to their work or goals. And once they are disrupted by such distracting events, they are far less likely to remember or to return to the work they were doing. But in addition to being more distractible, especially while working, children with ADHD have two problems that can make them appear to be even more distracted:

1. *Children with ADHD probably get bored with or lose interest in their work much faster than children without ADHD.* This leads them to go searching intentionally for something else that is more fun, interesting, stimulating, and active, even when their assigned work is not yet finished. Some scientists have argued that these children have a lower level of brain arousal and so need more stimulation to keep their brain functioning at a normal level than do children without ADHD. Other scientists have suggested that rewards lose their value faster over time for those with ADHD, meaning they are less sensitive to reinforcement. For now, the cause of this boredom isn't completely clear but may have to do with deficits in the motivational or reward centers of the brain. What is clear is that it exists to a great enough degree that some scientists call children with ADHD "stimulation seekers."

2. *Children with ADHD seem to be drawn to the most rewarding, fun, or reinforcing aspects of any situation.* Like magnets, they seem to be pulled toward these more immediately rewarding activities when there is work to be done that does not involve much reward. For instance, in 1992 Drs. Steven Landau, Elizabeth Lorch, Richard Milich, and their colleagues, all then at the University of Kentucky, studied children with and without ADHD while they were watching television. When there were no toys in the room, the children with ADHD watched the television show as much as the children without ADHD and were just as able to answer questions about what they watched, even though they tended to look away from the TV set more often. However, when toys were placed in the room, the children without ADHD continued to watch the TV program. The children with ADHD were more likely to play with the toys and less likely to watch the TV program. When the program was a typical situation comedy, the children with ADHD were able to answer as many questions about the show as the children without ADHD, but when the program was educational and conveyed the information more visually than verbally the children with ADHD were less likely to answer correctly. The children with ADHD were at a disadvantage only when visual attention was needed.

Why would children with ADHD have been drawn away by toys when children without ADHD were not? Perhaps children with ADHD simply lose interest faster. Or children with ADHD may find physical activities more fun, stimulating, and rewarding than passive activities such as watching TV.

Yet a third explanation comes from a study on curiosity in children with ADHD conducted more than 30 years ago by former colleagues of mine at Bowling Green State University, Drs. Nancy Fiedler and the late Douglas Ullman. They found that children with ADHD showed more physical curiosity during their play, and so they manipulated objects more, switched from one object or toy to another more frequently, and spent less time with any particular toy or object. Children without ADHD of the same age, however, showed more verbal or intellectual curiosity. They talked aloud about the object or toy, described a number of different things about the toy they found interesting, invented ways that the toy could be used in play, and even created stories about the toy. Thus the children without ADHD spent more time with a particular toy, given that its intellectual properties seemed to interest them.

Beginning in the 1980s, Drs. Ronald Rosenthal and Terry Allen at Vanderbilt University showed that whether or not children with ADHD are distracted more than children without ADHD seems to depend ultimately on how salient or appealing the source of the distraction happens to be. For instance, if a child with ADHD finds a video game on his desk when he goes to his room to do an hour of homework, you can imagine which activity he will be doing when you come to check on him 20 minutes later.

Even earlier, Drs. David Bremer and John Stern at Washington University found in a 1976 study that children with ADHD were somewhat more likely than children without it to look away from a reading assignment when a telephone rang with lights flashing or when an oscilloscope made patterns of unusual wavy lines on a screen in the same room. However, the groups differed much more dramatically in *how long* they were distracted by the event: an average of 18 seconds for the children with ADHD and 5 seconds for the other children. This indicated that the children without ADHD found it much easier to return to work after a distraction than the children with ADHD. And so it may be that children with ADHD are distracted from activities for longer periods of time than, and do not return to work as readily as, their peers without ADHD. Many studies have supported these conclusions since that time; children with ADHD are clearly more distractible than typical children and are drawn to activities or events around them that are more stimulating or interesting than what they may be asked to do at a particular time.

A Problem with Deferred Gratification

The inability to persist with a boring task is a sign of immaturity. As children grow, they become better able to resist appealing but inappropriate or competing activities. The children may talk to themselves about the importance of the work, reminding themselves of what rewards they may earn later by completing it or what punishment may result if they don't, and find ways to make the work more intellectually interesting. Children without ADHD also may learn to arrange consequences to reward themselves for sticking with a difficult task. We know that as children mature, larger but delayed rewards become more attractive to them, and they are likely to value them and work for them more often than they opt for smaller, more immediate rewards. Children with ADHD, in contrast, tend to opt for doing a little work now for a small but immediate reward, rather than doing more work now for a much bigger reward not available until much later.

This is clearly a problem with deferred gratification. Understanding this issue is crucial to helping children with ADHD. If we believe that people with ADHD are simply highly distracted by everything, we will use methods that have been recommended for over 40 years—removing sources of distraction—but such attempts to help may actually make these children more restless and less attentive. Reducing stimulation actually makes it even harder for a child with ADHD to sustain attention. In fact, Dr. Sydney Zentall and her colleagues at Purdue University showed more than 30 years ago in several studies that adding color to the work materials that were given to children and adolescents with ADHD reduced the errors they made during their work. Similarly, Dr. Mariellen Fischer, of the Medical College of Wisconsin, and I some 10 years later asked adolescents to watch a computer screen while numbers were flashed on the screen at the rate of one per second. They were to press a button when they saw a 1 followed by a 9. We found that adolescents with ADHD made more errors on this boring task than did those without ADHD. When we repeated this test with distracting numbers flashing to the right and left sides of the test numbers, the teens with ADHD matched the performance of the teens without ADHD. These and many other studies tell us that adding stimulation to a task may increase the ability of children and adolescents with ADHD to pay attention and complete their work with fewer mistakes. For instance, Dr. Howard Abikoff and his colleagues at the New York University Medical School determined more than a decade ago that teens with ADHD were able to get more of their math work done if they could listen to rock music than if they had to work with no music in the background. This again suggests that some stimulation may be beneficial to the ability of children with ADHD to concentrate better and control their attention span.

Returning to my point in this section, specifically, then, we should try to increase the novelty, stimulation, or fun involved in the tasks a child with ADHD is asked to do. We might also specify that certain desirable rewards or consequences can be earned immediately by completing the activity, rather than postponing them. We could also break the activity up into smaller segments, letting the child with ADHD take more frequent breaks while working. Of course, removing highly attractive, interesting, or very salient distractors from the child's vicinity while he or she is working is still a good idea. But as this information suggests, it should not be the only thing you do: increasing the fun or making the consequences associated with the task more enjoyable can be just as important.

Difficulty Controlling Impulses

Parents and teachers often describe children with ADHD as "blurting out answers to questions before the questions have been finished" and "wanting what they want when they want it." Children with ADHD have a lot of trouble waiting for things. Having to take turns in a game, line up for lunch or recess at school, or just wait until some activity (such as a religious service) is over may make them restless and "antsy." They may complain about the waiting and even start in on the activity they have been told to postpone. When parents promise to take them shopping or to a movie eventually, the children may badger the parents excessively during the waiting period. This makes those children appear to be constantly demanding, impatient, and very self-centered. So the second problem seen in ADHD is a decreased ability to inhibit behavior or to show impulse control. Those with ADHD have considerable problems with self-restraint, with holding back their initial response to a situation, so as to think before they finally act. They often blurt out comments that they would probably not have made had they thought first. They also respond to what others say or do to them on impulse, sometimes emotionally, and wind up being judged critically for doing so. They may act quickly on an idea that comes to mind without considering that they were in the middle of doing something else that should be finished first. They are excessive and loud talkers, often monopolizing conversations.

This behavior is often viewed as rude and insensitive, and it has negative consequences in both the social and educational arenas. Teachers note that children with ADHD often "blurt out comments without raising their hands" in class and "start assignments or tests without reading the directions carefully." They frequently are described as "not sharing" what they have with others and as "taking things they want that don't belong to them."

Since children with ADHD already have trouble sustaining attention, imagine how their inability to resist impulses—such as the impulse to abandon a boring task—will exacerbate their problems with working longer for later, larger rewards. More than 25 years ago, in 1986, Dr. Mark Rapport and his colleagues then at the University of Rhode Island gave a group of 16 children with ADHD and 16 children without ADHD some math work to do. When the children were told they would receive a small toy immediately for completing a small number of arithmetic problems, the groups completed the same number of problems. Then the children were given a choice: they could get a small toy for doing a small amount of work or could do larger amounts of work for a much larger and more valuable toy. But they would not get the bigger toy until 2 days later. Under these conditions, more of the children with ADHD chose the small, immediate reward for little work, whereas the other children were more likely to choose the larger, deferred reward for more work.

Dr. Susan Campbell and her colleagues at the University of Pittsburgh found similar results with preschool-age children with and without hyperactivity (present-day ADHD) a few years earlier, in 1982. They hid a small cookie under one of three cups while the children watched. The children were then required to wait until the experimenter rang a bell before they could pick up the cup and eat the cookie. The procedure was repeated for six trials, with the waiting period varying between 5 and 45 seconds. The children with ADHD made many more impulsive choices, taking and eating the cookie before the experimenter rang the bell, than did the other children. A number of other scientists have since replicated this problem with deferring gratification in association with ADHD in the interim, putting it on a solid scientific footing.

More recently, in 2001, Dr. Gwenyth Edwards and I and our colleagues then at the University of Massachusetts Medical School conducted a study in which we offered teenagers with ADHD varying amounts of money (hypothetical, not real, typically far less than $100) that they could have right now. We also offered them $100 if they were willing to wait a month, a year, or even longer. We found that teens with ADHD were far more likely than non-ADHD controls to choose the smaller amount of money now than the larger amount later. In such a study, we can actually estimate just how much the teens with ADHD discount the value of a reward if they have to wait for it. It was 20–30% less valuable to them than it was to the teens without ADHD. This implies that waiting for a later reward results in the child with ADHD devaluing the worth of that reward much more than do normal children—enough that it's just not worth his waiting for it. This helps us to better understand the thinking of children and teens with ADHD when they have to make choices about the various activities and outcomes they confront in their lives. They are more likely to opt for the small but immediate consequences in life than to work for the larger, later, and more rewarding outcomes.

Taking Shortcuts

Problems with attention and impulse control also manifest themselves in the shortcuts that children with ADHD are notorious for taking in their work. They apply the least amount of effort and take the least amount of time to perform boring or unpleasant tasks. For this reason, it is not clear that giving children or adults with ADHD extra time for examinations at school or in taking professional exams as adults actually benefits them. They may wind up just wasting the extra time they are given, rather than using it to full advantage to review their work, look for mistakes to correct, or tackle harder problems they initially passed over. Schools and testing organizations should probably not grant such requests for more time without structuring the task to better aid those with ADHD. Instead, they can give these students a stopwatch on their desk and let them have the same amount of "face time" with the task as others. But those with ADHD can stop the clock for brief periods to stand, stretch, get some water, and then return to the task, at which time they restart the watch. This strategy of "time off the clock" lets people with ADHD pace the task better and break the exam into smaller work quotas, all of which may be beneficial to doing better on the test.

Taking Too Many Risks

The impulsivity seen in ADHD may also show up in greater risk taking. Failing to consider in advance the harm that could follow an action may explain why people with ADHD—particularly children with ADHD, some of whom are also defiant and oppositional—are more accident-prone than others. It is not that children with ADHD do not care about what will happen. It is that they simply do not think ahead about likely consequences. Constantly "damning the torpedoes and proceeding full speed ahead," they are then surprised by the disasters that others foresaw clearly.

"Our daughter wants her driver's license. Yet she seems so immature and distractible. Are kids with ADHD at greater risk as drivers?"

Yes. Such shortsightedness may explain why Drs. Carolyn Hartsough and Nadine Lambert at the University of California at Berkeley found as far back as 1985 that children with ADHD were more than three times as likely to have had at least four or more serious accidents as children without ADHD. The greater risk for accidental poisonings had also been documented by Dr. Mark Stewart and his colleagues at the University of Iowa Medical School several years earlier. Then, in 1988, Dr. Peter Jensen and his colleagues then at the Medical College of Georgia found similarly that children with ADHD were nearly twice as likely to have had traumas requiring sutures, hospitalization, or extensive/painful procedures as a group of control children. As I found in my own subsequent research over the next 20 years, this accident-proneness of those with ADHD extends to their driving as well. In 1993, my colleagues and I then at the University of Massachusetts Medical School published a study in the journal *Pediatrics* that found that teens and young adults with ADHD had four times as many auto accidents (average of 1.5 versus 0.4) and were significantly more likely to have had at least two or more auto crashes (60% versus 40%) than youths without ADHD. The youths with ADHD were four times as likely to have been at fault in the accidents (48% versus 11%), were nearly twice as likely to have received traffic citations (78% versus 47%), and received four times as many such citations (four versus one) in their average of only 2 years of licensed driving experience. The most common citation they received was for speeding, and the second most common was for failing to obey stop signals. In a number of subsequent studies on teens and adults with ADHD and driving, Dr. Dan Cox at the University of Virginia Medical School and others and I have repeatedly found them to be higher risk drivers than those in our control groups. My colleagues and I also found that consuming even small amounts of alcohol resulted in a worsening of their driving-related abilities greater than in those without ADHD. Fortunately, we have also found that being on an ADHD medication appears to improve their driving performance, and therefore may reduce their driving risks. Finally, I found in studies jointly done with Tracie Richards and colleagues at Colorado State University that drivers with ADHD are significantly more likely to manifest "road rage," or anger, hostility, and even aggression toward other drivers, particularly when they are frustrated by the specific actions of another driver.

Lack of impulse control could also explain why teenagers and adults with ADHD may be more likely to take risks drinking alcohol, smoking cigarettes, and using illegal substances such as marijuana. In our study of teenagers with a history of ADHD mentioned earlier, Dr. Mariellen Fischer and I found that nearly 50% of these teens in our study had already used cigarettes by ages 14–15, compared to 27% of the teens without ADHD; 40% of the teens with ADHD had used alcohol, compared to only 22% of the other teens; and 17% had tried marijuana, compared to only 5% of the teens with no history of ADHD. These problems with drug experimentation and eventual abuse continued to ages 20 and 27 during our subsequent follow-up evaluations of these children into adulthood, resulting in more than 20% having a drug use disorder by adult follow-up.

Money Problems

The impulsiveness seen in ADHD may also explain why teenagers and young adults with ADHD have greater difficulties with managing money and credit. They buy things they see and want to have on impulse, without much regard for whether they can really afford them now. They do not consider what effects buying these items will have on their weekly budget or their ability to pay back the debts they already have. Teens and young adults with ADHD save significantly less income than others do; they also carry more debt (such as credit card debt), and are more likely to spend their money frivolously than others are.

Impulsive Thinking

The impulsiveness of those with ADHD apparently is not limited to their actions, but also affects their thoughts. Adults with ADHD have often told us during clinical interviews that they have as much trouble with impulsive thinking as with impulsive behavior. This was demonstrated elegantly in a study 20 years ago by Drs. G. A. Shaw and Leonard Giambra at Georgetown College, published in 1993. When college students were asked to press a button when they saw a certain target stimulus, the students with ADHD not only pushed the button more often when they were not supposed to than did the students with no history of ADHD, they also reported, when interrupted by the researchers, significantly more thoughts unrelated to the task than did the other groups of college students. Other studies have documented similar difficulties associated with ADHD. These studies provide clear evidence that those with ADHD find it harder to keep their mind on their work and to inhibit thoughts that are not related to the task at hand.

A Problem of Too Much Behavior

"Squirmy," "always up and on the go," "acts as if driven by a motor," "climbs excessively," "can't sit still," "talks excessively," "often hums or makes odd noises"—are these descriptions familiar? They define the excessive movement or hyperactivity that is a third feature of many, but not all, children with ADHD. This feature may appear as restlessness, fidgetiness, unnecessary pacing, or other movement, and also as excessive talking. It is difficult behavior to ignore, yet it is the behavior that lay observers are most skeptical about. Parents who consistently see their children shifting in their seats, tapping their fingers or feet, playing with nearby objects, pacing, and generally becoming quite impatient and frustrated by waiting periods know this behavior is not normal. Teachers who watch these children constantly getting out of their seats, wriggling or squirming when they should be sitting still, playing with a small toy brought from home, talking out of turn, and humming or singing to themselves when everyone else is quiet know that this behavior is not typical of most children. Yet others often persist in their opinions that parents and teachers are simply "making it up" or being "overly sensitive" about otherwise normal behavior.

Children with ADHD Are Hyperactive

The fact that children with ADHD really are more active than other children under many different circumstances has been demonstrated repeatedly over decades of research but no more beautifully than in a study published in 1983 by Drs. Linda Porrino, Judith Rapoport, and their colleagues at the National Institute of Mental

Health (NIMH) in Bethesda, Maryland. The children in the study wore a special mechanical device that monitors activity or movement. They wore it every day, all day and all night for 1 week as they went about their normal daily activities. The scientists found that the boys with hyperactivity (ADHD) were significantly more active than the boys without ADHD, regardless of the time of day (including during weekends and while sleeping). The greatest differences between the groups of boys occurred in school situations, which makes sense because such situations demand the most self-restraint and the most time sitting still.

In my own studies of children with hyperactivity (ADHD) very early in my career, published in 1976 and 1978, I determined that these children were moving about a room nearly eight times as often as other children, that their arm motions were more than twice those of children without ADHD, that their leg movements were nearly four times those of the other children, and that they were more than three times as restless while watching a short movie on TV (as described earlier) and more than four times as fidgety and wiggly during psychological tests while seated at a table. Clearly parents and teachers are not making it up when they say that children with ADHD are hyperactive.

For more than 45 years we have had studies that objectively document that children with ADHD are far more active, even during their sleep (and inattentive and impulsive), than typical or normal children—findings that have been repeatedly replicated in numerous studies since then. But the fact that children with ADHD do not regulate or manage their activity level to meet the demands of the moment is what causes them the most trouble. For instance, children with ADHD may have much trouble lowering their activity level as they move from the fast-paced, active play at recess on the playground to the restrained, quiet activity in the classroom. At these times, others may see them as loud, unrestrained, boisterous, rowdy, and immature. My early studies observing children with ADHD in a laboratory playroom, just described, showed that when the boys were told to stay in one corner at one table and play only with the toys on that table, the boys with hyperactivity (ADHD) reduced their activity level much less than the boys without ADHD. As far back as 1983 I published a study with Drs. Charles Cunningham of McMaster University Medical School and Jennifer Karlsson, then working in my lab at Milwaukee Children's Hospital, in which we audiotaped conversations between children and their mothers. We analyzed these conversations in detail and showed that children with ADHD talked about 20% more than children without ADHD. A surprise to us at the time was that the mothers of the children with ADHD also talked more than the mothers of the children without ADHD. We believed that the greater speech of the mothers of children with ADHD was a response to the excessive talking of their children. We proved this by giving the children with ADHD the stimulant drug Ritalin and finding not only an improvement in their ADHD symptoms but an immediate 30% reduction in their speech. The speech level of their mothers was also immediately reduced as well.

Children with ADHD Are Also Hyperreactive

What is most important to understand about children with ADHD is not simply that they move about too much, it is that they *react or behave too much.* They are much more likely to respond to the things around them in any situation than are children without ADHD of the same age. Their behavior occurs too quickly, too forcefully, and too easily in situations where other children would be more inhibited. Thus a better term for describing children with ADHD is *hyperreactive.* While such children are certainly more active than children without ADHD, the term *hyperactive* misses the larger point. Their greater activity level really seems, in large part, to be a by-product of their greater rate of behaving or reacting to things around them in a given situation.

This means that the hyperactivity and the impulsiveness seen in children with ADHD are part of the same underlying problem—a problem with inhibiting behavior (excessive reacting). I believe that much of their problem with sustaining attention is due to their poor inhibition as well. As the great psychologist William James wrote in 1898, it is not possible for humans to pay attention to any one thing for more than a few seconds. All of us keep adjusting our eyes and our bodies as we attend to things, and we often look away from things briefly before returning to them. It is this continual redirection of effort back to the task while resisting the urge to break off our attending to the task to do something else that creates our sustained attention. What those with ADHD have trouble with is not so much that they look away more than those without ADHD (although they do that too), it is that they have much more trouble returning to attend to the task they were doing before their attention was broken. Because the ability to keep returning attention to something requires that a person also be able to inhibit urges or tendencies to do other things, the problem with sustained attention in those with ADHD may actually also be part of their problem with inhibiting responses to things around them. So they look away more than others and fail to resist the temptation to leave an uninteresting task for something more interesting and stimulating to do. Those with ADHD find it much more difficult to resist distracting temptations and to sustain this type of inhibition over urges to do other things while they are working on a lengthy task. They also find that they are less likely to return to the task they were working on once they have been interrupted, since they cannot as easily inhibit the desire to respond to other things around them that may be more attractive or compelling. Hence sustained attention also requires sustained inhibition, and it is the problem with inhibition that may be one root of the attention problems in ADHD.

At its core, I believe that ADHD is primarily a problem of poor inhibition of behavior specifically and poor executive functioning more generally. This poor executive functioning will be described later in this book. Ultimately I would prefer to see the disorder renamed to reflect this new view, perhaps as *executive function deficit disorder.*

The problem with sustaining attention may even be evident on video games. It is commonly believed that children with ADHD are normal when they play such fast-paced, highly appealing, and immediately reinforcing games. That is not, however, what Dr. Rosemary Tannock and her colleagues at the Hospital for Sick Children in Toronto found in 1997 when they conducted two of the first studies on this issue. In their studies they compared children with ADHD to children without it, observing them while they played video games and also studying them while they were involved in two less interesting tasks. These scientists found that the children with ADHD were more active, restless, and inattentive than the children without ADHD during all of these activities, including the video games. They did find that all children were less active and more attentive when playing the video games than when watching TV or doing a monotonous laboratory task. The children with ADHD also did less well than the other children at the video games, experiencing more failure than the other kids. This was often because they failed to inhibit forward movement of their figures in the video games as readily as others, often crashing their action figures headlong into obstacles that cost them points or required them to restart the game. During a debriefing interview with parents, Dr. Tannock and her colleagues learned that, perhaps as a consequence of these difficulties, children with ADHD tended not to play video games in the presence of other kids but were more likely to do so alone. When they did play such games with others, more fights and tears often occurred. And so it seems that while children with ADHD may be more attentive and less restless while playing video games than when engaged in less interesting activities, their behavior and performance are not normal at these times; contrary to popular belief, their behavior remains distinct from that of normal children. More recent studies have extended these results to include Internet-based gaming and even Internet social networking, which those with ADHD appear more prone to engage in and have a higher likelihood of being considered Internet-addicted.

Difficulty Following Instructions

Those with ADHD are also said to suffer from an inability to follow through on instructions and adhere to rules as well as others of their age. Psychologists call this *rule-governed behavior*—when our behavior is controlled more by directions and instructions than by what is actually happening around us. Children with ADHD frequently end up being "off-task" or engaging in activities unrelated to what they have been told to do. For instance, the teacher gives a child with ADHD the simple instruction to return to her seat and start her math assignment. The child may start down the aisle, only to dawdle along the way, poke at other children, talk to others, and slowly wander to her desk, usually taking the long way to get there. Once at her desk, the child may take out a pencil and begin to draw pictures of flowers on paper or on her math assignment, to stare out the window at other children playing, or to take a toy from her pocket and play with it. The instruction given to the child in this case has clearly had little impact on controlling the child's behavior.

"My daughter won't do anything I ask. How can I get her to listen to me?"

This problem of following through on rules or instructions was made all the more evident to me when I first began studying the interactions of parents and their children with ADHD close to 25 years ago with Dr. Charles Cunningham, while both of us were in training at the Oregon Health Sciences University. Dr. Cunningham and I evaluated the interactions of a group of children with hyperactivity (ADHD) and their parents and compared these interactions to a group of children without ADHD and their parents. Each parent–child pair was required first to play together in a playroom with toys just as they might do at home. After this period, we gave each parent a list of commands to give the child to obey, such as to pick up the toys and put them back on the shelves. We observed these interactions from behind a one-way mirror and recorded how the parents and children interacted. We found that the children with ADHD were less compliant with their parents' instructions than the other children were and that this was especially apparent during the work period. Our findings have been confirmed in many other studies done over the past three decades.

One particularly revealing study was conducted as long ago as 1978 by Drs. Rolf Jacob, K. Daniel O'Leary, and Carl Rosenblad, then at the State University of New York at Stony Brook. They examined groups of children with and without hyperactivity (ADHD) in two types of classroom arrangements. In one arrangement the class was run in a rather informal way, with the children being given choices as to what activities they would do during class work periods. Little structure was provided by the teacher, except to encourage the children to select what they were going to do with their time from a number of academic activities. Then they changed the classroom procedures to resemble those of a more traditional, formal classroom. The teacher directed the children's academic work and either assigned them mimeographed worksheets or required them to listen to a lesson. The behavior of the children with and without ADHD did not differ very much in the informal classroom arrangement. But when the class arrangement changed to a more formal style, the children without ADHD were able to reduce their overall level of activity and inattentiveness and bring their behavior into line with the new rules operating in this more restricted type of situation. In contrast the children with ADHD were much less able to do so. This difficulty with following rules has been documented countless times in subsequent research up to the present, including my most recent survey of a cross-section of U.S. children published in 2012, and extends not just across school situations but to the home and community settings in which these children routinely participate.

The result of this inattentiveness, forgetfulness, and inadequate adherence to rules is that others frequently have to remind those with ADHD of what they are supposed to be doing. Those who supervise a child with ADHD end up frustrated and angry. Ultimately the child may fail, be retained in a grade, and eventually drop out of school. An adult with ADHD may even fail to get a desired promotion or be fired. The general impression left with others, at best, is that the person with ADHD is less mature and lacks self-discipline and organization. At worst, it implies that the person with ADHD is intentionally lazy, unmotivated, and indifferent or is intentionally trying to avoid his responsibilities.

I believe that these difficulties with following rules and directions are related to both the underlying problem with impulsiveness and to one of poor working memory—the capacity to hold in mind what one is supposed to be doing and use it to guide his ongoing behavior. It is less clear whether the impulsiveness creates the problem by disrupting the working memory and related rule following when urges to switch to competing activities arise or when the impulsiveness stems from an impaired ability of language to guide and control or govern behavior. Ample research exists to show that verbal ability, working memory, and impulsiveness are all interrelated. Individuals with better developed language and verbal skills typically have a greater capacity to keep in mind what they are supposed to be doing and are usually much less impulsive and more reflective in performing tasks than those with less well-developed verbal skills and working memory. The three problems are linked because young children learn to talk to themselves as one means of both remembering what they are supposed to be doing and for controlling their own behavior so as to be less impulsive, as mentioned earlier. Talking to themselves helps them keep things in mind and inhibit initial urges to respond a certain way. It also allows time for the children to talk over with themselves certain details of the task and various options for responding before choosing which one is the best response. We often refer to this as *thinking* or *reflection*. In either case, it is the use of self-directed speech that is a principal means of keeping our goals and plans in mind and is also involved in helping to control the children's behavior.

This problem of using self-directed speech to help actively remember what one is doing and to inhibit behavior was clearly demonstrated in a study conducted years ago and published in 1979 by my good friend Dr. Michael Gordon, then at the Upstate Medical Center (now Upstate Medical University) in Syracuse, New York. Dr. Gordon was studying the ability of children with and without hyperactivity (ADHD) to inhibit their responding to a task and learn to wait. He designed a small computer for this purpose and told the children to sit in front of the computer, press the button, and then wait a while before pressing it again. They earned a point only if they waited 6 seconds or more. The points could be cashed in for candies at the end of the experiment. The children were not told how long to wait each time before pressing the button, so they had to discover that interval through learning. Dr. Gordon found that the children with ADHD pressed the button much more often than the other children and were not as able to wait for the correct interval of time to pass. What was of more interest, however, was that while they were waiting for the time to pass before pressing the button, over 80% of the children without ADHD talked to themselves, counted, or gave themselves verbal instructions and strategies to help pass the time. The children with ADHD, by contrast, sang, hit the sides of the box, spun the button on the box, swung their legs a certain number of times, ran around the table, tapped their feet 16 times, stomped their feet 9 or 10 times, and the like. Only 30% of them reported the use of some verbal strategy like that used by the other children. The more the children used such physical behavior to help pass the time delay, the more hyperactive they were rated as being by their parents on a behavior rating scale. In other words, the children without ADHD were more likely to use verbal and thinking tactics to help them inhibit their behavior, stay on task, and wait, while the children with ADHD used more physical activity.

As you will see in Chapter 2, I now believe that the problem with inhibiting responses seen in ADHD arises first, interfering with the later development of the use of self-directed speech for self-control. However, because in later years they are not relying as much on such self-speech to help control themselves, children with ADHD are likely to be even more impulsive than children without ADHD. So the poor impulse control, though it arises first, prevents children with ADHD from using self-speech as effectively as other children do. This then hinders them further in their development of impulse control, self-control, and the use of plans and goals to guide their behavior.

Doing Work Inconsistently

Another symptom documented by research to be associated with ADHD is inconsistent and highly variable work performance. Because most children with ADHD are of average or greater intelligence, their inability to produce consistently acceptable work often perplexes those around them. On some days or at certain times, these children seem able to complete their assigned work easily, without help. At other times or on other days, they finish little if any of their work and may not get much done even with close supervision. Over time, this erratic pattern creates the impression that a person with ADHD is just lazy. As a child psychiatrist once said, "Children [with ADHD] do well in school twice and we hold it against them the rest of their life." Those times when children with ADHD complete their work unassisted can mislead people into thinking they have no real problems or disabilities. But the problem here is *not that they cannot do the work, but that they cannot maintain this consistent pattern of work productivity the way others can.* More than 35 years ago, this led Dr. Marcel Kinsbourne, a renowned child neurologist, to characterize ADHD as *variability disease,* or VD. Scientists now know that this rather striking pattern of inconsistency in their behavior and especially in their productivity is a clear sign that those with ADHD have a disorder of executive functioning. Using our language and self-directed speech to guide us is one of several of these executive functions and leads to much greater consistency in the way we act and work. Those with ADHD, as I have discussed, are influenced more by the moment than by a preconceived rule or plan. Consequently, their work will be highly variable, depending on the ever-changing conditions that day. It is quite possible that inconsistent work productivity is a by-product of the other symptoms described already, particularly of the core impairment of impulse control. Consistent work productivity demands the ability to inhibit impulses to engage in other, more immediately fun or rewarding activities, so the more limited and erratic one's impulse control is, the more variable work productivity will be. Productivity in children with ADHD will depend more on the circumstances of the immediate situation than on self-control, self-speech, and willpower, which eventually came to govern productivity in other children.

Where Is My Child's Self-Control?: A New View of ADHD

As this chapter has shown, the abilities to stop, think, inhibit, remember, plan, and then act, as well as to sustain actions in the face of distraction—the very things most of us do to help control ourselves—are problems for children with ADHD. Current scientific research, however, suggests that all of these surface problems may stem from a deeper core deficit in executive functioning—a developmental delay in self-regulation. It is my considered opinion that all of the primary characteristics of ADHD reflect a serious problem with inhibition and the other executive functions. This leads to a serious problem with self-control or the way in which the self acts as an executive to govern its patterns of behavior over time and especially toward the likely future. The self in a child with ADHD, in a sense, is not controlling, regulating, or executing behavior as well as it does in others. So the problems of those with ADHD do not stem from a lack of skill but from a lack of executive functioning or self-control. This means that *ADHD is not a problem with a child's knowing what to do; it is a problem with doing what the child knows*.

Unfortunately, most people believe that self-discipline, self-control, and willpower are entirely at our own command. Therefore children without self-control are viewed either as not wanting to control themselves (they are "bad seeds") or as not having learned to control themselves (they are viewed as simply "undisciplined" or poorly raised by their parents). Frankly, this view is grossly out of date relative to the science on the disorder. Science is showing us that there are neurological (brain) and even genetic factors that contribute to self-control and willpower, along with learning and upbringing. And when these brain systems are functioning improperly or become damaged, normal levels of self-control and willpower are impossible. Those with ADHD are such people. They have a biologically based problem with self-control and the execution of their willpower. This new view of ADHD as a disorder of executive functioning (self-control) is the subject of Chapter 2.

To study ADHD is to gain a glimpse of the will itself and how it comes to be so powerful as an agent in self-control. This power to show self-control for the sake of directing behavior toward the future is uniquely human; no other animal has it. Those with ADHD, I believe, have a developmental impairment in this power. As a result, *to have ADHD is to have a disabled will and consequently a future in doubt.* This is what makes you as a parent so concerned and alarmed about what you see going astray in your child's behavioral and social development. It may be why you are reading this book.

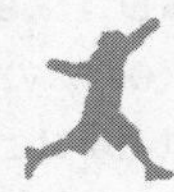

2 "What's Really Wrong with My Child?"

POOR SELF-CONTROL

ADHD is probably among the best studied of all psychological disorders of childhood. Still, our understanding of the psychology of ADHD is far from complete. While we now know that ADHD represents a problem in the manner in which children develop control over their impulses and their capacity to regulate their own behavior, these problems are not perfectly well defined.

How do children develop self-control? What are the behavioral or psychological mechanisms and processes that underlie our ability as human beings to control our own behavior better than any other species can? And which of these processes appears to be impaired or delayed in ADHD? As mentioned in Chapter 1, scientific studies have shown that the obvious symptoms associated with ADHD can be reduced to poor attention, impulsiveness, and hyperactivity and that the last two seem to be part of the same problem—impairment of behavioral inhibition. Since we have also learned that problems with attention may be part of childhood psychological disorders besides ADHD, it is important to identify precisely what kinds of attention problems link up with ADHD more than these other disorders. To date research shows that they are persistence over time toward goals or tasks (attention to the future) and resistance to distractions, which is obviously related to persistence. These occur alongside the problem with behavioral inhibition that also seems to be relatively unique to ADHD—these are the hallmark symptoms.

Even what we call problems with attention at times seem to be problems with inhibiting behavior—inhibiting the urge to do something a child would rather be doing than the task at hand. So when we say that children with ADHD have a short attention span, we really mean they have a short *interest* span. Similarly, when children without ADHD mature and become better at inhibiting the urge to shift to more rewarding or interesting activities, we say they have acquired a longer attention span, but what we should say is that they have a more developed ability to restrain their impulses and to stay with a plan or an instruction and not be so distractible. Children with ADHD are like younger normal children. Their problem does not seem to be only one of paying attention but also just as much one of sustaining inhibition. So it seems that all three problems thought to be the primary symptoms of ADHD—inattention, impulsiveness, and hyperactivity—can be reduced to a delay in the development of inhibition of behavior and of persistence toward goals and the future more generally.

Everything Comes to Those Who Can Wait: ADHD and the Brain's Executive Functions

I am not the first scientist to argue that the major problems of children with ADHD stem from a fundamental deficit in their ability to engage in self-control using the brain's executive functions or abilities. Chief among those executive mental abilities is the capacity to inhibit behavior, an ability to contemplate one's relevant past experiences, as well as to anticipate the future consequences that can be expected from such hindsight. This information is then used to decide how best to act at the moment and how to sustain one's actions toward achieving goals. The English physician Dr. George Still made this point as far back as 1902. What these scientists have not done, however, is explain how these problems with inhibition, self-contemplation, and poor persistence toward goals lead to the many impairments we find in the academic, social, occupational, mental, language, and emotional domains. Doing so would surely strengthen the theory that deficits in inhibition and the other executive functions are at the root of ADHD. I believe that this can now be done.

The commonly held view of ADHD as a problem with inattention and hyperactivity has, over the years, failed to explain many of the findings about children with ADHD—what I call "orphan" findings, since they have no "parent" theory to account for them. For instance:

- We know that children with ADHD do not benefit from warnings about what is going to happen later. They seem to base their behavior on what is at hand rather than on information about future events. How is this explained by the fact that they are impulsive or can't concentrate?
- Other studies have also found that the speech that children with ADHD typically use in talking to themselves while working or playing is less mature than that of other children. Why? What does that have to do with their not being able to inhibit their behavior?
- Dr. Sydney Zentall and her colleagues at Purdue University more than 35 years ago observed that children with ADHD do not do mental arithmetic as fast or as well as other children, despite the fact that they have no problem understanding math. Many other studies have found such deficits in being able

to hold information in mind and to manipulate it—deficits now known to be due to problems with working memory. How is this deficiency explained by their immature inhibition or inattention?

- Drs. Carol Whalen and Barbara Henker at the University of California at Irvine found more than 30 years ago that when children with ADHD play or work with other children on a task, the information they communicate to others is less organized, less mature, and less helpful in getting the activity done than the information communicated by children of the same age without ADHD. Other studies have routinely confirmed these initial results.

These and many other such orphan findings are the issues that must be resolved if we are to have a more complete account of ADHD. My belief that all of these problems can stem from a problem with inhibition and the other executive functions begins with my discovery of a theory advanced more than 40 years ago by Dr. Jacob Bronowski—the late philosopher, physicist, mathematician, and author of *The Ascent of Man,* the critically acclaimed book and public television series from the late 1970s. In a brief yet profound essay, in 1977 Dr. Bronowski discussed how our language and thinking came to differ so dramatically from the types of social communication used by other animals, especially our relatives, the primates. In his essay I found the seeds to understanding both the brain's executive (self-regulatory) abilities and what may be going wrong in the psychological development of those with ADHD.

Self-Directed Inhibition: The Mind's Brakes

In 1977 Dr. Bronowski proposed that everything that makes our language unique (and us human) flowed from the evolution of the simple capacity to impose a delay between a signal, a message, or an event that we experience and our reaction or response to it. We have the ability to wait for far longer periods of time than other species can before responding. This power to wait stems from our greater ability to inhibit immediate urges to respond, and because inhibition takes effort, waiting is not a passive act. Being able to inhibit our immediate urges to respond and instead wait for a while, wrote Dr. Bronowski, enables us to (1) create a sense of ourselves in our past, and from it a sense of our likely or possible future giving us a conscious sense of ourselves over time and what may be possible for us to become or achieve; (2) talk to ourselves and use such language to control our own behavior; (3) separate emotion from information in our evaluation of events and thus be more rational; and (4) break incoming information or messages into parts and then recombine those parts into new outgoing messages or responses (*analysis* and *synthesis*) and so engage in planning, problem solving, and goal-directed innovation. To these I would add one more: (5) the ability to self-regulate internal motivation to drive our behavior toward our goals. If ADHD is a problem with a person's ability to inhibit responses, then we might expect someone with ADHD to have problems with these five other mental abilities.

These five mental abilities are called executive functions because, like an executive running a corporation, they allow us to monitor and direct ourselves over time toward the future. They give us self-control. "Executive functioning" is a commonly used term these days in professional journals and in discussions with patients and their families. But there is no agreement as to its definition among scientists working in the field. To me, executive functioning is self-regulation, but it refers to types of self-regulation. Each type is considered to be such a function or mental ability. Recently, in my latest book on a theory of executive functioning and self-regulation, I specified that self-regulation can be thought of as involving three steps: (1) we direct some action back at ourselves, (2) in order to change our behavior from what it otherwise would have been, (3) so as to change our future in some important way (increase or decrease later consequences for ourselves).

With this definition of self-regulation in mind, I stated that there are six executive functions and each one is a type of self-regulation (an action we direct at ourselves to change ourselves in order to alter our future for the better). In other words, there are six things we do to change ourselves and our future. What are they? The first is (1) inhibition or self-restraint, as stated above. The others are (2) self-directed attention to achieve self-awareness, (3) self-directed visual imagery to achieve hindsight and foresight (awareness of ourselves across time), (4) self-directed speech to control ourselves by language, (5) self-directed emotions to manage them better and to achieve self-motivation, and (6) self-directed play, to solve problems and to invent solutions. I explain (2) through (6) below.

Self-Directed Attention (Self-Awareness): The Mind's Mirror

Our ability to delay responses and wait is one of three fundamental executive abilities. It is associated with the ability to direct our attention not only at the environment around us but at ourselves as well. We watch and so monitor ourselves as we behave, and so we have self-awareness. This means that inhibition (stopping) and self-awareness are two of our most fundamental executive functions. We use this awareness of ourselves and what we are doing to monitor our actions and to inhibit them when it seems wise to do so, such as in a novel situation or when we have made a mistake. Think of it as our mind's mirror on ourselves.

Self-Directed Imagery: The Mind's Eye

By storing in our memory our awareness of ourselves and our actions in prior situations, we can have a sense of ourselves now as well as of ourselves in that past. Doing so gives us a sense of who we are and what we have done; it is our personal history. Such stored awareness of our past can then be consciously remembered (usually visualized) at a later time, held in mind, and used to guide us in understanding and responding to the events of the moment based on whatever wisdom our past can shed on the situation. Thus our past learning informs our current behavior. We have *hindsight*. Using it, we learn from our mistakes and our successes far more rapidly and effectively than any other species can do. These images of our past can be used like a GPS (global positioning system) mapping device in our cars. The GPS shows us an image of the terrain we are in, where we have been, and where we are headed at the moment, which we use to get to our destination. Similarly, we hold images of our past in mind to guide us through situations that are similar to those past ones so we can get to our goals and be better prepared for what lies ahead of us.

Thinking about our past and contrasting it with our present also enables us to create what Dr. Bronowski called *hypothetical futures*. They are "what if" futures that arise from asking questions like "What if I did this or that now? What would it lead to later in the future?" It represents our sense of the likely future that may be in store for us if we continue to behave as we are doing or if we change our behavior and do something else. We make educated guesses about what will happen next because we have thought about our past and used any evidence of patterns from it to develop ideas about the future if that pattern were to continue or if we were to change it in some fundamental way. In doing so, we can both prepare better for those predictable events if we don't change and plan for the new events if we do change what we propose to do now. We now have *foresight*. Certainly our guesses about the likely future won't always be right, but we will be better off making educated guesses from our sense of our past than simply failing to think about the past and so about the future altogether. This way we use our sense of the past to create a sense of the likely future if we don't change course and of the possible future if we do change what we are doing. Eventually as children develop, along with that ability to recall memories of their past will develop their ability to manipulate and combine them, which forms their imagination. And also by recalling the past and using that to sense the likely future, we can share that sense of the future with others who have reasoned along with us; we can make plans with others and promises to them, using time as a benchmark for doing things as no other species can.

Referring backward (the past) and forward (the future) in time and our lives creates for us a mental window on ourselves across time as it applies to us. During our waking hours, we are almost continuously aware of this moving window of ourselves in time in our consciousness. From our sense of immediately past events, we are continuously inferring what is likely to happen in the immediate future. We use it to develop expectations, to create plans, and to anticipate likely future events. We seem to do this almost effortlessly, and so we take this foresight for granted. I consider this capacity for hindsight and foresight to be the third fundamental executive ability, alongside inhibition and self-awareness. Some researchers call it "nonverbal working memory," but I see it more simply as the ability to recall our past and from it to imagine our future.

If ADHD represents a deficit in inhibiting behavior and waiting, as I have suggested, then this theory predicts that people with ADHD should show a more limited sense of self-awareness and self-monitoring. This will eventually lead to a problem with having and using their sense of their past (hindsight) and, as a result, a more limited sense of anticipating their likely future (foresight) if they don't change their current behavior. They will also have less of a sense of the possible future that might occur for them if they would change the course of their current behavior. Their mental window on time and their sense of themselves across time should be much narrower. They would live in "the now" more exclusively than others who are thinking about themselves across time. Anyone who has lived with someone with ADHD knows that this is in fact the case. As parents often say, children with ADHD do not seem to learn from past mistakes, to act with a sense of their past, or to contemplate the future consequences of how they choose to behave. Rather than not learning, I think they respond too quickly, which prevents them from referring to their past experiences and so to consider what those might teach them about present events. In essence, this means that children and adults with ADHD have a "nearsightedness" to the future. They can see and deal with only those events that are very close at hand or imminent, and not those that lie further ahead. One could say that they are blind to time or the future, or have a sort of future neglect syndrome, in which they are less aware of and attentive to durations of time and the future that likely lies before them.

Those with ADHD will also be less prepared for the future. Because they do not "see" or contemplate events that are approaching from the future, they are likely to careen through life from crisis to crisis. When the inevitable catastrophe from such lack of foresight strikes, they are caught off-guard and react accordingly. They are far too much creatures of the moment.

The upside here is that they do not seem to be as limited by fear of the future as many of us are. We sometimes envy their almost child-like innocence, their happy-go-lucky nature, and their devil-may-care attitude about the moment. Those with ADHD may also take chances that might luckily pan out where others would hold back. Life for (and with) persons with ADHD may be more exciting as a result, both good and bad.

Lack of foresight, however, can have serious negative and even life-threatening consequences. At the least, the effects can be socially devastating. Promises broken, appointments unmet, and deadlines missed can bring down swift, negative, and unforgiving judgment by others. Reliability is, after all, one of the defining characteristics of a responsible adult in our society. Yet adults with ADHD or with a childhood history of hyperactivity report that they have problems with money management, household organization, management of children's schedules, and working independently on the job, with a commensurately slower upward movement in their social and occupational status—all related to their diminished sense of time and the future.

Because of the neurological deficit in the abilities to inhibit behavior, be self-aware, and use their hindsight and foresight, people with ADHD not only do not see what lies ahead of them as well as others, but they *cannot* do so as well as others. In essence, holding them responsible for their problem with anticipating and planning for the future is like holding a deaf person responsible for not hearing us or a blind person accountable for not seeing us—it is ridiculous and serves no constructive social purpose. Yet that is exactly what our society tends to do. We respond with disbelief when told that a person with ADHD did not fully understand the consequences of his behavior, calling it a cop-out to avoid accepting responsibility. We label these people careless, heedless, unreliable, or risktakers, and view them as immature or even immoral or irrational. We hold them responsible for their seeming carelessness and punish them accordingly, sometimes severely.

No wonder so many of those with ADHD are so demoralized upon reaching adolescence or young adulthood. By then they begin to adopt society's view of themselves, holding themselves as much to blame for their failures as do others. This sense of underachievement and of failing themselves and their families can be so serious in adults with ADHD as to require separate psychological treatment from what may be needed to deal with their ADHD symptoms alone.

The altered sense of time these deficits create in those with ADHD has several other interesting effects. First, it may make them feel as if time is passing more slowly than it actually does. This means most things seem to take longer than they expected, which is understandably frustrating. It's not surprising, then, that people with ADHD seem very impatient under many circumstances. Second, without a sense of the future, it's difficult to defer gratification. Studies that have followed children with ADHD into adulthood (see Chapter 4) provide clear evidence that they are not as likely to choose pathways in life that involve immediate sacrifice for longer term, much larger payoffs. Examples include sticking with higher education and saving money. Finally, there is some evidence that this diminished sense of the future causes those with ADHD to be less health-conscious than others. One price we pay for our sense of time is an accompanying sense of our own limited existence and eventual death. So the natural conclusion is that people with ADHD may not have the same sense of their own mortality that the rest of us have. Perhaps they are not part of the wave of increasing appreciation for the health-related consequences of our behavior.

Having less regard for the future consequences of any behavior, are individuals with ADHD more likely than others to engage in deleterious habits such as overeating, lack of exercise, smoking tobacco, drinking alcohol to excess, abusing illegal substances, and driving carelessly? Every indication that they may be so comes from follow-up studies that have found teenagers and young adults with ADHD to be more likely to smoke tobacco and drink alcohol, and to do so more frequently, than those who do not have ADHD. They also have a greater risk for speeding tickets and traffic accidents while driving than do others of their age group, as noted in Chapter 1. In addition, recent research suggests that teens with ADHD are likely to become sexually active somewhat earlier than normal teens, are less likely to employ birth control during sexual activities, and are more likely therefore to become pregnant or to contract sexually transmitted diseases. Young adults with ADHD may also be more overweight and less likely to exercise or engage in other forms of health maintenance and to use preventive medical and dental practices, and so be more prone to coronary heart disease. All of these risks illustrate the problems that can result from failure to give due deliberation to the future generally and the later consequences of current actions specifically.

Self-Directed Speech: The Mind's Voice

Another ability that is related to being able to inhibit behavior, show self-awareness, and have a sense of our past and future is the ability to talk to ourselves. Dr. Bronowski pointed out that all other species use their language to communicate with others. Only humans have developed the ability to use language to communicate with themselves as well. We see this ability developing in children. They progress from talking to others as toddlers to talking out loud to themselves while playing during their later preschool years to gradually talking to themselves subvocally (so that others do not hear) during the early elementary years. Finally they wind up talking to themselves in their "mind's voice" so that no one detects the self-speech at all. This is called *internalized speech.* It forms the fourth executive ability or function that allows us to control our own behavior. We can talk to ourselves.

The changes this self-speech brings about in behavior as it develops are quite remarkable. As speech goes from being directed solely at others to also being directed at ourselves and then being internalized, it also moves from just describing things to giving ourselves directions or instructions. That is, it becomes not just a way to talk about the world to ourselves, but a means of guiding and controlling our own behavior through self-directed instructions. Such self-instructions increasingly take over the guidance of our behavior, freeing it from the domineering control of immediate events around us. As a result, self-speech helps us stay on our course toward our plans and goals. It also helps us do better the next time we encounter a task because we have now formulated some instructions to follow, based on our initial experience with that task or situation. And it provides a means by which we can directly encourage ourselves to ride out the current situation, boring or unpleasant as it may be, so as to achieve the goal and the greater rewards often associated with such deferred gratification.

Psychologists have called the ability to use language to control behavior *rule-governed behavior.* When we develop plans for the future, set goals for ourselves, and then carry out our behavior according to those plans and goals, we are often using rule-governed behavior to facilitate it. These four executive abilities discussed so far largely underlie our sense of free will. We recognize that they free us from having our behavior controlled by the immediate and momentary circumstances that utterly control the behavior of other species. We can bring our behavior under the control of rules, instructions, plans, and goals so that our sense of the past informs our behavior in the present, but so does our sense of the future.

Current research on ADHD now gives us enough evidence to say with certainty that these four domains of executive functioning, including self-speech and rule-governed behavior, are deficient in those with ADHD. This may also help to explain why children with ADHD talk too much compared to others—their speech is less internalized or private. Certainly those of us who work clinically with these children, as well as many parents and teachers, have commented on the problems they have with using language and rules in the service of self-control.

Dr. Stephen Hayes, a psychologist who has written extensively about the human ability to use rule-governed behavior and its consequences, has identified a number of conditions that result from our ability to use self-speech and the rule-following behavior it permits. These conditions, being diminished in people with ADHD, support the theory that deficiencies in self-speech and rule-governed behavior are part of ADHD:

1. Our behavior in a given situation should be much less variable when we are following rules than when we are being influenced or controlled by the events of the moment. As mentioned earlier, inconsistent work performance and more variable behavior is a hallmark of ADHD.

2. A person who is following rules should be less susceptible to control by the immediate consequences or events in a situation and their momentary and potentially unpredictable changes. In ADHD, however, we constantly see people "going with the flow," apparently letting events control them rather than the other way around.

3. Where rules are in conflict with the desires of the moment, the rule is more likely to control our behavior. In other words, we are able to stick to a plan (such as a diet) even though the lure (the ice cream in the freezer) is more attractive right now. The person with ADHD is constantly being controlled by the promise of whatever seems more rewarding at the moment; she is more likely than most to give in to the craving for the ice cream, even though it means deviating from the diet.

4. At times rule-governed behavior makes us too rigid; the rule we are following is inappropriate for the specific situation we are facing, but we follow it anyway. For example, we prepare a recipe by a cook we trust, and the resulting dish is mediocre. Yet we follow it to the letter a second time, because the cookbook author is widely known and must be right. It still comes out less than great—because, unknown to us, there is a typographical error in the recipe; the rules are incorrect. A person with ADHD may taste the recipe as he goes along and modify it to his liking, even though such modifications are not part of the recipe. Because he breaks the rules and lets his tasting of the dish (the immediate feedback or consequences) guide him, the dish may turn out better. So under some circumstances, those with ADHD may actually have an advantage over people who are too rule-governed.

5. When we follow rules, we should be able to persist at what we are doing and behave "properly," even though any rewards for doing so will be long delayed. That is, we should be able to defer gratification. For instance, a child should be able to stick to the rules or plan to do homework because the more distant rewards—the

consequences of turning in the work the next day or not—are more important than the current reward of avoiding the boring assignment. The child with ADHD is more likely to get off-task (to lose track of the rule) during the homework and to pursue things that are more rewarding at the moment.

6. Finally, we should see a steady increase in the ability to use rule-governed behavior over time during a child's development into adulthood. Yet children with ADHD are consistently seen as immature precisely because they are more easily controlled by momentary events and immediate consequences than others their age, and because they lag behind in the ability to follow rules, to talk to themselves, to use rules to control their own behavior, and eventually to create their own rules when faced with problems.

Self-Directed Emotions: The Mind's Heart

This is the fifth executive function or ability. Being able to inhibit our urges to respond and to wait gives our brain time to split incoming information into two parts: the personal meaning of the event (our feelings or emotional reactions) and the information or content of the event. We can then deal with the content objectively, without introducing as much personal bias into our reaction based on our emotions. We certainly do not do this all the time, but we have the power to do it and to realize that exercising this ability enables us to deal more rationally, less emotionally, and so more effectively with a given situation. This is why we tell our children to count to 10 before reacting to an upset: it gives them time to settle down and begin to reevaluate what has happened more rationally and objectively.

We know from personal experience that responding impulsively with emotional behavior is clearly not always in our best interest. Neither is it always bad, but waiting and better evaluating what is happening to us allows us to formulate our reactions, even our emotional ones, so that they are better suited to the situation. This capacity to delay our response permits us to evaluate events more objectively, rationally, and logically, as if from the standpoint of an outside, neutral witness. It gives us the power to study our world more objectively than any other species can. In fact, if we could not separate our personal feelings about information from the information itself, we could not pursue science—our most rational human endeavor.

This is not to say that we develop to a point where we have no emotions or are entirely objective in our reactions to events. Nothing could be further from the truth. Our emotional reactions are an essential part of our ability to evaluate the world around us and make decisions. But how we respond to events and make decisions about them can be affected very adversely if we allow them to be governed by the first emotions we feel when something happens to us. It is this initial emotional urge that often requires some restraint and a period of moderation to make it not only more socially acceptable to others around us, but also more effective in helping us make the right decisions and to achieve our goals. This theory seems to explain why children with ADHD are so emotional compared to other children. By not inhibiting their first reactions to a situation, they do not give themselves time to separate their feelings from the facts. They usually live to regret these impulsive and raw emotional reactions because their behavior drives others away, resulting in social hostility, punishment, rejection, and eventually loss of friendships. It gives them a bad reputation with teachers and coaches, strains relationships with parents and siblings, and in adults can lead to even greater conflicts at home and especially at work, including a greater likelihood of being fired.

Their failure to inhibit their feelings as well as other children of the same age makes us see children with ADHD as emotionally immature. A 7-year-old child with ADHD may throw a tantrum when denied a snack just before dinner, for example. While we might accept this reaction from a 4-year-old, we would expect most 7-year-olds to be able to inhibit the angry reaction for long enough to cool off and evaluate the information conveyed by Mom: the reasons for denying the snack.

Unfortunately, we cannot push that 7-year-old to the maturity we'd like to see simply by telling her to inhibit reactions or wait before responding. As Chapter 3 explains, the power to do so is impaired because of a problem in the brain centers responsible for inhibition and the other executive abilities. Although people with ADHD may be able to learn consciously to inhibit their behavior in certain situations, this takes a great deal of effort.

Consequently, people with ADHD will have difficulty adapting to situations that require being cool, calm, and unemotional or objective. Unfortunately, our society seems to place us in many such situations. Indeed, our society highly values the ability to remain calm and rational, and often rewards it with greater status, prestige, responsibility, and even income than those without such ability can expect.

There is an upside, however: those with ADHD will be very passionate and emotional in their actions, and thus may do what they do with far more personal conviction and certainly less hesitation than the rest of us. Those with ADHD may very well match or surpass others in the performing arts (such as music or drama) or in the humanities (such as writing poetry or fiction), where strong emotional expression is advantageous. Where passionate conviction is desirable, such as in negotiation or sales, we might find that people with ADHD shine. Combined with their talkativeness and preference for socializing over solitary work, such passion can make for very good salespeople. Remember, it is not their intellect that is impaired. Nor is their *ability* to separate emotions from information completely lacking. People with ADHD simply do not exercise that ability as well or as efficiently or use it to guide their behavior as much because they respond too quickly. By not controlling their impulse to act, they do not leave time for emotional restraint and for the splitting off of facts from personal feeling. I do not mean to imply here that those with ADHD are better than other people in these particular professions. I only mean that they may be at considerably less of a disadvantage than they may be in other occupations that stress emotional restraint and objectivity. They will be less distinguishable from others in these walks of life and so may have a better chance to excel because of their other positive attributes.

Linked to emotional self-control is the capacity for *self-motivation*. When normal children develop emotional self-control, part of what they are doing is internalizing their emotions and keeping them from public display. The emotional reaction exists, but its public display is being restrained. This ability to keep emotions covert or inside while we experience them and attempt to moderate them can lead us to modify them as needed before displaying them to others. We may even be able to greatly reduce or eliminate these initial emotional urges by trying to calm ourselves down, thinking of something more positive, or talking to ourselves about why it would not be good to express that feeling.

This internalizing of emotion is important for another reason, however. Emotions tell us whether we find something positive, negative or unpleasant, or just neutral. As such, they can encourage us to continue what we are doing or stop it and switch to something better. That is, they motivate us toward some sort of action. So children who can internalize their emotions are automatically developing the ability to internalize their motivation. This facility is the origin of what many people call *intrinsic motivation* and what others might call *drive*, *persistence*, *ambition*, *determination*, *willpower*, or *stick-to-it-iveness*. When we create our own internal motivation, we don't need the encouragement, rewards, payoffs, or other incentives that younger children require as often as they do to stay the course. We can stick with our plans, follow through on our goals, and resist the things around us that may be distracting because we are using our own inner motivational state to drive our own behavior toward the goal. We can largely motivate ourselves in the absence of other incentives or inducements. Private, internalized emotions become the wellspring for our private motivations, and these can support our behavior directed toward goals and the future and help us stay the course toward them. This is a major part of the human will—will*power*.

This revelation helps us see why children with ADHD have so much trouble with persistence, willpower, or what others call a short attention span. It's not really attention that's the problem, but self-motivation. They cannot create private, internal, or intrinsic motivation as well as others, and so they cannot persist at activities, plans, goals, or instructions as well as others can do when there is little incentive or motivation in the setting or task to help them sustain it. The more boring and unrewarding an activity is, the harder it will be for them to do what normal children do: create their own motivation to help them stick with the task. This means that they must depend on external sources of motivation, and that when external consequences are not provided they will drift away from the work or activity at hand—not because of laziness, but because of a biological problem with the functioning of this part of the brain. Obviously, then, helping a child with ADHD complete a task often means arranging additional and at times artificial sources of motivation, such as rewards.

Self-Directed Mental Play: The Source of Problem Solving and Innovation

The sixth and final executive ability is related to our internal use of speech and consists of two parts: (1) the ability to break information or messages we receive into parts or smaller units (*analysis*) and (2) the ability to recombine these parts into entirely new outgoing messages or instructions (*synthesis*). We do not treat instructions or information as indivisible wholes. While we may treat a sentence as one grammatical unit, we recognize that it can also be broken down into nouns, verbs, adverbs, and other parts of speech. Likewise, we know that the idea conveyed can be broken down into the objects in the idea, the actions taken with the objects, the physical nature of the objects (colors, shapes, etc.), and so on. With this mental ability, we can first decompose and analyze the messages and information we receive, in the same way that we can parse a sentence. Second, we can reassemble those parts in a nearly infinite number of ways and then choose the outgoing message or behavior that may be most adaptive or successful at that moment. This ability endows us with tremendous powers of problem solving, imagination, and creativity. Unless we wait and allow enough time for it to happen, this process, called *reconstitution* by Dr. Bronowski, is unlikely to occur.

This ability constitutes yet another executive function: problem solving and goal-directed innovation or creativity. We can *invent* new ideas and new rules when we have no past experience or immediately available rule to follow. When we inhibit our response and wait, we can take old ideas and rules and break them apart, combining them with those of other ideas and rules to come up with entirely new combinations. We call this process *problem solving,* and as humans we are masters at it. People who cannot inhibit and delay their responses to what's happening around them will be less adept at devising solutions to problems they have encountered.

If ADHD involves a deficit in executive functioning, then those with ADHD should not be as good at this process of reconstitution or problem solving as people without ADHD. Very little research on this idea as it applies to ADHD is available, but what research does exist seems to support its being problematic for those with ADHD. The results of psychology experiments in which children with ADHD have been required to come up with as many solutions to a given problem as they can think of within a short period of time suggest that they are not able to do so as well as other children. Other studies examining the curiosity of children with ADHD during play have shown that they do not evaluate or explore objects as well as other children of the same age. The results suggest that children with ADHD do not analyze things they are doing into as many parts or dimensions as children without ADHD do. Such findings seem to hint that the process of problem solving or goal-directed innovation is not used as well in children with ADHD as in other children.

The Social Purposes of Executive Functioning and Self-Control

As I indicated earlier, these six executive functions are what give us our capacity for self-regulation and hence self-determination. We are the only species that possesses these mental abilities (though the first three of them may be evident in a very, very primitive form in our closest living evolutionary relatives, the chimpanzees). What is their purpose? How did they contribute to our survival and welfare in such important ways that they have evolved to their current far higher state of advancement in modern people? For more than a decade I have struggled to find answers to these questions. My search led me to not only review the existing science on what psychological and social deficits people have when they suffer injuries to their executive brain but also the major life activities in which we all engage to promote our survival and welfare and what research on human evolution might have to say on the matter. The results of my search were published in my 2012 book *The Executive Functions: What They Are, How They Work, and Why They Evolved,* which further develops my theory of executive functioning and self-control (and, by extension, of ADHD as well). The short answer to these questions was suggested in earlier books by clinical scientists studying the functions of the prefrontal lobes of the brain—those parts that have become the most highly evolved (and proportionally largest) in humans. These regions of the brain just behind the forehead have been called the "executive" brain because they direct the other parts of the brain and so other mental abilities for purposes of selecting, pursuing, and achieving our goals. Dr. Stuart Dimond, for instance, stated in 1980 that this part of the brain was the seat of our social intelligence. Fifteen years later, Dr. Muriel Lezak stated that they give us our sense of will and purpose and serve to meet our social responsibilities. Like other scientists before and after them, they saw the functions of this part of the brain as being crucial to our social life. I agree, and so I went on to create a model of executive functioning and self-control that identifies four important levels organized in a hierarchy that extend these mental abilities outward into the most important social and civilizing activities in which people engage in their daily life. This part of the brain, and hence these mental abilities, take 25–30 years to mature completely. I will very briefly describe these levels here so that you can understand what people with prefrontal lobe injuries or those with ADHD might be struggling with due to deficits in their executive mental faculties.

The Instrumental/Self-Directed Level

This first level of self-regulation consists of the six executive functions described above. They are called "instrumental" because they provide a means to an end—they consist of things we do to ourselves mentally to control, change, and adjust our behavior. We do that so that we not only can react well to the moment but, more importantly, so that we can improve our future. Specifically, we do so to maximize the later consequences for ourselves instead of always just focusing on the small immediate consequences, as other animals do. We generally cannot see people engaging in most of these self-directed actions because they are mental or private in nature, taking place in the head and forming the conscious mind of the individual; they are "cognitive." We cannot directly observe people engaging in self-awareness, hindsight, foresight, self-talk, emotion regulation, self-motivation, and mental play, but we know from research that they can do these things and do so throughout their waking day. When people think, this is what they are using to do so. These six instruments give us a set of "mind tools," like a Swiss Army knife that we can use to control our own behavior, and anticipate, prepare for, and maximize our future, and hence our longer term welfare and happiness. By themselves, they aren't much good until we see how they promote the next stage or level of self-regulation.

The Self-Reliant Level

When children are born, they are helpless and depend on others (usually parents and family) for their survival and welfare. They continue to be dependent, though progressively less so, for much of the next 10 to 20 years of their lives. With each passing year, however, we witness growth in their ability to care for themselves. This is not only evident in their growing ability to feed, dress, bathe, and otherwise care for their own immediate needs and survival. It is also evident in their growing self-determination, separation from others on whom they previously depended, and self-defense against being used by others to their own disadvantage. The first immediate purpose of executive functioning, then, is to promote the development of daily adaptive functioning (self-care), self-reliance (independence from others), and social self-defense against any pernicious influences of others (self-determination). I think of this as the Robinson Crusoe level of executive functioning—we care for ourselves and our needs while also protecting ourselves from others who may not have our own best interests in mind. As this stage matures, we will see an increase in five interrelated types of behavior and activities in the daily life of the individual: (1) time management, (2) self-organization and problem solving, (3) self-restraint, (4) emotional self-control, and (5) self-motivation. I have recently developed rating scales that can be used to assess these five dimensions of daily executive activities in children and adults. Once this level is well under way, it can facilitate the development of the next stage of executive functioning.

The Social Reciprocity Level

Although this stage begins in relationships within the family, it extends outward to eventually include reciprocal interactions with others. "Reciprocity" here means exchanging, sharing, taking turns, and otherwise trading with other people: we do something for someone, and that person returns the favor. This is the stage at which we make commitments to others, keep promises, trade things we have with others for things they have that we want, and share some of our bounty with others with the understanding that in the future they will do the same for us. People do this every day many times each day. It forms the basis not only for friendships with others but also for economics, division of labor and trade, social etiquette, and even civil and criminal laws. Unlike most other creatures, we are turn-takers, sharers, traders, and reciprocators. Social reciprocity is one of the principal means by which people survive. It spreads the risk of living in an uncertain world by using others in the group like an insurance risk-pool in which all assist each other as needed with the expectation of receiving similar assistance. We live in groups with others, and we have developed a means to depend on each other to promote our own survival and that of others we care for and live with. For this to succeed, we have to police our group and be quick to detect the cheaters among us, withdraw from future dealings with them, and even punish them for their cheating or freeloading without reciprocating. This is one of the major social purposes of the executive brain besides that of social self-defense and independence seen at the prior level.

The Social Cooperative Level

Although reciprocity or sharing and trading can be thought of as being cooperative, here I use the word *cooperative* as a noun to mean a group of people who come together to accomplish a goal that none of them could reach alone or through simply trading with each other. Here people who have a common goal get together to work to achieve it and divide up the benefits of doing so. By working as a team they can attain goals that are longer term, larger, more complex, and more beneficial than they could achieve by themselves. This is evident every day in many employment settings, community events, and other social activities that require a group of people to work together to achieve a common purpose or goal. If these groups stay together to accomplish multiple goals over time, they may even develop a type of behavior called *mutualism* seen among family members and close friends. This is where people look out for each other's longer term welfare and not just their own. They "have each other's back" so to speak in that they not only work together to achieve a specific goal but also relate to each other in myriad ways that place the other person's longer term welfare above their own immediate or near-term well-being. Neighborhoods, working groups, close friendship networks, military units, and other such groups that stay together long enough may eventually move up to this highest level of personal and social welfare.

When people experience injuries or developmental problems in their executive, prefrontal brain, these are the types of personal and social activities that are at risk of being deficient or impaired. Understanding executive functioning through this multistage model, we can see just how crucial it is to human survival, welfare, and everyday life and why disorders of executive functioning like ADHD are very serious.

The Development of Executive Functioning

We do not have this tremendous power to be aware of ourselves and to inhibit our behavior when we are first born or during our very early development. Studies of infants indicate that it begins to develop toward the end of the first year of life but continues for the next 20–30 years. As we mature, we can monitor our own behavior and delay it as needed in situations for increasingly longer periods of time so as to use our hindsight and foresight before we finally choose how to respond. Once these three executive abilities emerge (inhibition, self-awareness, hindsight/foresight), the other three mental abilities I have discussed here probably start to mature slowly and in a stepwise manner.

Dr. Bronowski seems to suggest that the ability to inhibit may develop alongside our emerging self-awareness. Perhaps it emerges during the first year of life. Within a few years, a sense of our past begins to mature and, along with it, a beginning sense of the future. The ability to talk to ourselves and to use self-speech likely develops next, between 3 and 5 years of age, and slowly becomes internalized so that others no longer hear us doing this. Research on early language development has indicated that the beginnings of self-directed and internal speech probably take 8–10 years to mature completely. Next to emerge, and dependent on the earlier stages, is the ability to create private emotions and from this self-motivation. The last to develop is the ability to analyze and break ideas down into units and then recombine or synthesize them into entirely new ideas. It is not clear when this ability begins to occur in child development, but it overlaps with the development of children's play.

In my opinion, future scientific studies of children with ADHD are likely to show that they develop all of these executive abilities somewhat later than children without ADHD do. Future research is also likely to show that they are less proficient at them than children of the same age without ADHD. Fortunately for most children with ADHD, some research is beginning to show that ADHD medications produce a temporary improvement in executive abilities such that children with ADHD behave and think much like their age-mates without ADHD while they are taking medication. They are now able to show self-control, to direct their behavior toward the future, and to free themselves from being controlled purely by events of the moment.

The Neurological Connection: Rethinking Our View of Will

We know that ADHD involves a deficit in the ability of the individual to inhibit responses to situations or events. That is, it is a problem of self-control. As such, the term *developmental disorder of self-control (executive functioning)* may be the most accurate name for ADHD. The term ADHD, focusing as it does on attention deficit and hyperactivity, clearly falls short. We also know from years of research that this ability to inhibit our behavior and self-regulate is controlled by the very front part of our brain, in an area known as the *prefrontal cortex*. Therefore, it has not been surprising to learn during the past 25 years of research that this part of the brain in people with ADHD is not as large, as mature, or as active as it is in those who do not have ADHD. This is also true of several other areas that are interconnected to the prefrontal cortex (see Chapter 3 for more on this subject). It is a tremendous advance in our understanding of ADHD to have a number of different studies that document this underdevelopment and underactivity of the brain and relate it to deficits in the executive abilities.

The theory I have discussed in this chapter indicates that this prefrontal part of the brain, or other parts closely related to it, must give us our powers of self-control and the capacity to direct our behavior toward the future. As Dr. Joaquim Fuster showed in his extensive research summarized in his 1997 book *The Prefrontal Cortex,* our knowledge from human patients and from primates with injuries to this part of their brain strongly suggests that it is likely to be so. Finally, our understanding of the brain and how it functions can now be fitted, like a piece of a puzzle, to what we have come to understand about the nature of ADHD, another piece of the puzzle. From this I believe we can safely conclude that ADHD involves a problem in the development and functioning of the prefrontal area of the brain and its connections to related brain regions.

The developmental–neurological nature of ADHD directly contradicts our strongly held beliefs that self-control and free will are totally determined by individuals and their upbringing. I believe that this contradiction is what underlies much of society's resistance to admitting this disorder into the class of developmental disabilities, for which we have great empathy and on behalf of which we make special allowances and rights. Society has struggled before with scientific advances that contradict the common wisdom of the time, and it has changed to accommodate them. It is my hope that society will come to do the same for ADHD.

Interestingly, while this understanding of ADHD should evoke empathy, it does not mean that we should stop holding children with ADHD accountable for their behavior. Those with ADHD are not insensitive to the consequences of their actions, but they have trouble connecting consequences with their own behavior because of the time delay between the behavior and the important delayed consequences of those actions. This means that to help those with ADHD we must make them *more* accountable, not less so. We must devise consequences that are more immediate, more frequent, and more salient than they would normally be in any given situation. Thus we can help them compensate for their deficit and live more normal, functional lives.

The perspective on ADHD presented here is the cornerstone of this book. The idea that ADHD is a disorder of self-control, executive functioning, willpower, and the organizing and directing of behavior toward the future more generally provides the rationale for almost every treatment recommendation that follows. It also provides a larger framework in which to understand the results of research on the developmental course of ADHD; the problems that are often associated with it; and the social, academic, and occupational problems that are caused by it over time.

This new outlook on ADHD can provide you with the fundamental rationale to accept your child's executive disability, to adapt the social and academic demands made on your child to the child's disability, to work to strengthen (where possible) your child's weaknesses in the processes involved in developing self-control, and to advocate for your child's need for and rights to services for this problem. This knowledge will empower you to act as the scientific, executive, and principle-centered parent that you will have to be to successfully raise a child with ADHD.

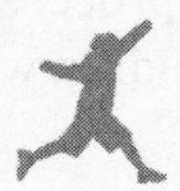

3 What Causes ADHD?

ADHD has multiple causes. Our knowledge of these causes and of how they influence the brain and behavior has increased dramatically over the past 30 years and especially the last decade. Just as important, we have learned that other things once thought to cause ADHD do not. This chapter reviews the chief causes of ADHD and debunks some widely disseminated myths.

As you read, keep in mind how difficult it is to produce direct and incontrovertible scientific proof that anything causes a problem with human behavior. The experiments required to give direct, conclusive evidence that, for example, ADHD is caused by damage to the frontal part of a child's brain during its development are simply unthinkable because they are unethical and inhumane. Scientists are not going to damage children's brains in various controlled ways and amounts just to see what happens. So behavioral scientists who wish to study the biological causes of ADHD are often left searching for information that is less direct than this but highly suggestive of a cause. As a parent attempting to keep abreast of the research, then, it is extremely important for you to understand the possible sources of information and their relative reliability.

One such source is studies that show a consistent *relationship* between a potential causal agent and ADHD or the behavior problems characteristic of it. For instance, smoking by a mother during pregnancy is associated with an increased risk of hyperactivity and inattention in the offspring of that pregnancy. The fact that two events or conditions occur together, however, does not prove that one causes the other. It is merely suggestive.

Another source is studies of accidents of nature involving the cause in which we are interested. For example, when interested in the role of brain injury in ADHD, we may study children who have suffered diseases that attack the brain or children who have had clear-cut head trauma or other neurological injuries. This type of evidence is somewhat stronger because we can see that an accident (a brain injury) changed something in a child (the child shows the behaviors of ADHD), but it still is not definitive proof that brain injury causes ADHD. Other factors associated with the process of being injured may be the real culprits, and we must remember that most children with ADHD have no evidence of a brain injury.

A third source of evidence comes from studies in which the causal agent is given directly to some animals but not to others in a true experimental test of that cause. To see if exposure of a fetus to alcohol during pregnancy causes hyperactivity, scientists give large doses of alcohol to some pregnant animals, such as mice, rats, or primates, and not to others. They then study the behavior of the animals born of those pregnancies to see how the offspring in these two groups may differ. The scientists may also sacrifice the animals and directly inspect the brain tissue for signs of abnormal development caused by the alcohol. Although such experiments prove more directly that some agent causes hyperactivity or ADHD in the animals, such conclusions cannot be generalized perfectly to humans. The brains of animals (especially primates) and humans are more similar than different, but they are not identical. So it is likely but not certain that what causes hyperactivity in animals may well cause it or ADHD in humans.

More recently, a fourth line of evidence has come from new technologies that allow scientists to gain an image of the structure and even the activity or functioning of the brains of children and adults with ADHD and compare it to those of people without the disorder. Such research often shows that certain areas of the brain in people with ADHD are a different size or have a different level of activity when engaged than is seen in others.

With few exceptions—such as direct tests of whether certain foods or chemicals in our diet may cause ADHD—behavioral scientists have had to depend on indirect evidence to show that any particular factor is a cause of ADHD. It is usually the combination of various lines of evidence such as the types discussed above that is taken to be sound proof that some toxin, agent, or event may cause ADHD. Scientists must consider the totality or weight of the evidence and whether it is logically consistent. They must consider all possible explanations for their findings and justify their conclusions to other scientists. This need to convince the widest possible audience of scientists working in the same field through objective evidence, logical explanation, and public debate is the basis of the scientific method. Through this method, evidence has been mounting that ADHD is the result of abnormalities in brain development and functioning and that these abnormalities are related more to neurological and hereditary factors than to social ones.

The Causes: Current Evidence

We now have extensive scientific research in hundreds of published studies on the causes of ADHD that it originates mainly in problems in the brain—resulting from either brain injuries or abnormal brain development. I begin this section by discussing the research pertaining to brain injuries. Since relatively few children with ADHD have been found to have actual brain injuries, however, I concentrate here on abnormal brain development. I first review the neurological findings regarding deficiencies in brain chemicals, lowered activity in certain brain regions, and structural immaturities or reductions in the size of the brain (smaller brain regions in five areas related to executive functioning). I then consider studies seeking to determine the causes of these abnormalities, which have centered on two groups of factors: (1) environmental agents, such as fetal exposure to alcohol and tobacco, and early exposure to high levels of lead; and (2) heredity (especially, in recent years, molecular genetics).

Research on Brain Injuries and ADHD

For almost 200 years, since Drs. Melchior Adam Weikard in Germany and Alexander Crichton of Scotland first wrote on the causes of attention disorders, scientists have suspected that what we now call ADHD is caused by some injury to the brain. They noticed striking similarities in behavior problems between children with ADHD and people who had suffered damage by injuries to the front part of the brain, just behind the forehead, known as the *prefrontal region.* This brain region is one of the most proportionately large in humans compared to other animals and is believed to be responsible for executive functioning and self-regulation, as discussed in Chapter 2—inhibiting behavior, sustaining attention, employing self-control, and planning for the future.

Research in neurology and neuropsychology is replete with case reports and studies of larger groups of patients who have experienced injury to the prefrontal part of the brain as a consequence of trauma, brain tumors, strokes, diseases, or penetrating wounds (such as gunshot wounds). Earlier in this century, this research convinced scientists that injuries to the brain from infections such as encephalitis and meningitis, trauma such as that caused by a fall or a blow to the head, or complications of pregnancy or delivery were the chief causes of ADHD symptoms. More than 35 years ago, however, scientists realized that most children with ADHD had no history of obvious or significant brain injuries from these sources. At most, perhaps 5–10% of children were likely to have developed ADHD from some sort of brain damage, by which I mean destruction of normal brain tissue. As discussed later in this chapter, children with ADHD tend to have had more pregnancy or birth complications than children without ADHD, but evidence that those complications have caused brain injury that in turn has caused ADHD is inconclusive.

Experiments with animals have served as a second line of research, producing evidence that ADHD may arise from brain injuries. There are many such studies, and they are quite consistent in their results. In these studies, primates such as chimpanzees are trained to perform certain psychological tests; then the scientists disable the prefrontal region of their brains through surgery or other means, and the tests are repeated. The animals' natural behavior in their environment may also be observed.

These studies have shown consistently that the primates' behavior patterns are quite similar or even identical to those seen in children with ADHD when these prefrontal brain regions are altered: the animals become more hyperactive, less able to pay attention for long periods of time, and more impulsive on the psychological tests. They are also less able to inhibit their behavior or delay their responding to events created in the experiments. These animals often develop significant problems in their social behavior with other animals as well. The studies also show that injuries created elsewhere in the brain do *not* produce these patterns of ADHD-like behavior. So the frontal area of the brain can be implicated in producing symptoms of ADHD in primates. Fewer than 10% of children with ADHD can be shown to have suffered brain *injuries,* however, so something must be disrupting the *development* or *functioning* of this part of the brain even if no tissue damage is evident.

Abnormal Brain Development in ADHD: Neurological Findings

The Structure of the Brain

Numerous studies attest to the involvement of the brain in ADHD. Consider that by 2007 Dr. Eve Valera at Massachusetts General Hospital and her colleagues were able to review and combine more than 21 studies that had been published to that date on the brain structure of individuals with ADHD (total of 565) compared to typical people of the same age (total of 583). This review concluded that at least five brain regions were significantly smaller in those with ADHD than in the control people: (1) the cerebellum, a very old structure lying at the back of the head and base of the skull; (2) the front part of the corpus callosum (the splenium), which is a large bundle of nerve fibers that connects the right and left hemispheres, allowing cross-communication between them; (3) the right side of the caudate nucleus, one of several structures forming the basal ganglia and the center of the brain; (4) the right hemisphere of the brain more generally; and (5) the frontal regions of the brain.

In 2011, yet another review was published, involving 14 separate studies measuring the gray matter volume of the brain. The review, called a *meta-analysis,* was done by an international team of scientists led by Dr. Tomohiro Nakao and combined and reanalyzed the data from all of these separate studies. They showed unequivocally that the brain volume of those with ADHD is significantly smaller and that the greatest size reduction was in the caudate region (part of the basal ganglia, as noted above). They also found that these differences in brain volume improved with age and with the length of time children had been taking stimulant medication (implying that taking medication does not harm brain development and may facilitate maturation in brain size). Further evidence for these conclusions has been found in other recent studies.

Among the largest, most unusual, and most fascinating studies of brain volume in children with ADHD published after this large literature review in 2007 was done by Dr. Philip Shaw and colleagues working at the NIMH in Bethesda, Maryland, in collaboration with researchers at Montreal Children's Hospital in Canada. These investigators initially compared the brain sizes and cortical structure of 223 children with ADHD and approximately the same number of normal children. They then repeated the scans on these groups of children every few years for up to 10 years. This allowed them to compare the pattern of growth or maturation of the brain between these two groups. They found that, on average, the children with ADHD were 2 to 3 years behind in their brain maturation, particularly in regions in the frontal lobes, but that brain size appeared to finally reach that of the normal children by their late teenage years. Note that while brain volume in children with ADHD may eventually become normal, this does not mean that brain functioning in these regions is necessarily becoming normal.

In general, the studies in this area of research have found that the prefrontal region, especially on the right side, several structures in the basal ganglia (the striatum and the globus pallidus), the midline anterior cingulate cortex (found at the midline of the prefrontal lobes), and the central area in the cerebellum, again, more on the right side, were significantly smaller and/or less active in children with ADHD than in normal children. These five brain regions are usually involved during tasks requiring inhibition, holding information in mind to guide behavior (known as working memory), and other executive functions. All of these results have led scientists to the conclusion that ADHD arises from delayed or impaired maturation of these regions that are significantly smaller, less mature, and less active than is typical of normal or non-ADHD individuals (prefrontal lobes, anterior cingulate cortex, caudate/striatum, cerebellum, and corpus callosum).

Brain Chemistry

Some scientists have suggested that certain *neurotransmitters* are deficient in those with ADHD. These are chemicals in the brain that permit nerve cells to transmit information to other nerve cells. Support for this idea comes from several sources:

1. Stimulant and nonstimulant drugs that are known to affect neurotransmitters (see Chapter 18) temporarily improve the behavior of children with ADHD.

2. Studies with animals suggest that these drugs increase the amount of the neurotransmitters, typically dopamine and norepinephrine, in the brain. These stimulants and nonstimulants produce significant improvements in the behavior of those with ADHD. This implies that the drugs are increasing the amount of these two chemicals in the brain, and so these two chemicals may be less plentiful in the brains of those with ADHD.

3. When the brain pathways that are rich in these neurotransmitters, such as dopamine, are selectively destroyed by a particular chemical in young animals, such as rats and dogs, these animals become quite hyperactive as they mature. Such studies

have also found that this hyperactivity can be reduced by giving stimulant medications to these animals—the same stimulant medicines used to treat children with ADHD.

4. Some studies have taken samples of spinal fluid from children with ADHD to see if it contains more or less of certain chemicals related to those in the brain. These studies have indicated the possibility that a lower amount of certain neurotransmitters, again like dopamine, may be related to ADHD. Evidence from other studies, however, using blood and urine samples, has not always agreed.

More recently, scientists have conducted hundreds of studies using various methods to identify particular genes that may be involved in ADHD. At least four genes that regulate dopamine have already been identified as having such an association. One is involved in the removal of dopamine from the *synapse* (the tiny gap between neurons) and is called the *dopamine transporter mechanism*. Another two are involved in determining the sensitivity of neurons to dopamine itself, and the fourth is involved in converting dopamine to another chemical transmitter called *norepinephrine*. (Note: Other genes have been identified that affect brain growth, how nerve cells migrate during development to arrive at their normal sites, and the way in which nerve cells connect to each other.) Children or adults with ADHD have been found to have different versions of these genes that affect these neurotransmitters from people without the disorder, suggesting that they are involved in the development of ADHD. Undoubtedly more genes will be found to be related to ADHD in the future (see "Heredity and ADHD," below).

What evidence there is seems to point to at least one possible problem in how much dopamine (and possibly norepinephrine) is produced or released in the brains of those with ADHD or how sensitive those brain areas are to this chemical when it is released during nerve activation. This evidence suggests that abnormalities in certain brain chemicals are likely to be involved in causing ADHD.

Brain Activity

Many studies to date have measured brain activity or functioning in people with ADHD and have found it to be lower in the prefrontal area of these people's brains than it is for people without ADHD.

Lower Electrical Activity. Dr. Sandra Loo and I reviewed a large number of studies in 2005 that compared the brain electrical activity of children with ADHD to that of children without ADHD using a device known as an *electroencephalograph* (EEG). Some of the studies we reviewed examined the children with ADHD while they were sitting at rest, and some studies did so also while the children were performing certain mental tasks. The totality of evidence we reviewed shows that the brain electrical activity of children with ADHD is less than that seen in children without

ADHD, particularly over the frontal area. The research to date shows that children with ADHD have an increased amount of slow-wave brain activity that is often associated with immaturity of the brain, drowsiness, and lack of concentration while having smaller degrees of fast brain-wave activity that is typically associated with focused concentration and sustained attention. Our conclusions have been strengthened by additional studies published since our review was done, making these findings some of the most reliable or robust in research on brain activity in ADHD.

Nearly 40 years ago, in 1973, in one of the first studies of brain electrical activity in ADHD, Drs. Monte Buchsbaum and Paul Wender, then at the NIMH, measured EEG activity in response to repeated stimulation in 24 children with ADHD and 24 normal children. The pattern they found in the children with ADHD was typical of younger children without ADHD; their responses reflected a less mature pattern of brain electrical activity. These researchers also found that giving stimulant medication to the children with ADHD reduced these differences. These findings have been replicated numerous times by other scientists such as Dr. Rafael Klorman working at the University of Rochester (New York). We now know for certain that this problem of brain underreactivity to stimulation is reasonably typical of children with ADHD. The results tell us that the problem here is not at the initial level of perception or in detecting the stimulus but at the level where the prefrontal lobes of the brain would enhance attention to that stimulus. This enhancing effect seems to be less in those with ADHD. Although children with ADHD show less activation in certain types of EEG activity, this does not automatically mean that training them to increase this activity is an effective therapy (see sidebar on p. 78).

Less Blood Flow. The more active certain brain regions are, the more blood they require. By measuring blood flow to various brain regions, one can therefore gain an idea of just how active those regions are. For instance, as long ago as 1984 Drs. Hans Lou, Leif Henriksen, and Peter Bruhn, working at the Kennedy Institute in Denmark, published a study comparing the blood flow in the brains of 11 children with ADHD (some of whom also had a learning disability) to the blood flow seen in nine children without ADHD. They found the children with ADHD had less blood flow to the frontal area and also in the *caudate nucleus*—an important structure in the pathway between the most frontal portion of the brain and the structures in the middle of the brain known as the *basal ganglia*. The caudate nucleus is made up of several bundles of nerve fibers, one region of which is known as the *striatum*. This region is important in inhibiting behavior and sustaining attention. In another study, these scientists compared the blood flow of nine children with ADHD to that of 15 children without ADHD and obtained similar results. In a third study, the same researchers and their colleagues compared 19 young patients with ADHD to nine children without ADHD. Again, the results showed decreased blood flow to the frontal brain areas, and especially to the striatum region of the caudate nucleus. When stimulant medication like that used to treat ADHD was given to these patients, the blood flow to these underactive areas increased to near-normal levels. These findings have been

Can EEG Biofeedback or Neurofeedback Help Treat ADHD?

If children with ADHD have low brain electrical activity, teaching them how to increase it might help them alleviate their ADHD symptoms. Over 30 years ago scientists began to test that theory using EEG biofeedback, and to this day some dramatic claims have been made for this kind of treatment. You may have seen advertisements stating that EEG biofeedback is an effective alternative to medication; that it results in permanent changes in the brain physiology underlying ADHD; that it improves IQ, social skills, and even learning disabilities; and that such improvements can last into adulthood in up to 80% of all treated cases. Those are fantastic claims for any treatment. How much of this should you believe?

Only some of it and only then with much greater caution. The term *biofeedback* means that a child is given back biological information about her brain activity through electrodes placed near the scalp that detect brain waves and a computer that classifies them. Over a great number of sessions, typically 40–80 sessions over 3–10 months or longer—at a cost of several thousand dollars ($100+ per session)—the child supposedly learns to improve her brain activity. She does this through mental exercises and some form of signal from the biofeedback equipment that she has been successful at increasing the desired brain activity related to sustained attention and decreasing the undesired activity associated with daydreaming or distraction. She is then rewarded as well for doing so. The result, supposedly, is that the child's inattention, hyperactivity, and impulsivity will then also improve.

Unfortunately, to date there have been only a few well-controlled studies, and they are contradictory in their results. Therefore, the evidence is mixed on the effectiveness of EEG biofeedback for children with ADHD, as reported in a 2012 review by Dr. Nicholas Lofthouse and colleagues.

Many of the studies that have been published by proponents of the treatment have not used sound scientific methods that would allow us to draw any straightforward conclusions from their results, even though they claim to have found this treatment to be effective. They do not clarify whether the biofeedback training or the academic tutoring and rewards program that accompanied it were responsible for the improved school and home behavior observed. So although we cannot rule out the possibility that EEG biofeedback training might be of some benefit, we cannot consider it a well-established and effective treatment at this time.

Furthermore, a child and family could receive 12 years of stimulant medication, 3 years of weekly group parent training, nearly 3 years of twice-monthly classroom consultations by a clinical psychologist, or almost 2 years of twice-weekly educational tutoring for the cost of 6 months of this treatment, based on current average charges. Which choice would you make for your child? My advice is to try the most effective and scientifically based treatments first (medication, behavior management techniques, classroom accommodations, etc.) and only after them, if more improvement is desirable, should you try neurofeedback and only then if you have sufficient expendable income to cover the cost of treatment.

replicated by other scientists since then and lend further support to the idea that abnormal brain activity in particular brain regions is associated with ADHD.

Lower Brain Activity on PET and fMRI Scans. Another approach to studying brain activity besides using blood flow relies on the amount of oxygen that is being used in various brain regions or on other tracers injected into the bloodstream and monitored as they enter the brain. The first evidence that a problem existed in the brain activity of adults with ADHD came from a study done more than 20 years ago, in 1990, by Dr. Alan Zametkin and his colleagues at the NIMH. In this study, the brain activity of 25 adults with ADHD was compared to that of 50 adults without ADHD using a very sensitive procedure known as a *positron emission tomography,* or PET, scan. In this procedure radioactive glucose, the sugar used as fuel by nerve cells in the brain, is injected into the bloodstream. A PET scan device then takes pictures of the brain as it uses this glucose. Dr. Zametkin and colleagues found that adults with ADHD had less brain activity, particularly in the frontal area. The low level of activity was temporarily corrected when the adults took stimulant drugs like those commonly used clinically to treat children with ADHD. Dr. Zametkin repeated this study with 20 adolescents with ADHD and again found reduced activity in the frontal region, more on the left side than on the right side. The results were especially obvious for teenage girls with the disorder compared to girls without ADHD and less so for the teenage boys with ADHD relative to boys without it. Since then, many other studies using this and other neuroimaging technologies have found similar results, all implying that underfunctioning and even underdevelopment of certain brain regions contributes to ADHD.

Another way to study brain activity is through *functional magnetic resonance imaging,* or fMRI. Like PET, the devices and procedures involved in fMRI can show how well or poorly different brain regions are activating, typically in response to some mental task the individual must perform while in the scanner. Many studies using this technology have also demonstrated that various regions of the brain in those with ADHD are not functioning normally or optimally relative to the brains of people without the disorder. Most of these studies were reviewed in 2007 by Dr. Yannis Paloyelis and colleagues at the Institute of Psychiatry in London, who commented that *all* studies using fMRI had found differences in the brain activity between cases having ADHD and typical individuals of the same age. Again, much of this reduced activity appears to be occurring in one or more of the five brain regions discussed above.

Comparing Brain Activity in ADHD and Other Psychiatric Disorders. In a study using similar brain-imaging techniques, Dr. Karl Sieg and colleagues at the University of Kansas reported as early as 1995 that they had also found significantly reduced brain metabolic activity in the frontal regions of 10 patients with ADHD, compared to six patients with other psychiatric disorders but not ADHD. This study is important because it provided some evidence that the reduced frontal brain activity is specific to patients with ADHD and does not just accompany any psychiatric disorder.

Many other studies since then have supported such distinctions between brain structure and functioning in ADHD in comparison to other disorders, such as studies in the past decade by Dr. Joseph Biederman and colleagues (see above) that compared cases of bipolar disorder with those having ADHD or those having conduct disorder to those with ADHD that showed different brain regions associated with these various disorders. For instance, a study in 2009 by Dr. Katya Rubia and colleagues, then at the Institute of Psychiatry in London, found reductions in brain activity in those with ADHD and also patterns of underactivation that were distinct from those patterns seen in patients with conduct disorder.

Conclusions

In summary, the scientific findings from many lines of scientific research to date clearly indicate that at least five interconnected areas of the brain are involved in ADHD, especially that area in the very front part of the brain, known as the *prefrontal region.* This region connects to an area at the midline of the prefrontal lobes called the *anterior cingulate cortex.* This region is connected to the amygdala and limbic system, which are very old brain structures that govern our emotions. This pathway has come to be known as the "hot" executive circuit because of its role in the "top-down" executive control of our primary emotions. The prefrontal lobes also send connections through a pathway of nerve fibers into a structure called the *caudate nucleus* (which is part of the *striatum*). This pathway is known as the "what" or "cold" executive circuit because it is responsible for how well what information we are holding in mind is likely to guide our actual behavior. The prefrontal lobes also send connections farther back into an area at the back part of the brain known as the *cerebellum.* This path has been called the "when" executive circuit because it appears to be involved in the timing and timeliness of our thoughts and especially the actions guided by our thoughts. Substantial evidence now exists to show that these three executive circuits may be responsible for the development of ADHD. Variation among people with ADHD in how poorly each of these circuits is functioning probably helps to explain some of the individual differences we see in the types of symptoms people with ADHD may express.

As I have described earlier, these brain areas are those that create our executive functions or abilities. They help us inhibit our behavior, be aware of ourselves and our actions, contemplate the past and future, sustain our attention and actions toward our goals and the future, and inhibit responding to distractions when we are pursuing tasks and our goals. They also let us inhibit and control our emotions and motivation, as well as help us use language (rules or instructions) to control our behavior and plan for the future. These scientific findings are very consistent with my view that a problem with executive functioning or self-control is the hallmark of ADHD and that this arises from abnormal levels of activity in the regions of the brain responsible for these human abilities.

How is it, many parents still ask, that children with ADHD, who are more active and energetic than children without ADHD, could have brains that are *less* active? Remember that the areas of the brain that are not as active as they should be are the parts that *inhibit* behavior, delay responding to situations, and permit us to think about our potential actions and consequences before we respond—the executive brain. The less active these inhibitory and executive centers are, the less "top-down" self-control a child will be able to demonstrate.

Some Causes of Abnormal Brain Development

We now know that certain brain chemicals seem to be altered, and that certain brain regions are underactive and underdeveloped, in people with ADHD. We still need to discover why. Among the possible explanations, two stand out from the evidence available: hazardous agents and events that affect early brain development and genetics of the brain.

Environmental Agents

Substances Consumed during Pregnancy. Nicotine from cigarette smoking and alcohol from drinking during pregnancy have been shown to cause significant abnormalities in the development of several of these brain regions, such as the caudate nucleus and the prefrontal regions of the brain. Nearly 40 years ago, in 1975, a study showed that the mothers of 20 hyperactive children had consumed more than twice as many cigarettes per day during pregnancy as mothers of 20 reading-disabled and 20 control children.

A much larger 1992 study found that direct exposure to cigarette smoke during pregnancy or indirect exposure after pregnancy increased the odds of behavior problems in the children of these pregnancies. The combination of exposure both during and after pregnancy created the greatest likelihood that the children of that pregnancy would have significant behavior problems. Subsequently, in 1996, Dr. Sharon Milberger and her colleagues, then at Massachusetts General Hospital and Harvard Medical School, found a significant relationship between the quantity of cigarettes smoked during pregnancy and the risk for ADHD in the children of those pregnancies, even after the researchers controlled for the family history of ADHD that might have existed. Many other studies done since then have found this link between maternal smoking during pregnancy and risk for ADHD in the offspring of that pregnancy. Thus, substantial scientific evidence suggests that exposure to cigarette smoke is related to a higher risk for behavior problems similar to those in ADHD. Mothers who smoke at least 10 cigarettes per day or more during their pregnancies increase the risk of ADHD in their children by 2.5 times the risk seen in the nonsmoking population.

Research indicates that children born to alcoholic mothers are more likely to have problems with hyperactivity and inattention and even clinical ADHD. Many studies support this association. The amount of alcohol consumed by their mothers when pregnant appears to be related directly to the degree of risk for inattention and hyperactivity in their children at ages 4–7. The risk of having a child with ADHD increases 2.5 times for women who drink during pregnancy over women who do not.

Keep in mind, however, that all of these studies merely provide evidence of an *association* between these substances and ADHD, and associations can be misleading. Again, however, Dr. Milberger and colleagues did control for family history in their research on smoking and ADHD, and so we can have more confidence in the possibility that smoking during pregnancy is probably related to ADHD.

Similarly, we know that adults with ADHD drink more alcohol than others whether they are pregnant or not. We also know that ADHD is highly likely to be inherited (as discussed below). Therefore it may very well be genetics alone and in interaction with the alcohol or tobacco smoking that caused ADHD in the children in these studies. Research by Dr. Rosalind Neuman and colleagues found persuasive evidence of just such gene × toxin interactions that showed that each increased the risk of having ADHD but that in combination the risk genes for ADHD and maternal smoking made the risk to the children for developing ADHD markedly worse.

Supporting a direct causal connection between these toxins consumed by mothers during pregnancy and ADHD symptoms, animal studies *have* shown fairly conclusively that tobacco smoking and alcohol cause abnormal development of certain brain regions and that these abnormalities lead to increased hyperactive, impulsive, and inattentive behavior. So perhaps the most significant conclusion is that a mother may increase the risk of ADHD in her child by smoking or drinking during pregnancy, and this risk may be increased further if the mother herself also has ADHD.

Exposure to Lead. As discussed by Dr. Joel Nigg of the Oregon Health Sciences University in his 2006 book *What Causes ADHD?*, there is some scientific evidence that high levels of lead in the bodies of young children may be associated with a higher risk for hyperactive and inattentive behavior. This relationship seems to exist especially when the lead exposure occurs between 12 and 36 months of age. The relationship is rather weak, although it is found consistently in many studies. For instance, on a scale of 1–100, the relationship between body lead and hyperactivity rates only 6–15. But even at high levels of exposure, a 1979 study found that fewer than 36% of children with elevated lead levels were rated by teachers as inattentive, distractible, impulsive, and hyperactive. High levels of lead in the body may well cause some cases of ADHD because animal and human studies do show that lead exposure at moderate to high levels injures brain tissue. So lead is a toxin to the brain, just as alcohol and tobacco are; it may therefore be viewed as a potential cause of inattention, hyperactivity, or even full-fledged ADHD in some cases. But like the other toxins discussed above, consuming it does not guarantee that a child is automatically going to develop ADHD as a consequence.

Heredity and ADHD

Only a minority of children (25–35%) appear to have acquired their ADHD as a consequence of toxins or other hazardous events that may have disrupted early brain development, according to Dr. Joel Nigg in his 2006 book *What Causes ADHD?* What else could be causing the altered brain chemistry, brain underactivity, and smaller brain regions? One highly likely reason has been found in the substantial research on the role of genetics and heredity in ADHD—for one thing, the disorder clearly runs in families. For many years we've had evidence that the biological relatives of children with ADHD have more types of psychological problems—particularly depression, alcoholism, conduct problems or antisocial behavior, as well as hyperactivity/ADHD—than relatives of children who do not have ADHD. Such a family contribution to ADHD was evident as long as 40 years ago in initial studies on the families of hyperactive children conducted by Drs. James Morrison and Mark Stewart, then at the University of Iowa Medical School, as well as Dr. Dennis Cantwell and colleagues at the University of California, Los Angeles, Neuropsychiatric Institute. Such research strongly supports the idea that a genetic predisposition contributes substantially to this disorder.

Family Studies. Clearer and stronger evidence that ADHD may be inherited comes from studies that directly evaluate all members of an immediate family for ADHD and determine the risk to other family members if one of them is diagnosed with ADHD. As an example, consider the large study by Drs. Joseph Biederman, Stephen Faraone, and their associates at Massachusetts General Hospital. Published in 1990, the study evaluated the 457 first-degree relatives (mothers, fathers, and siblings) of 75 children with ADHD and compared their results to their evaluation of the family members of 26 control children (that is, children with no psychiatric disorders) and 26 children with psychiatric disorders other than ADHD. They found that over 25% of the first-degree relatives in the families of children with ADHD also had ADHD, whereas this rate was only about 5% in each of the other groups. This 5% is what you would expect by chance to find in any sample of children, since it is the prevalence of the disorder in the population at large. Notice that if a child has ADHD, then, there is a five times greater increase in the risk to other members in that family. Many other subsequent studies have found similar results.

Twin Studies. Research using twins is even more persuasive. Scientists have found that if one twin has symptoms of ADHD, the risk that the other will have the disorder is as high as 75–90%. This risk is two to three times greater than the risk to one sibling if another one has the disorder (25–35%) and 9–15 times greater than the risk seen in the general population of children (5–8%). For example, consider the results of a study published in 1992 by Dr. Jacquelyn Gillis and associates at the University of Colorado. They found that 79% of identical twins both had ADHD when one of the twins had already been diagnosed. For fraternal twins the figure was only 32%, but that is still 6–10 times greater than that seen among unrelated children, where the prevalence of ADHD at the time was only 3–5%.

Besides comparing the risk between two identical twins if one has the disorder, scientists can also study large samples of identical twins compared to nonidentical or fraternal twins and mathematically compute the degree to which differences among all of the people in the sample are a result of differences in their genetic makeup. More than 40 very large studies of twins have been done in various countries to date. They have been able to determine that differences in genetic makeup explain between 55 and 97% of the differences among people in their level of symptoms of ADHD, with an average of about 78% of such individual differences being due to genetics.

These studies can also determine the extent to which unique environmental events or factors contribute to variation in ADHD traits in the population. Such events are called "unique" because they happen to just that child (and not others in the family)—such as toxins like lead poisoning, maternal infections that occurred during just that pregnancy, maternal use of tobacco or alcohol that occurred in just that pregnancy, that child being born highly premature, or other complications occurring during that pregnancy and birth. Such unique hazardous biological events seem to explain only between 6 and 15% of the differences among people in level of ADHD traits. This clearly supports a very large role for heredity in the expression of ADHD. Yet it also supports the discussion above that a small degree of ADHD can arise from nongenetic sources, like brain injuries or maternal alcohol and tobacco consumption during that child's pregnancy.

Twin studies can also be used to calculate the amount of variation in ADHD traits among people that arise from shared environmental events or factors. These are things that all children in a family are likely to have experienced, such as a similar diet, amount of exposure to TV and video games, problems in parenting, psychological difficulties in one or both parents, the neighborhood in which they are all being raised, and so on. What is so surprising and important in these studies is that they have consistently shown that these shared or within-family events do not explain much if any of the variation in ADHD traits among children. This is why we can now safely conclude that bad parenting or other things occurring in a family to which all of their children are exposed does not contribute to causing ADHD. Besides the strong genetic contribution to ADHD found in all of these studies, this finding of little or no role for the within-family environment in ADHD is one of the most reliable findings in scientific research on ADHD to date.

What Exactly Is Inherited? The specific factors inherited in ADHD probably include a tendency toward problems in the development of the prefrontal cortex of the brain, the caudate nucleus, and the other brain regions discussed above. Scientists are now carrying out studies that evaluate all members of a family that include a child with ADHD and are scanning the entire human genome (all active gene sites in humans) to determine just how many genes are involved in the disorder and their locations. Subsequent research can then investigate the nature of the genes located at these sites and help us begin to understand how that gene functions in the human brain (build nerve cells, help with their normal migration, support the cells, determine their sensitivity to neurotransmitters, create the neurotransmitter chemical itself, etc.). So far 22–40 or more sites have been identified in these initial genome scans. The genes at some of these sites are already known, while others remain to be identified.

Suffice it to say here that this is one of the most exciting and most rapidly developing areas of research in ADHD at this time. What all this means is that ADHD is caused by multiple genes. Each gene makes a relatively small contribution to the risk for having the disorder. But a child who gets enough of those ADHD-risk genes will manifest symptoms severe enough to be diagnosed with the disorder. Family members that have fewer numbers of these genes may show a few and milder symptoms of the disorder but not enough to be diagnosed with it or to be necessarily impaired by it. They show what researchers call the "family phenotype" of the disorder even if they don't show the full spectrum or severity of the disorder itself. We are also learning that the genes that may be involved in causing ADHD are really not an abnormal one or a "disease" gene. Typical people without ADHD are likely to have this gene. But the version of the gene related to ADHD may be different in some way, typically being unusually longer or shorter than that seen in people without the disorder.

For instance, a number of studies have confirmed that at least two genes involved in the neurotransmitter dopamine mentioned earlier may be related to ADHD. One of these, called the *DRD4,* is related to the personality dimension known as *novelty seeking*. Children and adults with ADHD are more likely to have a longer version of this gene. The gene may make their dopamine nerve cells in the brain less sensitive to normal amounts of dopamine. They require more of it than other people to make the cells activate. This effect on the nerve cells may make them more likely to seek out novelty because it stimulates their brain and especially the release of dopamine. They are therefore said to have novelty seeking in their personality. That is, they exhibit more sensation-seeking behavior, risk taking, impulsiveness, and restless behavior than is typical for the normal population.

A second gene, the *DAT1* gene, also has a longer form that is more commonly associated with ADHD than would be expected to occur in the general population. This gene may help to regulate dopamine activity in the brain by influencing how quickly dopamine is removed from the synapse, the small gap between neurons (see "Brain Chemistry," above). Besides these two genes, at least seven others have been identified as likely risk genes for the disorder. And as the genome scans found above, ADHD results from even more genes than these nine. Be sure to watch for news reports about new scientific discoveries related to the genetics of ADHD.

Is ADHD Simply an Extreme Form of a Normal Human Trait? The genetic explanation of ADHD has an important implication that can easily go overlooked: *ADHD may simply represent an extreme form of a normal human trait and not a grossly pathological condition in most cases.* As we have just seen, which of us end up with ADHD seems to be determined much more by genetics than by environmental factors. In that sense, ADHD may be viewed in the same way as height, weight, intelligence, or reading ability, to name a few traits that are dimensional (people vary in degree) and that are largely (but not wholly) genetically determined: the trait of executive functioning and the self-control related to it represents a dimension or continuum of a human ability, and we differ in how much of it we inherit, just as we differ in how much height, weight, intelligence, or reading ability we inherit. What is considered "abnormal" for any trait is simply a reflection of where we draw a line on the continuum. When people fall near the extreme lower end of the continuum for a dimensional trait like ADHD and that deficiency results in their suffering impairment in their major life activities (social relations, education, work, etc.), we label them as having a disorder. Such labels make it appear that the disorder is like some category that some people fall into while most do not. It can obscure the fact that those with ADHD fall along a dimension of normal abilities differing only from typical people as a matter of degree, not as being a different kind of person. The difference here is a quantitative one, not a qualitative one. To put it another way, we all have a degree of this ADHD trait because we all have executive functioning and self-regulation. Those who are diagnosed with ADHD simply represent the extreme lower end of the dimension(s) related to self-regulation and executive functioning.

Understanding that ADHD is just an extreme form of a trait we all possess and that it is something people "come by naturally" should help everyone view ADHD from a kinder perspective, I hope. Your child was born with this problem; it is through no fault of his own that he lies at that position on the continuum. Likewise, you should neither assign blame to yourself nor accept it from others.

The Myths: What Does *Not* Cause ADHD

No doubt you've encountered claims that factors other than those just discussed cause ADHD. Some of these were originally founded in sound hypotheses but have since been disproven. Others are sheer falsehoods; there is not now and never has been any scientific support for them. As we continue to make conclusive findings about ADHD, let us hope that quackery surrounding the subject will greatly diminish if not vanish altogether. In the meantime, use what you know about the scientific method to sort fact from fiction.

It's Probably Not Something They Ate

In the 1970s and early 1980s, it was very popular to view ADHD as resulting from chemical food additives. This theory stemmed mainly from the widespread media attention given to Dr. Benjamin Feingold's claim that over half of all hyperactive children got that way from eating foods that contained additives and preservatives.

Most of the substantial amount of research done over the next decade was simply unable to support Feingold's claim. In fact, only a very small number (5% or fewer) of children, mainly preschoolers, showed a slight increase in activity or inattentiveness when consuming these substances. No evidence has ever been provided that normal children develop ADHD by consuming such substances or that children with ADHD are made considerably worse by eating them. In 1983, Drs. Kenneth Kavale and Steven Forness of the University of California–Riverside published a review of 23 studies investigating the Feingold diet. They concluded that diet modification was not effective for treating hyperactivity.

Despite that view being shared by many scientists studying ADHD, the popular media continued to tout this now unfounded belief. In 1986, in fact, Ann Landers published and personally supported a letter from a parent making such an erroneous claim and directing parents to write to the Feingold Association of the United States (*Worcester Telegram and Gazette,* September 19, 1986). Unfortunately for parents who may have read such nonsense and taken the advice, nothing could be further from the truth. More recently, scientific interest in this theory has diminished greatly, and so has that of the general public.

"Is it sugar that causes ADHD, as I so often hear?"

However, in its place, the public then adopted a popular view that sugar causes ADHD. So widely accepted was this idea that in January 1987 it was paired as the correct response to the statement "The major cause of hyperactivity in North America" on the popular television game show *Jeopardy.* Not a single scientific study has been provided by proponents to support these claims. Since 1987 a number of scientific studies of sugar have been conducted, and these have generally proven negative. As an example, a study published in 1988 by Dr. Lee Rosen of Colorado State University and colleagues showed that even when given a beverage with the equivalent of two candy bars' worth of sugar, normal preschool- and elementary school-age children may have slightly increased their activity level, but not so as to be detectable by their teachers or the experimenters throughout the school day. No effect of sugar was found on the academic work of the children. Only the girls showed a slight decrease in their attention and learning on one of the psychological tests done within 20–30 minutes after they had the drink, but this was a very small change and not noted on any of the teacher ratings or observations. No child developed the disorder of ADHD. The conclusion of the authors was that sugar does not cause clinically significant or dramatic changes in children's behavior, much less the clinical disorder of ADHD.

Drs. Mark Wolraich, Richard Milich, Phyllis Stumbo, and Frederick Schultz at the University of Iowa Hospital School then conducted two studies of hyperactive children published in 1985. They intensively studied 16 boys in each study who were admitted to the hospital school for 3 days, during which the sugar content of their diet was directly manipulated. To keep the children and other staff from knowing what days the sugar was in the diet, the investigators used aspartame (Nutrasweet) as a placebo. These scientists took 37 different measures of behavior and learning and found no significant effects of sugar on either behavior or learning. In 1986, Drs. Richard Milich, Mark Wolraich, and Scott Lindgren published a review of all of the research conducted up to that time on the adverse effects of sugar on children's behavior. They concluded that "most studies have failed to find any effects associated with sugar ingestion, and the few studies that have found effects have been as likely to find sugar improving behavior as making it worse" (p. 493).

How could this be the case when nearly half of the parents and teachers queried in one of these studies stated that their children appeared to them to be quite sugar-sensitive? One answer has been known to psychological research for decades, and that is the power of psychological suggestion. To evaluate this possibility, Drs. Daniel Hoover and Richard Milich at the University of Kentucky published a study in 1994 using 31 boys ages 5–7 whose mothers reported them to be behaviorally "sugar-sensitive." When each mother and child came to the clinic, the mother had been told that on the day of the appointment their child would be given either sugar or aspartame (as a placebo, again) in Kool-Aid. Actually, though, none of the children were given any sugar in their drink. On the morning of the appointment, half of the mothers were told their children were getting sugar and the other half that the children were getting aspartame. The mothers and children were then observed interacting during a period when they played freely and then during a period when they performed work together. The mothers also rated their children's behavior at the end of these periods. Direct measures of the children's activity level were also taken. The scientists found that the mothers who had been told their children received sugar rated their children as being more hyperactive than the mothers who were told the truth (that aspartame was given). The mothers who thought their children received sugar also were more critical of their children's activities, maintained closer physical proximity to their children (hovering), and talked more frequently to their children than the mothers who knew the children had aspartame. This study clearly shows that what parents believe about a dietary cause of hyperactivity (in this case, sugar) not only can bias their reports but also can change the way the parents treat their children. This study is worth keeping in mind the next time someone tells you that something children eat makes them hyperactive or causes ADHD. But despite research over the past 25 years showing no significant link between sugar and ADHD, it still remains today as one possible cause of ADHD in the minds of some in the general public.

"I saw a doctor on a talk show who said that food allergies cause ADHD. Can you test my son for that? If not, where can I go to have him tested?"

Over the years other unsubstantiated claims have been made about the influence of diet on ADHD. Almost 40 years ago, several professionals claimed that large doses of vitamins, particularly vitamins B_3, C, and pyridoxine, would be of benefit to severely mentally ill patients. Nearly 20 years later, another professional published statements that hyperactive and children with learning disabilities could benefit from so-called *megavitamin therapy* or *orthomolecular psychiatry*. None of these claims has been verified by scientifically rigorous research. In fact, one reasonably well-done study found that the behavior of children with ADHD actually became worse on the megavitamin treatment program. Similar claims have been made for large doses of minerals. There is no evidence that megadoses of vitamins or minerals can help children with ADHD, or that vitamin or mineral deficiencies in any way cause the disorder. *Parents should also be aware that large doses of vitamins (especially fat-soluble vitamins) and minerals can actually be harmful to children.*

You may also have read (or seen on TV talk shows) that allergies to substances in foods besides the chemical additives targeted by Dr. Feingold can cause ADHD symptoms (and, incidentally, a raft of other symptoms). One very large study conducted in The Netherlands by Dr. Lidy Pelsser and colleagues that was published in 2010 compared a large general population sample of children not receiving a controlled diet and another group that had various substances controlled or eliminated from their diet. It reported that children in the controlled diet improved in their inattention, activity level, and other symptoms of ADHD. These improvements were noted primarily by parents and might well have arisen in part because the parents could tell which children were receiving the controlled diet and which were not. While this study suggests that some children may benefit from removal of certain chemicals, colorings, or flavorings from the food in their diet in improving their behavior, the results of this study go against most other studies recently reviewed by Dr. Joel Nigg and associates that found a much smaller effect of treatment. As always, more and better research is necessary to completely rule in or out the possibility that some children may be adversely affected in their behavior by certain food additives. But the evidence is not compelling to me as of this writing that this is a major cause of ADHD, even though some small effects have been seen in some studies. Also the American Academy of Allergy and Immunology does not advocate investigating allergies when ADHD symptoms appear. Americans have been so fascinated for the last 35 years with how foods affect human health that it should come as no surprise when links between diet and ADHD continue to be proposed, but at this point most such claims cannot be taken seriously.

Are Hormones Involved in ADHD?

A study published in early 1993 (by Dr. Peter Hauser and colleagues) showing a link between low thyroid hormone levels and ADHD received a great deal of publicity from the media. Some stories even claimed that the "gene" for ADHD had been discovered because the gene for thyroid deficiency is known and it was assumed that the two must be related in some way. These hormones, chemicals produced in the thyroid (a gland in the neck), are important in controlling human growth and may have other functions that are not fully understood. A few people may have a rare condition of thyroid deficiency that may be genetically determined. The study found that 70% of children and 50% of adults who were deficient in thyroid hormone had ADHD. Since then this link has been studied in three additional published papers, and none has found any significant link between problems with thyroid hormone functioning and hyperactivity or ADHD. Thus the initial study appears to have been flawed in some way. Children with ADHD should not be routinely tested for thyroid deficiencies, nor should thyroid hormone treatments be considered to hold any promise for the treatment of ADHD at this time.

No other hormones have been shown to have any relationship to ADHD.

Motion Sickness and ADHD

For many years Dr. Harold Levinson of Great Neck, New York, has been garnering media coverage for his theory that ADHD, learning disorders, and other behavioral and emotional problems can occur because of a problem within the vestibular system of the brain, which affects balance, sense of gravity, and head position. This system is located in the inner ear and makes connections with parts of the brain, especially the cerebellum, located at the lower back portion of the skull. Contrary to what most scientists believe, Dr. Levinson claims that this system also regulates our energy levels, so that any impairment in this system can lead to hyperactivity and impulsive behavior. He recommends that children with ADHD or learning disorders take Dramamine or dimenhydrinate (an anti-motion-sickness medicine available over the counter) because it is known to have some effects on the vestibular system. He provides patients with other medicines as well, some of them powerful psychiatric drugs, other vitamin supplements, or herbal extracts.

In their 1994 review of the evidence available on Dr. Levinson's theory and treatment recommendations, two psychologists, Drs. Barbara Ingersoll and Samuel Goldstein, concluded that the theory is surely inconsistent with what is known about ADHD and the vestibular system and its functions. The vestibular system does not seem to be involved in any way with impulse control, attention span, or regulation of activity level. Dr. Levinson claims to have used this approach to treat thousands of patients with ADHD and learning disorders, with at least 70–80% of patients responding well. Even so, he has never published a well-controlled scientific study on this issue. Thus we have only his word to take on how useful this treatment program is for those with ADHD. As with the dietary treatments discussed earlier, parents should avoid this treatment program and view it as entirely unsubstantiated by legitimate scientific research.

Can Yeasts Cause ADHD?

Dr. William Crook, a pediatrician and allergist from Jackson, Tennessee, has been a vocal proponent of yeasts—particularly those such as *Candida albicans* that can live in the body—as a major cause of many different learning, behavioral, and emotional problems, especially ADHD. These yeasts are typically kept in check by other bacteria in the body as well as by the body's immune system. Dr. Crook believes that toxins given off by the yeasts can irritate the brain and nervous system and can weaken the body's immune system. He recommends that children with ADHD be placed on low-sugar diets, because sugar can stimulate the growth of yeasts. Like Dr. Feingold, he also believes that additives and other chemicals in foods may contribute to a yeast problem in the body, and so these should be eliminated from the diets of ADHD children. He believes that some children may even need to be treated with an antiyeast medication such as nystatin, and that others may need vitamin, mineral, or other dietary supplements to control their behavior problems.

Presently, not a shred of sound scientific evidence supports Dr. Crook's theory. Given that the American Academy of Allergy and Immunology has found the theory of yeast sensitivity unproven, parents are encouraged to ignore any advice based on it. Certainly Dr. Crook's recommendations that children take large doses of vitamins and minerals, as noted earlier, can be potentially harmful to children.

Can Bad Parenting or Chaotic Family Life Cause ADHD?

Theories that blame the social environment as the major cause of ADHD have not received much support in the scientific literature. Some writers have claimed that ADHD symptoms such as hyperactive behavior can result from poor parental management of the children; these parents are thought to be too permissive or too disorganized in their parenting or do not provide enough training, structure, or discipline. No studies support this view. Yet even in the January 28, 2012, *New York Times* an op-ed piece was published by L. Alan Sroufe, PhD, a psychologist at the University of Minnesota, in which a similarly baseless claim was made about parenting causing ADHD. There simply is no evidence available to support such parent bashing in explaining ADHD, while there is much evidence that refutes it, raising questions about the motives of those who would continue to make such outlandish and strongly scientifically contradicted assertions that certain behaviors of parents toward their child can cause ADHD. Earlier in my career, I studied family life and particularly the interactions between parents and their children with ADHD for more than 24 years. My own research did show that the parents of children with ADHD are more likely to give commands to their children, to be more directive and negative toward them, and in some instances to be less attentive and responsive to their children than are parents of children without ADHD. My colleagues and I also have found that the children with ADHD were less compliant with their parents' commands and directions, were more negative and stubborn, and were less able than children without ADHD to keep complying over time with the parents' commands. Many other studies have noted these and other differences in the parent–child interactions of families having children with ADHD. Is it the parents' fault that the children are acting this way, or the children's fault that the parents are reacting this way?

"My parents think that I spoil my son too much, that I don't discipline him the way I should, and that this is why he acts this way. How do I convince them he really has a disability?"

To evaluate this question further, we gave stimulant medication (Ritalin) on some weeks and placebos on the other weeks to children with ADHD. Then we observed what happened in mother–child interactions. Neither the mothers nor the children knew which weeks the children were on the real medicine and which weeks they were taking the placebo. We found that when the children were on the real medicine, their behavior toward their mothers was much improved. But we also found that the mothers' behavior toward the children was improved. It even resembled the behavior of the mothers of children without ADHD. This indicates that much of the negative behavior of the mothers seemed to be *in response* to the difficult behavior of these children and not the cause of it. After all, by directly changing the ADHD symptoms of the children with medication, we showed that the behavior of their mothers became much more "normal."

You may also have read claims that a chaotic family life or a "dysfunctional" family can cause ADHD, based on the fact that parents of children with ADHD are somewhat more likely to have psychological problems or even psychiatric disorders. Studies have found that the parents (and immediate relatives) of children with ADHD are more likely to have problems with alcohol and substance abuse, antisocial behavior, and depression, and to have had school problems and hyperactivity when they themselves were children. Parents of children with ADHD also report more stress in their role as parents and more marital or couple problems than other parents. Moreover, the families of children with ADHD move more frequently than families who do not have such children. Such things can easily influence how well a household runs, how organized the parents are in managing their personal and family life, and how well they are able to manage their children. These disruptive influences can also create much more stress for the children than may be experienced in the family life of children without ADHD.

In the minds of many people (including some professionals), this line of reasoning justifies the claim that ADHD can arise out of disorganized, dysfunctional family life. But several lines of reasoning clearly disprove this view. First, the greater problems seen in family members of children with ADHD are easily explained by the hereditary evidence described earlier. We should expect to see more ADHD and its symptoms in the biological parents and family members of children with ADHD, even if the children with ADHD were adopted away at birth; and we do. This explains why the family members of children with ADHD may be having more trouble themselves, may move more often, and may have more marital or couple problems and a higher divorce rate than families without such children. It is not the psychiatric problems of these family members and the resulting "bad" family environment that cause ADHD in the children, but the ADHD risk genes that the parents and children have in common.

Second, later research contradicts this theory. Studies found that these psychiatric problems among the family members of children with ADHD occurred most often in only a subgroup composed of children who also have serious problems with aggressive, defiant, and antisocial behavior. The parents and relatives of this subgroup are the ones who are more likely to have problems with drug and alcohol abuse, depression, and antisocial behavior. Children who have only ADHD, without significant aggressive behavior, do not seem to have these serious problems among relatives any more frequently than do children without ADHD. This tells us that these parent and family problems are linked to the development of aggressive and antisocial behavior in the children and not to the children's ADHD. In other words, chaotic or dysfunctional family life due to psychological problems in the parents may be contributing directly to children's risk of having very aggressive and antisocial behavior. Thus, although chaotic family life and parental psychiatric problems are associated with and may well cause serious defiant and aggressive behavior, they are not causative of ADHD.

Finally, there are the findings from my own research that have been replicated since by others: my colleagues and I videotaped interactions between parents and their children with ADHD and compared these to the interactions of children without ADHD and their parents. But we also subdivided the children with ADHD into those who were very oppositional, defiant, and aggressive and those who were not. We discovered that the interactions in the group of children with ADHD who were not aggressive were no different from the interactions of the families of normal children in most respects. It was only in the aggressive group that we found more negative interactions between the parents and their children. Both the aggressive children with ADHD and their parents used more insults, putdowns, and commands with each other. They also were less positive in their interactions than were the other two groups of children (nonaggressive children with ADHD and children without ADHD). These families of aggressive children reported the greatest amount and intensity of conflicts with each other at home. The parents of these aggressive children also reported more personal psychological problems in themselves than did the parents of the other groups of children. This finding is in keeping with the results that parental psychological problems are more common in the families of aggressive children with ADHD. Also, recall the point made earlier that twin studies have found that the home or rearing environment of children does not make a significant contribution to the expression of the disorder.

All of this evidence makes it highly unlikely that any purely social cause, such as "bad parenting" or a disruptive, stressful home life, creates ADHD in the children of such families. Instead, the research suggests that children with ADHD can create stress for their parents and cause some disruption of family life. In cases where poor parenting and disruptive family life have some influence on children, it seems to be one of contributing to aggressive and defiant child behavior, not to ADHD.

Is It Due to Too Much Television?

Some years ago, the syndicated newspaper columnist and family therapist John Rosemond, among others, argued that ADHD resulted primarily from children spending too much time viewing TV—much more than was typical in earlier generations.

This idea has some superficial appeal because it is consistent with popular folklore that watching too much TV surely must shorten a person's attention span. To my knowledge, no scientific studies have ever shown this folklore to be true. While some studies have found that children with ADHD watch more TV than normal children do, such studies do not prove that watching TV causes ADHD. Even these studies have not been consistent in their findings; just as many found no association between TV viewing and ADHD symptoms as have noted such an association. I and other scientists believe that it is more likely that people with ADHD watch more TV because it requires less effort and a shorter attention span than other leisure pursuits, such as reading. For instance, in my own research in which we followed children with ADHD into adulthood, we asked them as adults how they spent their leisure time. We found that the young adults who had ADHD watched more TV, played more video games, talked on the phone more, and went joyriding more often in their cars than the control young adults did, while the latter spent more time reading, studying for work or college, and exercising than the young adults with ADHD. Such studies tell us only what those with ADHD like to do with their spare time, not that the things they do during that time are directly causing their ADHD. But the greatest evidence against Rosemond's idea comes from twin studies that have found that the rearing environment that twins and siblings share growing up in the same family makes *no* significant contribution to differences among children in their degree of ADHD symptoms. TV viewing is a part of that shared environment, so these studies indicate that too much TV does not contribute to ADHD.

Who Is at Risk for Developing ADHD?

Even before a child is born, certain parental or family characteristics increase the odds that the child will have ADHD. These risk factors may not necessarily directly cause ADHD, but their presence signals that a child born into that family may be more likely to have ADHD than children born into families without those risk factors.

Features of the Parents and Family

As you know, studies tell us that parents who have ADHD are about eight times more likely to have children with ADHD. This is obviously because of the strong hereditary role in the disorder as reported above. In fact, any family history of ADHD increases the odds of a child's having ADHD. For instance, having a sibling with ADHD increases the likelihood that another child in the family will have ADHD to 25–35% overall. Scientists estimate this risk to be approximately 13–17% for girls and 27–30% for boys, regardless of the gender of the sibling with ADHD. It is not clear why boys have a greater risk of having ADHD than girls within the same family. The reasons may lie in the realm of genetics—we know, for example, that it is possible for a characteristic inherited in the genes of both boys and girls in the same family to become manifest only in the boys. Maleness, you might say, has some greater biological risks associated with it, and ADHD may be one of them. Such sex differences are evident not only in ADHD but also in mental retardation and learning disabilities such as dyslexia (reading disorder). Whatever the explanation, it is not likely to rest on purely social factors, such as differences in the ways in which parents treat boys and girls within the same family.

As seen above, if a child has ADHD, the risk goes up significantly that other family members may also have ADHD. But what if it is the parent who has ADHD? Then the risk to the children of that parent is between 20 and 54%. In other words, a parent with ADHD is 8 to 10 times more likely to have a child with ADHD than a parent who does not have ADHD. This clearly shows how strong the genetic contribution is to the disorder. Other family risk factors associated with the early development and persistence of ADHD are (1) less education of the mother, (2) lower socioeconomic status of the parents, (3) single parenthood, and (4) abandonment of the family by the father. However, these factors produce only a very small elevation in risk for ADHD and obviously do not *cause* ADHD in the children of such parents. They are simply associated with a greater risk for ADHD, most likely because of some third condition that explains both these risk factors and the ADHD itself—again, possibly due to the shared genetics for the traits of ADHD.

Features of the Pregnancy

Several studies have shown that mothers who experience complications of their pregnancies or deliveries are more likely to have children with ADHD than mothers without such complications are. This is also true for repeated infections experienced by the mother in her pregnancy. The type of complication or infection does not seem to be as important as the total number of such complications. These complications may cause ADHD by interfering with the normal brain development of the fetus, or a third factor may be involved: ADHD in the mother. In this case, the mother's ADHD would lead to poorer prenatal self-care and thus greater complications; the cause of the child's ADHD would be genetic inheritance. This is an example of noncausal association, discussed earlier in this chapter.

The fact is that there is little evidence that these complications actually cause ADHD. Even 40 years ago, evidence was accruing that pregnancy and birth complications might contribute some risk to causing ADHD in the offspring of those pregnancies. For instance, in a large study by Dr. Nichols and colleagues known as the Perinatal Collaborative Project, conducted by the federal government in the 1970s, the following complications before or during birth were found to increase (by a small degree) the risk that a child might have symptoms of ADHD: the number of cigarettes smoked by the mother per day, seizures in the mother, the number of times the mother was hospitalized during pregnancy, breathing problems in the child during and after delivery, and the weight and health of the placenta when inspected after delivery. A higher incidence of problems in these areas increased the odds that a child would have symptoms of ADHD; the worse the mother's problems, the worse the child's symptoms.

Studies of babies born prematurely and with low birth weights have frequently shown that these infants have a markedly higher likelihood of developing ADHD in later childhood—sometimes five to seven times higher than that of the general childhood population. A study from 20 years ago suggested that this may be due to the fact that such babies have a high risk of having small hemorrhages in their brains. Over 40% of such babies who had these small bleedings in their brain were found to have ADHD (among other developmental and learning problems) later in childhood, whereas those without such bleedings were far less likely to have these problems.

Features of Infancy and the Toddler Years

Scientists have also identified some features in the early development of children that may predict a greater risk for the later appearance of ADHD in those children. Delays in motor development, smaller head size at birth and at 12 months of age, amniotic fluid stained by *meconium* (material from the intestine of the fetus), signs of nerve damage after birth, breathing problems after birth, and low birth weight were found in the Perinatal Collaborative Project to be related to risk for later hyperactivity. The risk was still quite low, however, even when these signs were present. Children who are less healthy during their infancy or preschool years, and who are slow to develop in motor coordination, have also been found to be at a higher risk for early and persistent ADHD symptoms later in childhood.

Young children who are excessively active as babies may have a higher risk for having ADHD later in childhood. Also, children who attend to objects or toys for short periods of time, who cannot persist as well in pursuing objects in their field of vision, or who show a strong intensity of reaction to being stimulated may be at higher risk for having ADHD. Infants or toddlers who are very demanding of their parents are more likely to display ADHD later on. We do not believe that these features of children or their early development cause the ADHD symptoms to occur later. Instead, many psychologists believe that these are just the early signs of the ADHD itself, which may not be fully formed in its expression at so early an age as infancy or toddlerhood. Very young children display only the behavior that is possible for them to show at that early stage of the brain's development. The "seeds" of ADHD may be within these children, but will not appear until the stages of development where attention span, inhibition, and the other executive functions that help with self-control over activity and behavior normally emerge. At those points, children with ADHD will fall behind other children.

Features of the Preschool Years

During the preschool years (ages 2–5 years), the development of early and persistent problems with overactivity and with getting along with other children can mark a child as being at risk for ADHD. Also, not surprisingly, young children with excessive inattention and emotional difficulties (such as frequent anger or temper outbursts, or a proneness to becoming easily upset by things) may be more likely to have ADHD as they grow up.

Once again, young children whose early temperament is negative and demanding are more likely to be diagnosed as having ADHD later on. *Temperament* refers to an early and persistent pattern of personality characteristics, including activity level, intensity or degree of energy in a response, persistence or attention span, being demanding of others, quality of mood (irritability or quickness to anger or display emotion), adaptability or capacity to adjust to change, and rhythmicity or the regularity of sleep–waking periods, eating, and elimination (bowel and bladder control). As predictors, these features appear to be as important in the preschool years as they are in infancy. These characteristics, especially overactivity, high intensity, inattention, negative mood, and low adaptability, have also predicted the continuation of ADHD into later childhood once it develops. Certainly children whose inattentive or hyperactive symptoms are sufficiently severe to get them a diagnosis of ADHD in early childhood are quite likely to continue to receive this diagnosis up to 5–10 years later.

The presence of these personality characteristics early in life is a very strong predictor of later risk for ADHD. For instance, even 30 years ago, in 1990, Dr. Susan Campbell and colleagues at the University of Pittsburgh found evidence of this when they studied 46 children who were reported by their parents to be excessively active, inattentive, and defiant at ages 2–3 years. They also studied 22 children who had no significant behavior problems of this sort. They then followed all of the children until age 6 and reevaluated them. At age 6, approximately 50% of the children with early behavioral problems were still hyperactive or had a formal diagnosis of ADHD, which suggests that children who are hyperactive and difficult to manage at age 2 have at least a 50% chance of being labeled as ADHD or hyperactive by entry into school at age 6.

Still, 50% of the children did *not* persist in their behavior problems. Dr. Campbell and colleagues found that in cases where this pattern of early hyperactive and defiant behavior was combined with other factors in a child's life, ADHD was more likely to develop. What were these other features? Among the important ones were the characteristics of the parents' personality, especially the presence of psychiatric or psychological problems that may have interfered with caregiving and raising the child. Dr. Campbell and colleagues studied this issue and found that a negative, critical, and commanding style of child management by mothers of young children with hyperactivity was likely to predict persistence of those problems into later years. Parents who are very hostile or who are having marital/couple problems may also contribute to the risk for ADHD in preschool children with negative temperament. Thus it appears that child temperament, while an important early risk factor, can be either improved or worsened by the type of home environment parents create and the manner in which they respond to a difficult child. This environment can combine with a child's early temperament problems to increase the risk for *later* ADHD. These problems with parents are not necessarily causing the child's ADHD. It is possible (1) that they may exacerbate it somewhat; or (2) that the parent is simply reacting to a child who has more severe symptoms of ADHD, and it is that severity that determines the persistence of the child's ADHD over development, and not so much the parents' behavior. More important, such parenting factors may increase the risk that the child may develop oppositional defiant disorder (discussed in Chapter 1).

I along with Dr. Terri Shelton and other colleagues did a 5-year study of preschool children at risk for ADHD at the University of Massachusetts Medical School in the 1990s. We screened most children from 4½ to 6 years of age entering the public school kindergarten program in Worcester, Massachusetts, for those having high levels of ADHD symptoms and aggressiveness. We then gave these children a thorough psychological evaluation and found that over 65% of them qualified for a diagnosis of ADHD—a figure that changed very little over the next 3 years that we followed and annually reevaluated these children.

Taken together, these research findings suggest that it is possible to identify children at risk for developing an early and persistent pattern of ADHD symptoms prior to their starting kindergarten, and perhaps even as early as 2 or 3 years of age. A combination of child and parental variables seems the most useful guide to making such predictions. The following factors, listed in descending order of importance, would appear to be useful as potential predictors of the early emergence and persistence of ADHD in children:

1. The early emergence of high activity level and demandingness in a child's infancy or preschool years.
2. Family history of ADHD.
3. Smoking and alcohol consumption by, and poor health of, the mother during pregnancy.
4. A greater-than-normal number of complications during pregnancy (especially premature delivery and/or low birth weight that is associated with bleeding in the brain).
5. Being a single parent and having less education than normal (which may be an indication of possible ADHD symptoms in the parents).
6. Poor health of the infant, and delays in motor and language development.

Summary

To summarize, biological factors (abnormalities in brain development) are most closely associated with and may perhaps be causes of ADHD. Studies so far indicate a very strong genetic contribution to ADHD symptoms—one that is much greater than the contribution of environmental agents or purely social factors. Everything we know points to the idea that children with ADHD have delayed brain development and less brain activity, especially in the prefrontal regions—precisely those brain centers known to be involved in executive functioning and self-control, such as inhibition, persistence toward tasks and goals, resistance to distraction, and control of one's activity level. The precise cause of this delayed maturation and underactivity is not known but appears to likely be due to genetics: people with ADHD have different versions of genes that build and operate these brain regions, and these variations may be contributing to altered brain development and functioning.

Where purely social factors seem to be important, as in the case of poor child management skills by parents, is in predicting which children may have more aggressive and defiant behavior. Even the existence of this relationship, however, does not mean that how parents are managing a child with ADHD is the cause of the ADHD, only of the defiant and aggressive behavior.

We have much more to learn about ADHD and its potential causes. Nevertheless, great advances have been made in the last decade in understanding the possible causes of ADHD. All of the evidence to date points to genetically based neurological factors as being the most important in explaining the extent of ADHD in the population. A smaller percentage of cases of ADHD appear to be due to acquired injuries to the developing brain, such as through toxins consumed by the mother during pregnancy or child after birth. When we fully comprehend what causes this disorder, perhaps we will also discover how to cure it. In the meantime, the information that is available, along with what we know about the nature of ADHD (see discussion in Chapter 4), has brought us a long way toward successful management of ADHD—the subject of Parts II through IV (Chapters 6–19).

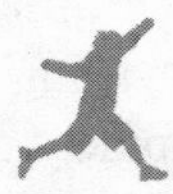

4 What to Expect

THE NATURE OF THE DISORDER

As parents of children with ADHD know, ADHD is a perplexing disorder that can make day-to-day coping a unique challenge. By its very nature, it seems to create adversarial relationships between a child with ADHD and everyone else. The mundane routines of a normal day can seem like a series of battles. It is possible to make life easier, and a good way to begin is to stop fighting the inevitable. Know all you can about the nature of this disorder—what you can and cannot change.

ADHD is found in about 5–8% of all children worldwide (about 7–8% of U.S. children). That means more than 3 million of all those under age 18 in the United States could have the disorder. In several ways, though, the label "ADHD" is relative. In Chapter 3 I discussed the idea that most cases represented just one end of a continuum for a normal trait that we all have. This means that there are degrees of the disorder in the population; some people have mild or even borderline ADHD, whereas others have moderate or severe ADHD. Typically people today are diagnosed with ADHD when their symptoms occur more frequently and with greater magnitude than in 93–95% of those of their age and sex. But even within that group, the frequency and severity of symptoms will vary. How professionals determine the severity of the condition in any given case is explained in Chapter 7.

"I've heard that other countries don't have as much ADHD as we do. Is that true? Why is it that in Great Britain or France they hardly ever diagnose ADHD and don't use medications at all?"

We also know that the definition of ADHD is constantly evolving. Other countries may not even recognize the disorder as such (France, Russia). It used to be called a *conduct problem* in Great Britain, or children simply may be branded *undisciplined* in Eastern Europe, the countries of the former Soviet Union, or China. Even in these regions, the increased information available through the Internet and scientific journals about ADHD is resulting in a growing awareness of ADHD as a distinct and legitimate disorder of children and adults. It's unfortunate that such labels as "behavior problem" or "undisciplined" perpetuate the misperception of ADHD as a problem of personal character or bad parenting. The fact remains that ADHD is a neurologically and primarily genetically determined disorder and is found throughout the world. When it comes to diagnosis, however, methods of quantifying the symptoms vary across countries.

ADHD Is Difficult to Quantify

To arrive at a figure for total cases of ADHD, a common approach is to conduct surveys of parents and teachers about children under their care, using behavior rating scales that measure the symptoms of ADHD. The number of children in that population who probably have the disorder is then determined by establishing a certain cutoff score for the questionnaire, above which a child will be considered to have ADHD. This is not the same as doing a careful evaluation of all the children in a given region, which would not be feasible and would be too costly. But it is one way of getting a rough idea of how many children might qualify for the disorder. These studies have turned up a range of less than 1% to as high as 14%. Obviously, though, where researchers place the cutoff score on these rating scales will determine how many children get labeled as having ADHD.

Of course ADHD should never be diagnosed simply on the basis of a child's score on a behavior rating scale completed by a parent or teacher. As explained later in this book (Chapter 7), a more thorough evaluation is required to make the diagnosis, and a child must meet all of the recommended criteria for the disorder before the diagnosis should be rendered by a professional. Not only must the child's behavior be very deviant from the behavior exhibited by other children of his or her age and sex (as might be indicated through use of a rating scale), but these problems also must have developed during childhood or early adolescence (by 12), have lasted for at least 6–12 months, and be producing impairment in one or more domains of major life activities, such as home, school, or peer-group functioning. When all of these criteria are used to make a diagnosis, studies indicate that the prevalence of ADHD is about 5–8% of school-age children. The disorder is three times more common in boys than in girls.

Stories about ADHD in the popular media have sometimes suggested that ADHD is found only among American children, that other countries have little or no ADHD. Such stories often state that the diagnosis is not used in other countries or is not used as often as it is here. These statements can be highly misleading. The fact that a foreign country does not use the diagnosis to the extent that we do in the United States does not mean its children do not have the disorder. If you don't look for it or measure it, then it doesn't seem to exist in those regions. But that reflects ignorance, not the true state of affairs. More often it means that professionals in that country lack knowledge about the disorder or are uninformed of the scientific literature that supports its existence and legitimacy. Parents should bear in mind that the United States is the world leader in the amount of research done and published on mental health disorders in children; more research is done on children's psychiatric disorders in the United States than in the rest of the world combined. As a consequence, professionals in the United States are more likely to be abreast of the latest research and clinical management of children's disorders than are professionals in many other countries. Recent developments in Canada, Australia, Great Britain, Holland, Spain, Italy, the Scandinavian countries, and Japan support such a conclusion: as professionals and parents in these countries have become more knowledgeable about the nature and existence of ADHD in their children, the rates of diagnosis and of the use of medications to treat the disorder have risen sharply.

Studies done in many other countries over the last 15–25 years have found that ADHD exists in every country and in every ethnic group studied to date. These studies have produced, for example, these figures for prevalence: New Zealand, 2–7%; Germany, 4-6%; India, 5–29%; China, 6–9%; Japan, 7–8%; The Netherlands, 1–3% of teenagers (children not studied); and Brazil, 5–6%. Many other studies have now been published that find ADHD to exist in other countries, often at the level seen in the United States. It is safe to conclude, then, that ADHD is a universal disorder that is found in all countries.

The average of the rates produced by the many studies done worldwide is approximately 5% of school-age children. Remember, though, that the figure is higher for boys and lower for girls. The estimate means that roughly one out of every 20–30 children is hyperactive or has ADHD. This makes ADHD one of the most prevalent disorders seen in children. Given that 50–65% of these children will continue to have the full disorder into adulthood, ADHD should be present in about 4–5% of adults, or one in every 33–50 individuals. That is precisely what has been found in actual surveys of adults, such as one done by Kevin Murphy and me in our study of a large sample of adults from central Massachusetts in 1996. We found that 3–4% of adults met the criteria for having ADHD. In a larger survey of U.S. adults representative of the entire country done in 2011, I found it to be about 5%, a result very similar to that from a study conducted by Dr. Ronald Kessler, his colleagues, and me in 2005 at Harvard Medical School. The problem of estimating the percentage of adults with ADHD is made more difficult by recent findings that the criteria that were used for diagnosis—those of the *Diagnostic and Statistical Manual of Mental Disorders*, fourth edition (DSM-IV)—may not be as sensitive to the disorder as they are in detecting cases in childhood. That's because the criteria were developed largely for use with children, and so the symptoms described in the DSM-IV are mainly those problems of self-control that children might display, not so much those that adults would demonstrate. ADHD is seen in all social classes, ethnic groups, and nationalities in the United States. As just mentioned, it is seen more often in males than females during childhood—three times more frequently. But by adulthood this gender difference is nearly gone and males and females have the disorder in nearly equal percentages. Mental health clinics that specialize in the disorder may see as many as six to nine boys for every girl who comes into their clinic because of a referral bias: people tend to refer children who are more aggressive and difficult to manage to such clinics, and boys with ADHD are typically more aggressive than girls. One obvious lesson from this is that more girls with ADHD until recently have gone unrecognized and untreated, but that situation is changing rapidly as professionals come to understand this problem.

ADHD Changes with Development

One of the most vexing aspects of ADHD for parents is that it evolves as a child grows up. What worked at age 6 may not work at age 16. Up to 80% of school-age children given a clinical diagnosis of ADHD will continue to have the disorder in adolescence, and between 50 and 65% or more will have it into adulthood, depending on how recovery or normalization is defined in any particular study. Parents are likely to notice ADHD first when a child is 3–4 years old or younger. Some children with ADHD, however, may have been difficult to care for, active, and irritable or temperamental since infancy. Others may not have shown such difficulties until entering preschool, kindergarten, or even first grade. In these latter cases, the child probably had some features of the disorder earlier, but these either did not create problems for the parents or did not interfere with the mastery of relatively simple developmental tasks.

Preschool Children with ADHD

A great deal of research has shown that up to 57% of preschool-age children are likely to be rated as inattentive and overactive by their parents by 4 years of age. As many as 40% of these children may have sufficient problems with inattention to be of concern to their parents and teachers. Yet the vast majority of these children improve in their behavior within 3–6 months. Even among those children whose problems may be severe enough to receive a clinical diagnosis of ADHD, only half will have the same diagnosis by later childhood or early adolescence. This tells us that the appearance of symptoms by age 3–4 by itself does not guarantee that ADHD will persist. However, in the majority of those in whom this early pattern of ADHD lasts for at least a year, ADHD is likely to continue into the childhood and teenage years. This means that both the degree of early ADHD symptoms *and* how long they last in early childhood determine which children are likely to show a chronic course of ADHD.

Children with this durable pattern of ADHD in this age group are described by their parents as restless, always up and on the go, acting as if "driven by a motor," and frequently climbing on and getting into things. Persistent in their wants, demanding of parental attention, and often insatiable in their curiosity about their environment, preschoolers with ADHD pose a definite challenge to the child management skills of their parents, particularly their mothers. Such children require far more frequent and closer monitoring of their ongoing conduct than do other preschoolers. Sometimes a few of them are so active they even have to be tethered for their own safety to allow parents to complete necessary household chores that require their undivided attention. Those children with ADHD who also exhibit excessive moodiness, quickness to anger, and low adaptability are likely to prove the most distressing to their mothers. Disobedience of mothers' instructions is common, and at least 40–80% may be seriously defiant or oppositional, especially if they are boys. Even though temper tantrums may be common even for normal preschoolers, they occur more often and with greater intensity in young children with ADHD.

Although the mothers of preschoolers with ADHD are likely to report feeling competent in managing these children, this confidence will decline progressively as these children grow older and parents find that the typical techniques used to manage other children are less effective with their child with ADHD.

Placing a young child with ADHD in day care or preschool is likely to bring additional distress to parents. The staff members are likely to begin to complain about the child's disruptive behavior, and it is not uncommon to find the more active and aggressive of such children "kicked out" of day care or preschool. So begins the course of school adjustment problems that afflict many of these children throughout their compulsory schooling. Other children with ADHD, especially those who are not oppositional or aggressive and who have milder cases of ADHD, and perhaps those who are intellectually brighter, may have no problems in day care, particularly when it is only a half-day program for a few days each week.

Many mothers of young children with ADHD have also told us how difficult it can be to find babysitters, which severely limits the parents' mobility and opportunities for much-needed leisure—a particularly difficult problem for single parents. No wonder parents of children with ADHD tell us that the preschool years were often the most stressful and demanding in their life as parents.

School-Age Children with ADHD

Once children with ADHD enter school, a major social burden is placed on them that can last for at least the next 12 years. It will prove to be one of the most severely affected domains of major life activities adversely affected by their disability and will create the greatest source of distress for many of them and their parents. The abilities to sit still, attend, listen, obey, inhibit impulsive behavior, cooperate, organize actions, and follow through on instructions, as well as to share, play well, and interact pleasantly with other children, are essential to negotiating a successful academic career. It is not surprising that the vast majority of children with ADHD are identified as deviant in behavior by entry into formal schooling or within a year or two of doing so. Parents will now have to contend not only with the ongoing behavioral problems at home, but also with the burden of helping their child adjust to the academic and social demands of school. Regrettably, these parents must also tolerate the complaints of many teachers, who naively see the child's problems at school as stemming entirely from home problems or poor child-rearing abilities in the parents.

Often at this stage parents must confront decisions about whether to retain a child in kindergarten or a later grade because of "immature" behavior and possibly slow academic achievement. The fact that many schools now assign homework, even to first-graders, makes an additional demand on both the parents and the child to accomplish these tasks together. Homework time becomes another area of conflict. For the 20–35% of children with ADHD who are likely to have a reading disorder, this will be noted as the children try to master the early reading tasks at school. Such children are doubly hampered in their academic performance by the combination of these disabilities. For those who will develop math and writing disorders, these problems often go undetected until several years into elementary school. Even without learning disabilities, almost all children with ADHD will be haunted by their highly erratic educational performance.

At home, parents often complain that their children with ADHD do not accept household chores and responsibilities as well as other children their age. They need help with these daily chores as well as with dressing and bathing. While the frequency of temper tantrums is likely to decline, as it does in children without ADHD, children with ADHD will show such behavior when frustrated more frequently than normal children. Often, children with ADHD are barely tolerated or ejected outright from social activities such as clubs, music lessons, sports, and Scouts. Their overall pattern of social rejection will start emerging during the school years if it has not done so already. Overwhelming, intrusive, emotionally impulsive, impatient, and even aversive to others, children with ADHD who are attempting to learn appropriate social skills become confused by peers' avoidance, and by late childhood some are developing low self-esteem. Not all children with ADHD have low self-esteem, however. In fact, many may present an image of themselves to others that is unrealistically positive, in the sense that they have been found to overestimate their abilities and likelihood of succeeding at a task when asked about it beforehand. While this could simply be bragging, research by Drs. Mary Beth Diener and Richard Milich at the University of Kentucky suggests that it may be self-protective. That is, children with ADHD wish to present a more positive view of themselves to others than is realistic in an effort to be more liked and positively evaluated by others, and out of fear of admitting that they are not as good as they believe they ought to be at the task. Nevertheless, many children with ADHD will place the blame for these difficulties on their peers or on parents and teachers because of their own limited self-awareness and reduced willingness to accept responsibility (social immaturity).

By later childhood and preadolescence, patterns of social conflict are well established for many children with ADHD. Between 7 and 12 years of age, at least 30–50% are likely to develop symptoms of conduct disorder and antisocial behavior, such as lying, petty thievery, and resistance to authority. Twenty-five percent or more may have problems with fighting with other children. Those who have not developed some other psychiatric, academic, or social disorder by this time are in the minority, and it is these children who are likely to have the best adolescent outcomes, experiencing problems primarily with academic performance and eventual attainment. The majority of children with ADHD by this time will have been placed on a trial of ADHD medication, and over half will participate in some type of individual and family therapy. Approximately 30–45% will also be receiving formal special educational assistance by the end of sixth grade.

Adolescents with ADHD

Numerous follow-up studies published since the late 1970s have done much to dispel the idea that ADHD is typically outgrown by the adolescent years. From 70–80% of children clinically diagnosed with ADHD are likely to continue to display significant symptoms and qualify for the diagnoses by age 16, and as many as 25–45% of the adolescents display antisocial behavior or conduct disorder. As many as 20–30% may be experimenting with or frankly abusing substances, such as alcohol, nicotine, and marijuana. Up to 58% have failed at least one grade in school, and at least three times as many teenagers with ADHD as those without ADHD have failed a grade, been suspended, or been expelled from school. Almost 35% of children with ADHD quit school before completion. Their levels of academic achievement are well below normal on standard tests of math, reading, and spelling.

The same issues that make these years difficult for individuals without ADHD—identity, peer-group acceptance, dating, and physical/sexual development—erupt as a second source of demands and distress as well as new domains of impairment for adolescents with ADHD. Sadness or even depression may arise in a minority of cases; others may show poor self-confidence, diminished hopes of future success, and concerns about school completion and social acceptance. My own follow-up study with Dr. Mariellen Fischer at the Medical College of Wisconsin in Milwaukee mentioned earlier in this book has also demonstrated that teens with ADHD may start having sexual intercourse by as much as a year earlier than other teens and may be less likely to employ birth control when they do so. Consequently, we found that more than 38% of our sample had been involved in a teen pregnancy and more than 17% had been treated for a sexually transmitted disease by the time they were 19 years old. By age 20, the ADHD group had 37 children to just 1 born to a person in our control group. We have also documented a greater risk for driving problems in teens with the disorder, finding them three to four times more likely to get speeding tickets and two to three times more likely to have auto accidents. The accidents they have are also more serious in terms of both dollar damages and bodily injuries sustained in the crashes. Parents may need to be more vigilant about monitoring their teens' activities in both of these areas and about discussing ways of preventing these negative outcomes, such as using ADHD medications while driving.

Adults with ADHD

Research to date suggests that 50–65% of children with ADHD continue to have symptoms as they reach adulthood. Although many of them will be employed and self-supporting, their educational level and socioeconomic status tend to be lower than those of others, even their own siblings. Antisocial behavior is likely to be troublesome for at least 20–45%, with as many as 25% qualifying for a diagnosis of adult antisocial personality disorder—a pattern of repetitive antisocial and irresponsible behavior beginning in early adolescence.

Only 10–20% of children with ADHD reach adulthood free of any psychiatric diagnosis, functioning well, and without significant symptoms of their disorder. The rest continue having many of the same problems they had as children and then as teenagers, even if they don't meet all the criteria professionals use to give a diagnosis of ADHD. Dealing with those problems for so long can take a tragic and irreparable toll. It is fair to say that perhaps 25% are persistently antisocial in adulthood: adults with ADHD are four times as likely as others to have committed acts of physical aggression toward others within the last 3 years.

In the undemanding part-time jobs typically held by teenagers, adolescents with ADHD function as well as their peers without ADHD. In the adult working world, however, they are likely to have problems that add up to a poorer work record and lower job status than those of other adults. My own follow-up study of children with ADHD as they move into adulthood has shown that they are likely to change jobs much more often than those without ADHD, and that they are more likely to be fired from their jobs as a consequence of their misbehavior and poor self-control. Like their performance in high school, occupational functioning for those with ADHD in adulthood is marked by significant problems with the capacity to work independently of supervision, to be punctual for deadlines and even work schedules, to be persistent and productive in getting assigned work done, and to interact cordially with fellow workers.

Like the children, the adults with ADHD have considerable problems with inattention, poor inhibition, difficulties resisting distractions, poor emotional control, and generally poor self-regulation or self-discipline. While they may not be as overtly hyperactive as they were in childhood, they often describe themselves as feeling restless and needing to always be on the go, doing things; always needing to be busy. Some even say they feel more internally restless, more tense and jittery than others. What makes the adults different, of course, is the impact of these symptoms on their functioning in adult settings and handling adult responsibilities. Young children with ADHD do not have trouble with driving, sexual activity, money management, health maintenance, their marriages or other relationships, or their jobs because they cannot engage in these activities at their tender age. So the effect the disorder has on the handling of daily responsibilities and life's demands changes more than the underlying nature of the disorder itself. The consequences for ADHD symptoms in adulthood are more widespread and serious, but that is because of the increase in the types, diversity, and importance of the major domains of responsibility they must meet.

In general, the approach to treatment is much the same with adults with ADHD as with children with the disorder. Getting properly diagnosed and then educated about the disorder is always the first step in treatment. Then using the same types of medications we use with children can be helpful, although doses may need to be larger for some adults. And of course combining the medications with the most appropriate accommodations and psychological treatments will be important, just as it is for the children. The settings where these accommodations may be needed are different, of course (for example, work instead of school). But the nature of the accommodations is generally the same as what I have recommended in this book for home and classroom management strategies.

For instance, we may not put an adult with ADHD who has trouble in the workplace on a poker chip token system to help him get more work done, as that would seem childish if not impossible in the workplace. But following the same principle behind that recommendation, we would seek to increase his accountability to his supervisors on a more immediate, frequent, and salient basis. We would have the adult break down his work into smaller steps, state his goals for the morning work period to his supervisor beforehand, have his supervisor meet with him periodically through the morning to review progress, and even try to arrange consequences at work contingent on meeting the goals.

We have known for a long time that children diagnosed with ADHD have a number of significant additional problems to contend with as they get older. Some of these may be preventable with prolonged treatment, but keep in mind that children with ADHD should not be dismissed as having little or no future risk. What determines who will outgrow ADHD is not clear at this time. Certainly children with quite mild ADHD who have no other disorders seem to have a better chance of outgrowing it. We do know that children with ADHD benefit from the same advantages that children without ADHD do: intelligence, lack of aggression or defiance, good care and supervision from parents who do not have their own serious psychological problems to deal with, and sufficient affluence to have access to various economic, medical, psychiatric, and community resources.

The Symptoms of ADHD Change with the Situation

To make life even more challenging for parents of children with ADHD, all of the primary symptoms of ADHD change not only with a child's growth but also with the situation: where the child is, what she is asked to do, and who must care for the child. Table 1 shows the results of a study I did in the late 1970s to examine those situations in which children with hyperactivity (present-day ADHD) were most likely to have problems when with their parents. The table illustrates that the less restrictive the setting and the less demanding the tasks required, the less distinguishable children

TABLE 1. Percentage of Hyperactive- and Control-Group Children Displaying Problems in 14 Home Situations and the Average Severity Rating in Each Setting

	Hyperactive group		*Control group*	
Situation	*Percent*	*Average severity*[a]	*Percent*	*Average severity*
While playing alone	40.0	4.3	0.0	0.0
Playing with others	90.0	5.4	10.0	1.6
Mealtimes	86.7	4.7	13.3	3.0
Getting dressed	73.3	6.1	10.0	2.3
Washing/bathing	43.3	5.1	16.7	1.2
When parent is on phone	93.3	6.6	33.3	1.3
While watching television	80.0	5.0	3.3	2.0
When visitors are in home	96.7	6.1	30.0	1.6
When visiting others	96.7	5.4	13.3	1.5
Public places	96.7	5.4	23.3	2.7
When father is at home	73.3	3.9	6.7	2.5
When asked to do chores	86.7	5.6	36.7	2.0
At bedtime	83.3	5.0	20.0	1.5
While riding in the car	73.3	4.8	20.0	1.7

Note. From Barkley, R. A. (1981). *Hyperactive Children: A Handbook for Diagnosis and Treatment.* Copyright 1981 by The Guilford Press. Reprinted by permission.

[a]Severity was rated by parents on a scale from 1 (mild) to 9 (severe).

with ADHD are from children without ADHD. Other studies have since gone on to replicate many of these differences.

Interestingly, Table 2 also indicates that children with ADHD are more compliant and less disruptive with their fathers than with their mothers. There are several possible reasons for this, discussed in Chapter 5.

Research that I reviewed in my 2006 handbook for the diagnosis and treatment of ADHD also has shown that children with ADHD do better under the following conditions.

TABLE 2. Percentage of Hyperactive- and Control-Group Children Having Medical Problems

Medical problems	*Hyperactive group*	*Control group*	*Significantly different?*
	Pregnancy/birth problems		
1. Poor health of mother	26.4	16.2	Yes
2. Young mother (under 20 years of age)	16.3	6.7	Yes
3. At least one previous miscarriage	21.1	24.4	No
4. First pregnancy	42.7	32.8	Yes
5. Rh factor (blood) incompatibility	14.9	12.4	No
6. Premature delivery (under 8 months)	7.9	5.4	No
7. Postmaturity (over 10 months)	7.9	1.5	Yes
8. Long labor (13 or more hours)	24.8	15.7	Yes
9. Toxemia or eclampsia during pregnancy	7.8	2.5	Yes
10. Fetal distress during labor or birth	16.9	8.0	Yes
11. Abnormal delivery	26.6	20.2	No
12. Low birth weight (under 6 pounds)	12.2	7.8	No
13. Congenital problems	22.1	13.2	Yes
14. Problems in establishing routines during infancy (eating, sleeping, etc.)	54.6	31.7	Yes
15. Health problems during infancy	50.9	29.2	Yes
	Developmental milestones		
16. Delay in sitting up	0.4	0.0	No
17. Delay in crawling	6.5	1.6	Yes
18. Delay in walking	1.5	0.5	No
19. Delay in talking	9.6	3.7	Yes
20. Delay in bladder control	7.4	4.5	No
21. Delay in bowel control	10.1	4.5	Yes
	Childhood illness and accidents		
22. Chronic health problems	39.1	24.8	Yes
23. One or more acute illnesses or diseases in childhood	78.0	79.0	No
24. Four or more serious accidents	15.6	4.8	Yes
25. More than one surgery	27.3	19.5	No
	Childhood health status		
26. Poor general health	8.9	2.4	Yes
27. Poor hearing	11.1	7.6	No
28. Poor vision	21.6	13.4	Yes
29. Poor coordination	52.3	34.9	Yes
30. Speech problems	26.6	14.8	Yes

Note. Adapted from Hartsough C. S., & Lambert, N. M. (1985). Medical factors in hyperactive and normal children: Prenatal, developmental, and health history findings. *American Journal of Orthopsychiatry, 55,* 190–201.

Unfamiliar Surroundings or Novelty

Children with ADHD do much better at the beginning of the academic year, when teachers, classmates, classrooms, and even school facilities are novel. Their behavioral control deteriorates over the initial weeks of school as their familiarity with school increases and boredom starts to set in. Similarly, they may be less troublesome when visiting with grandparents whom they have not seen frequently. These grandparents are likely to provide them with more one-on-one attention than their parents and are unlikely to make as many demands concerning the children's self-control as do parents. At such times, it is likely that children with ADHD will be better than usual. Research also suggests that more colorful, highly stimulating, bright, cheerful, fun educational materials presented differently from the usual dry textbook or workbook format may be important in helping children with ADHD to work better at school.

Immediate Rewards for Complying with Instructions

Children with ADHD are often better able to pay attention and persist in situations that give them immediate and frequent feedback for how they are doing, such as in video games, than they are in such tasks as homework or schoolwork, where such feedback is infrequent or quite delayed. Even during video game performance, however, their behavior is distinguishable from that of normal children, as discussed earlier. They are still more distractible and inattentive, less able to inhibit impulsive actions, and less coordinated in maneuvering within a video game than are normal children. They perform better when special rewards such as money are promised immediately upon completion of a task, perhaps even as well as children without ADHD do. However, when the timing and amount of the reward are decreased, the behavior of children with ADHD worsens significantly. These dramatic changes have led scientists to question whether ADHD is actually a deficit in attention at all, as discussed in Chapter 2. They fit better with the view that ADHD involves deficits in self-regulation (executive functioning) and so is at its worst in settings that place heavier demands on these abilities.

Individual Attention

During one-to-one encounters with others, children with ADHD may appear less active, inattentive, and impulsive. In group situations, children with ADHD may appear at their worst. Again, they may be at their best with grandparents, who are likely to give them this individualized attention. They work more effectively under close supervision and when instructions are repeated frequently.

Most Demanding Schedule in the Morning

Fatigue or the time of day may determine how problematic a child's ADHD symptoms are likely to be. Children with ADHD seem to do better on schoolwork in the mornings, more so than they will be able to do later in the day. This means not only that educators would do well to schedule repetitive, boring, or difficult tasks requiring the greatest powers of attention and self-control for morning, but also that trying to do homework with a child with ADHD in late afternoons after school is sure to result in trouble unless the child is on an extended-release type of ADHD medication.

Other Problems Are Associated with ADHD

It is rare in a clinical practice to see children who have only one disorder; probably fewer than 20% of the children who come to an ADHD clinic have only ADHD. Being diagnosed as having ADHD raises the odds of having several other disorders as well—a phenomenon called *comorbidity.* In particular, people with ADHD may be more likely than others to have additional medical, developmental, behavioral, emotional, and academic difficulties.

Intelligence

Children with ADHD are likely to represent the whole spectrum of intellectual development, ranging from being gifted to being typical to even being intellectually delayed. Some but not all studies have found that children with ADHD are more likely to be slightly behind the general mental or intellectual development of children without ADHD, to a not very large, but scientifically significant, degree. Children with ADHD may score an average of 7–10 points below others on intelligence tests. Some of the difference here may be more a reflection of the problems ADHD imposes on the test-taking abilities than of intelligence. But some of it has also been shown to be related to the degree of deficits the child has in executive functioning because the latter ability is also required for parts of IQ tests.

School Performance

One area of tremendous difficulty for children with ADHD is academic *performance*—the amount of schoolwork they are able to perform and their general behavior in the classroom. (*Achievement*, in contrast, means the level of difficulty of work they are able to accomplish, as usually reflected in test scores, such as on reading tests.) Almost all children with ADHD who are referred to clinics are doing poorly at school;

it is one of the chief reasons for the referral to the clinic. They seem to have at least two main problems with academic work: (1) They are not getting as much done as other children are during the same amount of time (underproductivity) or as would be expected from their known abilities, and so have lower grades and are retained more often in their grade levels. (2) Their achievement skills are also somewhat below those of children without ADHD and may even decline somewhat over their years in school. Consequently, it is not surprising to find that 40% or more of children with ADHD may eventually be placed in special educational programs for children with learning disabilities or behavior disorders. Nor is it unexpected that as many as 40% will have been retained in a grade at least once before reaching high school. Being inattentive and impulsive in a setting where self-regulation and sustained effort are crucial for success, such as in school, can be devastating for these children.

Children with ADHD are also more likely than children without ADHD to have learning disabilities (LDs). An LD is a significant delay in a child's academic achievement, such as in reading, spelling, math, writing, and language. Between 20 and 30% of children with ADHD have at least one type of LD, in math, reading, or spelling; in some studies the prevalence of LDs is even higher.

Why do nearly three to five times as many children with ADHD as children without it have LDs? Scientists are not sure, but possible explanations are emerging from studies on the genetics of ADHD and LDs. Both disorders have a strong hereditary predisposition. Recent studies suggest that at least for reading disorders the two do not tend to be inherited together; that is, most of the genes for ADHD are not the same as those for a reading disorder, but a few of the genes may be shared between the disorders and perhaps help to explain the inattentiveness and slow response speed seen in both disorders. A study done more than a decade ago by Dr. J. Gillis and his colleagues at the University of Colorado suggests that a few of the genes for ADHD may also occur in some LDs, like writing and spelling. Much more research is needed on this issue before this relationship can be taken as proven, however. No one has yet looked at the inheritance of math disorders, so we have no clues as to how these come to coexist with ADHD. Although most children with ADHD are not seriously delayed in the development of language, they are more likely to have specific problems in speech development than normal children. Children with ADHD also are more likely to have problems with expressive language and fluency.

Although scientists are still not certain why LDs occur more often with ADHD, an intriguing hypothesis was supported by a study conducted by Dr. Joseph Biederman and colleagues at Massachusetts General Hospital and Harvard Medical School. They found that adults with ADHD were more likely to have children with mates who had LDs, such as reading disorders, and vice versa. This is known as *nonrandom mating,* in that people with certain characteristics have a higher probability of mating with people having other particular features. Humans generally do not mate randomly, but are selective in their choice of partners for the purposes of having children. This is particularly true of women. Among the characteristics that people seem to use in mate selection is education, most likely because it is a general, though imperfect, indicator of intelligence. Both ADHD and LDs are largely hereditary. And both hinder how far a person is likely to progress in schooling. As a consequence, people with these disorders are more likely to find themselves in the same social circles, since they are likely to have comparable levels of education. This raises the probability that a person having one disorder will choose someone with the other disorder as a potential mate, and that raises the likelihood that their offspring will get the genes for both disorders. Certainly more research on this fascinating explanation is in order before it can be accepted as accurate, but it does provide a reasonable explanation in addition to that of there being some shared underlying genes for why LDs and ADHD often co-occur in children.

Other Mental Abilities

Children with ADHD also tend to be less skilled in the use of complex problem-solving strategies and the organizational skills needed for solving intellectual or social problems. Their impulsiveness and poor sustained attention are a disadvantage to them in most problem-solving situations, as discussed in Chapter 2. They also use less-efficient strategies in searching their memory when they need to think about how to react to a situation. We often refer to this as *hindsight*, and again Chapter 2 discusses how I believe ADHD precludes the use of adequate hindsight. Children with ADHD do not have difficulties with memory, in the sense that they can readily store and retrieve information as well as others. However, as noted earlier, they do have problems with a special kind of memory known as *working memory*. Working memory is the ability to hold information consciously in mind that you need to get something done. Think of it as remembering to do something, especially something later in time. In this type of memory those with ADHD have substantial problems. Their problems in doing mental work come when they must apply thoughtful strategies in that work—when they must inhibit the urge to respond too quickly and reflect on the problem. Little wonder, then, that many studies also show that children with ADHD are less organized or planful in their approach to learning and performing schoolwork in general.

Physical Development

Several relatively large studies have indicated that children with ADHD have more problems with physical development than children without ADHD. Table 2 summarizes one done more than 25 years ago by Drs. Carolyn Hartsough and Nadine Lambert of the University of California at Berkeley that is still relevant today. In 1985 they published their findings on the medical histories of 492 children with hyperactivity (present-day ADHD) from the East Bay area of San Francisco. The percentages of the hyperactive and the control or normal children having each developmental problem are shown in this table. If a "Yes" appears next to the item or problem, then that difference is considered to be statistically significant—this simply means that the groups can be considered to be reliably different on that item. Where a "No" appears, even though the numbers are not quite the same, the groups should be considered to be the same. This study found that the hyperactive children were more likely to have problems than the other children with 19 of the 30 problems listed in the table, but we should keep in mind that other studies have disagreed. Let's look at some individual problems.

Congenital Problems

Table 2 shows that mothers of hyperactive children were much more likely to have experienced complications of their pregnancies than mothers of control children. The hyperactive children were also more likely to have experienced medical problems shortly after birth (congenital problems) and to have had general health problems during infancy.

Hearing and Speech

While there is no evidence that children with ADHD are any more likely than children without ADHD to have difficulties in the development of their hearing, some studies show that more will have otitis media, or middle ear infections, than other children; these infections can episodically reduce hearing and create problems with speech development. The findings are not very consistent across studies, however. But as noted above, children with ADHD are more likely to have delays in speech and language development. This is especially so in what is known as the executive use of language—how they organize and use language to accomplish tasks and goals effectively.

Vision

Children with ADHD seem somewhat more likely to have vision problems than children without ADHD, but again research findings are inconsistent.

Motor Skills

Drs. Hartsough and Lambert found their sample of hyperactive children to be slightly more likely to be delayed in crawling than the control children (6.5% versus

1.6%), but over 93% of the hyperactive children had no such delays. Nevertheless, as many as 52% of children with ADHD, compared to up to 35% of children without ADHD, are likely to have poor motor coordination—especially fine motor coordination, such as buttoning, tying shoelaces, drawing, and writing. These findings have now been replicated many times by studies in the United States and in other countries, like Sweden.

Physical Appearance

One fascinating finding is that children with ADHD seem to have more minor or slight deformities in their physical appearance than children without ADHD. These may include an index finger that is longer than the middle finger, a curved fifth finger, a third toe that is as long as or longer than the second toe, ears that are set slightly lower on the sides of the head than normal, no earlobes, or a furrowed tongue. However, recent research shows that all children with psychiatric disorders tend to have more such anomalies, so these anomalies are not just a sign of ADHD alone.

Health or Medical Problems

Children with ADHD seem to have more problems with their general health than do children without ADHD. Up to 50% were described by their mothers as having been in poor health during infancy, compared to less than half this number in children without ADHD. We do not yet understand why children with ADHD are more likely to have medical problems, but children with other psychiatric disorders also have a greater tendency toward general health problems.

Similarly, nighttime bed-wetting (enuresis) and problems with toilet training plague children with ADHD more than other children, but the same can be said of all children with psychiatric problems.

Parents often complain that their children with ADHD do not sleep well, and several studies have confirmed that these children take longer to get ready for bed or to fall asleep, wake up more frequently during the night, are more restless during sleep, and may be unusually tired upon awakening. Such sleep difficulties have been found in as many as 40% or more of children with ADHD. While some of these are technically bedtime behavior problems (not staying in the bedroom at bedtime as requested), others may signal actual sleeping disorders, such as frequent night waking, labored breathing or other signs of sleep apnea, and exceptional tiredness on awakening. In those cases, an evaluation at a sleep lab may be indicated. While many children with sleep problems have inattention, some of which may rise to the level of ADHD, these sleep problems are not comparable to a clinical diagnosis of ADHD.

Many studies have found that children with ADHD are more accident-prone than children without ADHD. This research shows that children with ADHD are more likely to experience all forms of accidental injury, including burns, accidental poisonings, lacerations, closed head injuries, pedestrian–auto accidents (usually while bike riding), and other trauma. No wonder then that the medical costs alone associated with raising a child with ADHD have been found to be more than double those for raising a normal child, with much of this cost associated with more frequent visits to the local hospital emergency room. Recent studies using much larger groups of children have found this to be even more problematic for children who are also defiant and stubborn than for those who have only ADHD.

Adaptive Functioning

Dr. Mark Stein, now at Seattle Children's Hospital, and his colleagues demonstrated more than 18 years ago, in 1995, that children with ADHD have significant delays in development of adaptive functioning: meeting day-to-day responsibilities for caring for themselves, interacting and communicating well with others, and becoming independent of their parents. Adaptive functioning includes self-help skills (such as dressing, bathing, feeding, and toilet training), language and interpersonal skills (such as sharing, cooperating, keeping promises, following directions, and attending to personal safety), and skills related to becoming an independent member of the community (such as understanding money and economic exchanges, following social rules, and knowing community resources and how to use them). Dr. Stein and colleagues found that children with ADHD were markedly below their expected levels of development in these areas despite having normal intellectual development. Dr. Terri Shelton and I, along with other coworkers, examined this finding in our kindergarten screening project mentioned earlier, when we both worked at the University of Massachusetts Medical School. Like Dr. Stein, we also found that children with ADHD were generally well behind normal children in developing adaptive functioning skills. When we examined those children with ADHD who were in the lowest 10% of normal development in this area, we discovered that these children had the highest risks for developing conduct disorder and other forms of aggressive and antisocial behavior, that they were also more delayed in their academic skills at school entry, and that their parents were reporting far more stress at home and more conflict in their interactions with these children than in children with ADHD who were developing normally in these areas. After following these children over a 3-year period, we found that being low in adaptive functioning at the beginning of the study continued to predict the same sorts of problems with antisocial behavior, poor school performance, and greater parental problems and family conflict. This tells us that preschool children with ADHD who are not developing well in their adaptive functioning may be much more likely than other children with ADHD to experience significant problems in their later school, home, and community functioning.

Behavioral and Emotional Problems

ADHD is often associated with other behavioral and emotional disorders. From early infancy, children with ADHD are often reported to be more demanding and difficult to care for in their general temperament and more stressful than are children without ADHD (see Table 2). Up to 80% of children with ADHD have at least one other psychiatric disorder besides ADHD, and many have two or more additional disorders. Children with ADHD also display more symptoms of anxiety and depression that do not always qualify for a formal psychiatric diagnosis of those conditions than do other children.

It is widely accepted by scientists that children with ADHD have more difficulties with oppositional and defiant behavior. Up to two-thirds (or more) can be very stubborn and argue with their parents more than other children. Many of these defiant children are also aggressive toward others. They may be quick to get angry, verbally attack others, or even physically assault others more often than other children of their age. These conduct problems can progress to more severe forms of antisocial behavior, such as lying, stealing, fighting, running away from home, destroying property, and other delinquent or criminal behavior. My own follow-up study noted earlier shows that up to 65% will eventually have a diagnosis of oppositional defiant disorder (see Chapter 1), and as many as 45% may progress to the more severe diagnosis of conduct disorder.

How Do Children with ADHD Get Along with Other Children?

Children with ADHD do not usually get along very well with their peers. More than 30 years ago, Drs. William Pelham and Mary Bender, then at the University of Pittsburgh Western Psychiatric Institute, reviewed research on the social relationships of children with ADHD. They estimated that over 50% had significant problems in their peer relationships. Research shows that the inattentive, disruptive, off-task, immature, and provocative behaviors of children with ADHD quickly bring out a pattern of controlling and directive behavior from their peers when they must work together. And, despite talking more, children with ADHD are less likely to respond to the questions or verbal interactions of their peers. My own theory of ADHD discussed in Chapter 2, as well as some recent research on peer relations, suggests that children with ADHD are less able to cooperate and share with other children and to make and keep promises regarding the mutual exchange of favors. This is known as *reciprocity* or *social exchange*, and it is at the very heart of developing friendships and demonstrating effective interpersonal dealings with others. Given their deficits in the executive abilities needed to support such reciprocal and cooperative social activities, it is easy to see why many children with ADHD have few, if any, friends with whom to play.

This can be very painful for parents to witness. We all want our children to be liked by others, to have friends, to be invited out with other children, and to develop close relationships with their peer group. We know that such relationships can sustain us through other difficulties we may experience as we grow up. When parents notice that their children with ADHD are having great troubles in forming and keeping friendships, they have reason for concern.

A Final Note

This chapter should have shown you that children with ADHD are not all alike. They will vary in the severity of their ADHD and even in its associated disorders or impaired major life activities. Some will exhibit different patterns of behavior, development, and later risks than others. Some will have only ADHD; others will have this disorder as well as learning problems, aggression, antisocial conduct, and poor peer relations. All share the problem of reduced ability for self-regulation, that is, to inhibit their behavior and to sustain their efforts toward activities, goals, and the future more generally. And, of course, all are children in need of our care, support, guidance, nurturance, and love, though they can be challenging to raise and do not always appear grateful for our efforts to guide and raise them to adulthood.

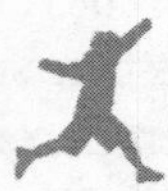

5 The Family Context of a Child with ADHD

Children with ADHD do not exist in a vacuum. They occupy specific places within various social networks or systems, the most significant of these systems being the most immediate one, the family. Forgive me for stating the obvious, but traditionally our theories, assessment, and treatment of these children focus so heavily on them as individuals and their behavior in isolation from others that we forget this important point. No one can fully appreciate the disorder—its causes, impairments, course, and outcome—without recourse to this social environment and a child's interactions with others within it. The very diagnosis of ADHD hinges on our understanding this point. The reports of others within this social network are what determine which children get referred, diagnosed, and treated. The prognosis of ADHD for any given child surely revolves around this factor as well. To understand who develops ADHD, who continues to have ADHD over time, which children with ADHD develop additional problems, which children will fare well despite these problems, and which individuals will fare poorly in adulthood requires reference to this social network. Therefore, knowing that children have ADHD is of limited importance in predicting their future or in designing treatment for them. We must consider further the various contexts in which specific children live and interact, with whom they interact, and who in turn act on them.

Knowing what impact children with ADHD have on their families, how their families act on the children, and how their behavior is managed by parents will help you understand not just your child but also yourself, and even your family as a whole. The journey of discovery that led you to this book must also be a journey of self-exploration for you as a parent. As you read this chapter, consider how you typically respond to your child's appropriate behavior, and especially to inappropriate, disruptive, or demanding behaviors. Also consider how your child treats you, what reactions your child brings out in you, and the overall quality of your relationship. Then examine, in turn, how your child affects others in the family and how they treat this child. Are you married or living with a partner? If so, do you have marital or cohabiting problems that spill over into your relationships with your children, particularly the child with ADHD? Or is your marriage or other intimate relationship a source of strength for you in dealing with the day-to-day demands of raising children and managing a household? Do you work outside the home? Does this bring stress into your home and affect your relationship with your children? Or is your job also a source of personal growth and success that feeds your strength as a parent? Although I describe here the results of research on the family interactions of children with ADHD, the ultimate purpose of this chapter is to encourage you to examine your own family relative to these scientific findings. See if there are things about *your* family that you would like to change. Then make a commitment to change them. The later chapters of this book are intended to help you with that goal. In any case, it should be obvious that you are at least seeking to change the quality of your relationship with your child, or you probably would not have started reading this book.

The family context of a child with ADHD is critically important in understanding the child, for several reasons. First, the parent–child and sibling–child interactions in a family of a child with ADHD have been shown to be inherently more negative and stressful for all family members than the typical interactions in other families. Despite the view taken in this book that the development of ADHD has a strong biological (largely hereditary) predisposition, not even the strongest advocate of this view could deny the powerful effects this difference in social interaction must produce on the additional problems a child with ADHD is likely to experience.

Second, much evidence exists that the parents and siblings of a child with ADHD are more likely to be experiencing their own psychological distress and psychiatric disorders, including their own ADHD symptoms, than parents and siblings of a child without ADHD. In fact, there is about a 25–40% chance that at least one of the parents of a child with ADHD also has the disorder. These difficulties that other family members are experiencing surely have some influence on the manner in which the child with ADHD is perceived, managed, reared, loved, and then launched into adulthood. This influence acts in unique ways that seem to have long-lasting effects for the adolescent and adult outcomes of such children. Perhaps it starts a vicious cycle much like the following:

1. Parents who are having personal problems often perceive their child with ADHD as showing more disruptive behavior, and that behavior is perceived as more demanding of their time and more difficult for them to manage than it is for parents without such problems.

2. These perceptions affect the way the parents react to the child's behavior, sometimes resulting in unnecessarily high levels of expressed negative emotion, harsh punishment, or a general irritability toward the child no matter what the child does.

3. The child may also receive much less encouragement, praise, approval, and general warmth than would otherwise be given.

4. This treatment of the child in turn influences how the child behaves toward the parents, perhaps increasing the level of defiance, stubbornness, argument, and general conflict.
5. This behavior may reinforce the parents' view that the child is a problem or difficult to manage.
6. The cycle starts anew.

This does not mean that one or both parents are the chief cause of the child's disruptive or defiant behavior; it only suggests that the parent–child relationship can affect the severity of a child's behavioral problems and a parent's perceptions of how stressful the child is to raise.

Since 1980 or so, a large number of scientific studies have been published on the way in which children with ADHD behave toward their parents and the reactions of their parents to them. I devoted much of my own early scientific career to understanding these interaction patterns and how they are changed by various treatments. What does the research tell us?

The Interactions of Children with ADHD and Their Mothers

The first studies to directly observe the interactions of mothers and their children with ADHD were done more than 40 years ago. For instance, in 1975 Dr. Susan Campbell and her colleagues at the University of Pittsburgh observed that boys with hyperactivity (present-day ADHD) initiated more interactions than other boys when working with their mothers to complete a task. These children also talked more with their mothers and requested more help. In short, these children seemed to require more attention from, talk more to, and seek more help from their mothers during interactions with them. The mothers of the children with ADHD gave them more suggestions, approval, disapproval, and directions on impulse control than the mothers of the other children. In other words, mothers of children with ADHD had to manage the behavior of their children more and involve themselves in their children's self-control more than mothers of children without ADHD did. Extended over time, this degree of interaction and supervision can be quite stressful and exhausting to mothers.

In my own early studies, I found that children with ADHD were much less compliant, more negative, more likely to get off-task, and less able to persist in complying with their mothers' directives. Their mothers gave more commands, were also more negative, and at times were less responsive to their children's interactions than I observed in the relations of other children. I also found, as did Dr. Campbell, that children with ADHD talked more during these exchanges.

Later I found that these interaction conflicts changed with age (but were the same problems for boys and girls with ADHD). Younger children both with and without

ADHD had far more mother–child conflicts than older children in both groups. However, at none of the ages studied did the children with ADHD behave like their peers without ADHD—and, of course, the two groups of mothers did not behave alike either. So there is hope that these family relationships improve somewhat, but there is some evidence that they do not become fully normal or typical.

The Interactions of Children with ADHD and Their Fathers

"I have a lot of problems in managing my child, but my husband has far fewer problems. Why?"

One of the things I have heard repeatedly from mothers of children with ADHD is that the children seem to behave better for their fathers. When Dr. James Tallmadge and I were working together at the Medical College of Wisconsin more than 30 years ago, we compared videotaped interactions between mothers and children with ADHD to those between the fathers and children. Overall we did not find much difference. We did notice, however, that the children were less negative with their fathers and were more likely to stay on task than when with their mothers.

I am not sure why this should be so. It might have to do with the fact that mothers still typically carry more of the responsibility than fathers for interacting with children with ADHD at home—especially in getting work and chores done, even when the mothers work outside the home. A parent who taxes the self-control deficits of a child with ADHD will clearly have greater conflicts with that child (an illuminating example of this problem is related in Chapter 17). Mothers also appear to rely somewhat more on verbal explanations, reasoning, and affection in gaining their children's compliance with instructions. Because children with ADHD cannot use their language as well as others for following through on instructions and are not as sensitive to praise, this approach is less likely to manage or motivate them to behave well. Fathers may reason and repeat commands less and may impose swifter punishment for noncompliance. So perhaps a parent who talks less and acts quickly to provide some consequence for a child's good and bad behavior may get more compliance. We also cannot rule out the fact that the greater physical size and strength of the father may be more intimidating to a child with ADHD.

Regardless of why the discrepancy exists, the fact that it does exist can cause problems in the parents' marriage or relationship. The father in such a case may attribute the mother's reports of serious problems with the child to exaggeration or decide that the child's worse behavior with her results from her being too permissive. He may then conclude that it is the mother, not the child, who needs professional assistance. I have also heard of similar scenes being played out in the pediatrician's office: when a male physician has no difficulty managing a child with ADHD, he labels the mother as hysterical and incompetent. It is time for fathers and male professionals to realize that children, especially children with ADHD, differ in their responses to mothers and fathers. Any parents who doubt this assertion should let the father assume greater responsibility for the day-to-day care of the child with ADHD for a while and see if his view of the child's behavior problems begins to resemble the mother's more closely.

The Interactions of Children with ADHD and Their Siblings

The relationship of children with ADHD to their brothers and sisters also seems to differ from that seen in other families. Children with ADHD argue more, play more disruptively, yell at siblings more, and are more likely to encourage inappropriate behavior or mischief, so it's no surprise that conflict is greater than normal. Again, this difference is more marked when children with ADHD are younger.

"How do we get our other kids to understand why their sister acts the way she does, that she is different from them? They think she's lucky for all the help she gets."

How do the siblings without ADHD feel? Brothers and sisters tend to grow tired and exasperated by living with such a disruptive—and baffling—force, with some coming to resent the greater burden of work they often carry, compared to a child with ADHD. Certainly the greater time and attention the child with ADHD receives from the parents is often a source of envy, especially when the siblings without ADHD are younger. Little additional research exists to tell us how these sibling interactions might contribute to problems for both the child with ADHD and the siblings. But let's not forget that the siblings of a child with ADHD have approximately one chance in three or four of having ADHD themselves. When they do, it exacerbates the situation for the whole family.

How Does ADHD Affect Parent–Child Interactions?

What effects does ADHD have on parent–child interactions? An obvious starting place is the ADHD symptoms themselves. The inattentive, impulsive, and overactive behavior patterns of children with ADHD and their general deficits in self-regulation often conflict with the demands all parents must make on their children. Many daily tasks place heavy demands on a child's ability to show self-restraint, sustain attention, persist in effort, manage time well, organize materials, and ignore things that might be more fun to do at the moment. When a child with ADHD has trouble complying with instructions or getting routine work completed, the parents cannot help reacting with greater direction, control, suggestion, encouragement, and ultimately anger. But even when no task is required of the child, the excessive behavior, activity, speech, emotion, and vocal noises are likely to be viewed as intrusiveness and aversive by others, especially over extended periods of time.

So who is causing this cycle-of-interaction conflict? Both the child and the parents contribute to the upward spiral of conflict, but the child contributes more than the parents may realize. Keep in mind, of course, that the child does not do this intentionally. Research on the interactions between children with ADHD and other adults and children outside the family, such as teachers and peers, shows that when the children with ADHD are placed in a classroom, teachers, like mothers, are likely to increase their commands to, reprimands of, and discipline of the children. Likewise, when children with ADHD first enter a new play group, the other children will start to act like "little mothers"—giving more commands, directions, and help to the children with ADHD. When this doesn't squelch the hyperactive and disruptive behavior, the other children may get angry, tease, or insult the children with ADHD. Failing this, they will pull away to find some peace from this unruly, intrusive, and domineering child with ADHD.

Studies have shown that when children with ADHD are placed on ADHD medication, the use by mothers, teachers, and peers of commands, disapproval, and general control diminishes to that seen with children who do not have ADHD, and the interactions become generally more positive. If the parents of children with ADHD were the major cause of the conflict, medicating their children should produce little change in the parents' behavior or little decline in the conflicts. This was hardly the case in our studies, which suggested that the chief origin of the interaction problems rested with the child's ADHD.

How Parents Seem to React to Child Misconduct over Time

Although there is little research on the issue, I have been impressed clinically that the parents of children with ADHD may move through several steps in their efforts to control their children's disruptive behavior. When one strategy fails to work, they move on to the next step in this sequence. My experience suggests that parents initially try to ignore or withhold attention from their children when the children show disruptive behavior. Perhaps they believe that some of this behavior is intended merely to get attention and therefore ignoring the children should decrease the problem. But the children's behavior is not merely the result of bids for attention, so these techniques are unlikely to succeed. As the disruptive behavior continues or intensifies, parents give more commands and directives, especially those aimed at controlling the children's impulses. These commands are often restrictive, calling for the children to stop what they are doing, and parents will find themselves repeating them frequently. It is as if the parents have to take over the child's self-regulation and become the child's executive abilities, sort of a proxy for the child's immature prefrontal "executive" brain.

At some point, frustration and exasperation may result in the parents issuing threats along with these repeated directives. When this approach fails (as it often does) to get the children with ADHD to listen and obey, parents may move on to the actual use of physical discipline or other forms of punishment (loss of privileges or time-out) to regain control over their children's unruly behavior. Some parents may simply give up at this point, giving in to the children and perhaps even doing the children's task themselves or simply walking away, leaving the task undone. If the children have begun to comply but the quality of compliance is poor, parents step in and assist the children in doing the chore. In general, the parent is getting frustrated with the child's noncompliant behavior and the child is learning that stalling in compliance leads to someone stepping in to help get it done, doing it himself, or just walking away, leaving the job undone.

Over time, parents do not start at the beginning of this sequence whenever they have to step in to control their children with ADHD. Instead, they may proceed straight to the last strategy of management that produced some partial success. This can readily lead to immediate negative reactions or harsh physical discipline when the children start to show even minimal disruptive behavior. Some parents appear to have reached such a severe state of failure in their management of their children that they could best be described as being in a state of "learned helplessness." They make no, or minimal, effort to give or enforce commands to their children, leaving them to do as they please. They begin to withdraw from the children, ultimately providing little if any supervision. At this point many such parents report depression, low self-esteem in their role as parents, and little satisfaction with or involvement in their parenting responsibilities. In some cases such parents may shift between complete disengagement and overly harsh reactions to their children's misbehavior, depending on their own mood and irritability at the time. The parents may even start to spend progressively less time in leisure activities with the child because the interactions can be so stressful or unpleasant. In short, living with a child who has ADHD can seriously tax a parent's mental health and commitment to parenthood. If that parent is already experiencing personal emotional problems, it can make them far worse.

Parental Psychiatric Problems

Parents and relatives of children with ADHD are in fact more likely to have psychological problems than those of children without ADHD. Some of these come about from the difficulty of living with someone who has ADHD; others are rooted in the parents' own psychological and even biological makeup.

Parenting Stress

There is no question that parents of children with ADHD, especially mothers and particularly when the children are young, experience greater stress than caretakers of children without ADHD. Mothers of children with ADHD tell us that they have lower levels of parenting self-esteem and experience markedly more depression, self-blame, and social isolation than mothers of children without ADHD. The more severe are a child's behavior problems, the more severe the mother's stress. Obviously, other factors that are affecting a mother's psychological well-being can distort how she views her child and thus how much stress she feels, but our studies show that the major source of parenting stress comes from a child's ADHD and especially its associated defiant and disruptive behavior, rather than from other sources in the family.

"I'm at my wits' end with him. I'm afraid I'm going to hurt him. He's driving me crazy and won't listen. I can't cope with him anymore. I may have to send him away."

We also have found that both the stress of raising a child with ADHD and the greater risk for personal emotional problems in the parents can greatly strain a marriage or relationship, especially when the child has serious oppositional, defiant, or aggressive behavior. My associates and I have found that over an 8-year period, during which we followed a large number of families of children with ADHD, their parents were three times more likely to have separated or divorced than in families of children without ADHD.

Parents of children with ADHD also may be deprived of the encouragement, warmth, and assistance of a supportive family. They tell us that they have fewer contacts with their extended family members than in families without children with ADHD and that these contacts are less helpful to them as parents and more aversive or unpleasant. So parents of children with ADHD may experience a form of social isolation that is detrimental both to their caretaking abilities with their children and to their own emotional well-being.

Psychiatric Disorders

As I have said, the biological parents of children with ADHD are themselves more likely to have ADHD or at least some of the residual characteristics of the disorder. About 15–20% of the mothers and 20–30% of the fathers of children with ADHD may have ADHD at the same time as their children. The biological siblings of these children also share this risk: approximately 26% of brothers and sisters may have the disorder. In general, the risk of ADHD among the first-degree biological relatives of children with ADHD is between 25 and 33%.

Parents of children with ADHD are more likely to experience a variety of other psychiatric disorders as well, the most common being conduct problems and antisocial behavior (25–28%), alcoholism (14–25%), mood disorders like depression or excessive emotional responding to distress (10–27%), and learning disabilities. Even if they are not abusing alcohol, parents of children with ADHD consume more alcohol than do those of children without ADHD. Recall, though, that these psychiatric problems are associated mainly with aggressive and antisocial behavior in the children and not so much with the children's ADHD itself. The more aggressive and antisocial a child is, the more numerous and severe are the psychiatric problems among the relatives. Only ADHD and a history of school problems seem to be more common in the family members of children with ADHD who are not seriously aggressive or antisocial. This certainly suggests that parent and family psychiatric problems may be giving rise to aggressive and antisocial behaviors in cases where a child with ADHD exhibits these. They do so by the influence the parental problems have on the child-rearing skills of the parents and the emotional climate of family life in the home.

What Does All of This Mean for You as a Parent?

All of the preceding information can be boiled down to the simple fact that having a child with ADHD places great stress on parents, particularly mothers. This stress is as great as or greater than that experienced by parents who have children with autism, a far more serious developmental disorder than ADHD. The excessive, demanding, intrusive, poorly self-regulated, and generally high-intensity behavior of children with ADHD, as well as their clear impairment in self-control, naturally elicit greater efforts at direction, help, supervision, and monitoring by parents—efforts far in excess of what parents of children without ADHD need to do. Parents with more than one child with ADHD are assured that their stress levels will be more than twice those of any other family with just one such child. It therefore is easy to see how you could become overwhelmed by the demands the child or children place on you as a parent. I am sure you are aware that when people are exposed to high levels of chronic stress they are more likely to have medical problems, especially those related to immune disorders, such as colds, flu, and other infections. They are also more likely to have mental health problems, such as depression. So you may find yourself similarly affected and find your overall energy level lower since having a child with ADHD.

Short of placing your child with ADHD up for adoption, which no one would suggest, there are many ways to make life at home easier that we consider in Parts II, III, and IV of this book (see Chapters 6–19). Above all, do not give up as a parent. Children with ADHD do have a positive side, and raising such a child to adulthood can give you tremendous satisfaction, provided you learn to cope with the extra stress such parenting brings with it. Draw on the seven principles of effective parenting discussed in the Introduction, and, particularly, do not ignore opportunities for your own personal renewal (see Chapter 10). Strive to be a principle-centered, executive, and scientific parent, and you should find that the stress of raising a child with ADHD is substantially diminished.

Part II

Taking Charge: How to Be a Successful Executive Parent

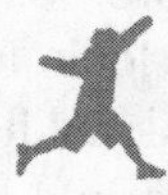

6 Deciding to Have Your Child Evaluated for ADHD

Deciding to seek a professional evaluation for a child is a major decision for any parent. Most parents reach this turning point when they realize that their child's problems exceed the capacity of family and school resources to solve them, and when their frustration in trying to help and get help has reached a peak. Consequently, many parents who are taking that first tenuous step toward help already feel overwhelmed. The goal of this chapter is to make the transition from self-help to professional help a smooth one.

When Should You Consider Getting a Professional Evaluation?

Many parents notice on their own during the preschool years that their child seems to behave differently from other children. Excessive activity, lack of attentiveness and control over emotions, aggressiveness, excitability, and the other symptoms described in Chapter 1 become difficult to ignore. Sometimes it's also obvious that the tried-and-true methods used to manage other children's more typical levels of disruptive and temperamental behavior are not having much impact on this more severely uncontrollable child. It's often when these two factors converge, and parents perceive the continuing need to help their child more than other parents do, that they conclude something is wrong.

In many other cases, the child's problems are pointed out by school staff members. Parents often learn that their child is behaving differently and disruptively before reaching kindergarten from day care or preschool personnel. Sometimes, however, staff members don't say anything, so the parents, who may only suspect a problem, do not seek immediate assistance. It is in fact in the formal school setting, usually during the first year or two, that the vast majority of parents learn that their child has a behavior problem that needs attention. In the more demanding setting of the primary grades, a child who can't sit still or be quiet when appropriate, follow rules, and demonstrate age-appropriate self-regulation is impossible to overlook. In a small but significant minority of cases, the parents have not sought professional help for their child's ADHD or have not been advised to do so by the time the child has gone through several years of school. At some point these parents encounter media stories depicting children with ADHD, and this sparks the recognition that their own child may well have this disorder. Frequently parents call an ADHD clinic after seeing or hearing an expert on ADHD on a TV or radio program or reading an article, desperate for help now that they finally have an idea of what may be wrong with their child.

At whatever point in their child's life parents begin to suspect a problem in development, they are likely first to confide in friends or relatives. They may also make a trip to the library or bookstore to get the latest paperback on child development or use an Internet search engine like Google to see what they can learn on their own. Invariably, they begin to hear a lot of the folklore surrounding ADHD. This is especially true of information on the Internet where more than 4 million hits will be found just by Googling "ADHD," much of which is dated or biased information. They may try cutting back on the child's sugar intake, taking the child for allergy testing, exercising firmer discipline—all to no avail.

If they're lucky, they stumble across an informative, factual article on ADHD, on a website like *www.chadd.org, www.help4adhd.org, www.WebMD.com, or www.ADHDlectures.com,* or just happen to find an astute preschool or primary-grade teacher who recognizes the signs of ADHD. As a result, these parents seek the advice of their family physician, who may recognize the hallmark characteristics of the disorder and make a diagnosis of ADHD. More often, the physician suspects that the child may have ADHD and refers the child to other professionals in the community—child psychologists or psychiatrists, developmental pediatricians, or child neurologists—who may be more expert at the assessment and diagnosis of the disorder. The doctor may also suggest, for school-age children having significant behavioral problems at school as well as at home, that the parents apply for a school evaluation to determine whether the child should receive special educational assistance.

If you're beginning to suspect that your child has a problem that may be ADHD, don't ignore it in the hope that it will go away. Consider seeking a professional evaluation when any of the following conditions exist:

1. For at least 6 months the child has displayed activity, inattentiveness, and impulsiveness far greater than other children of the same age.
2. For at least a few months other parents have been telling you that your child has much poorer self-control or is far more active, impulsive, inattentive, and just poorly self-regulated when with other children than is normal.
3. Far more of your time and energy is required to manage and keep the child safe and out of trouble than other parents invest.

4. Other children do not like to play with your child and avoid the child because of excessively active, impulsive, emotional, or aggressive behavior.
5. A day care staff member or schoolteacher has informed you that your child has been having significant behavioral problems for several months.
6. You frequently lose your temper with this child; you feel as if you are on the verge of excessive physical discipline or might even harm the child; or you are greatly fatigued, exhausted, or even depressed as a consequence of managing and raising this child.

What Type of Professional Should You Call?

Generally, the professional to call is the one in your area who seems to know the most about ADHD. Whether you consult a pediatrician, child psychologist, child psychiatrist, child neurologist, social worker, school psychologist, family practitioner, or other mental health professional seems to matter less than finding someone who is familiar with the substantial scientific and professional literature on ADHD. Parents' support groups, such as CHADD or ADDA (see "Support Services for Parents" at the back of this book), can provide recommendations based on their experience in your region. If no local chapter exists, ask your child's teacher or physician for a referral to someone who has a solid reputation in the area for dealing with ADHD. Or if there is a university nearby, contact the psychology department to see who they may recommend; if it is a medical school, check with the psychiatry department seeking the same information. If you live in a major city of the United States, many have specialty clinics for ADHD affiliated with hospitals, universities, or medical schools, so check the Yellow Pages directory for one. In specific circumstances, however, you may need the services of a particular type of professional.

Physicians

Any child who is to be evaluated for ADHD should first have a standard pediatric checkup to rule out the rare medical causes of the symptoms. Epilepsy is relatively rare, even in children with ADHD, so you should not routinely seek out a neurological evaluation just because a child has ADHD. But if there are other indications that your child may be having medical problems such as seizures, you will want to call a pediatrician or child neurologist for an appointment. If it is already clear that seizures are occurring, you can take your child to a local emergency room for an evaluation.

Sometimes you might need to consult a physician after your child has already been diagnosed as having ADHD. If you've been working with only psychologists, social workers, and educators, you'll need to find a physician who knows ADHD and how to use medications with the disorder in cases where you're considering a trial of medication for your child (see Chapters 18 and 19). Not all pediatricians, child neurologists, and child psychiatrists are knowledgeable in this area, so your best bet may be to contact either a child psychiatrist who specializes in medications for children, a developmental and behavioral pediatrician, or a behavioral neurologist who knows about ADHD and specializes in developmental and behavioral problems. Then when you call for the appointment, ask the office staff whether the doctor sees a lot of children with ADHD or knows a lot about medications used with ADHD.

Psychologists and Other Therapists or Counselors

Psychologists are trained not only to evaluate psychological problems in children, but also to give psychological, learning, or neuropsychological tests that can help pinpoint the type of learning or behavior problem a child has. For this reason, the majority of parents seeking an evaluation of their child consult a licensed psychologist.

If you have already had your child evaluated and diagnosed properly but are seeking a particular kind of treatment, then of course you will want to seek out a professional specializing in that type of therapy. There are, to name just a few, cognitive-behavioral therapists, family counselors, psychotherapists, group therapists, and school counselors.

Before You Choose . . .

Again, just be sure that the person you contact knows something about ADHD and its treatment. Ask these questions of the office receptionist, the nurse, or the professional him- or herself:

- "Is the professional licensed?" (If necessary, contact the state licensing board to be sure.)
- "Does he or she see children with ADHD frequently?"
- "Is he or she well informed about the disorder and well trained in how to manage it?"
- "What types of treatment for ADHD does he or she routinely provide?" (If the answer does not include the ones you are after, try again elsewhere.)
- "Have any malpractice complaints been filed against the professional?"

Don't be embarrassed to ask such pointed questions. Find another professional if the one you ask is offended.

What about the Cost?

You'll want to get the very best professional help that suits your unique situation, but on a purely practical level you have to consider the expense. Take these steps to avoid unpleasant surprises:

1. When you're calling a professional's office for an appointment, ask what the cost is likely to be. Most professionals accept insurance payment, but a few do not, so be sure to inquire.

2. Then contact your insurance carrier to be sure that it will cover this type of evaluation. Most insurance companies classify an evaluation for ADHD as a mental health service and will limit how much they will pay for such services, usually to $500 or $1,000 per year. A rare few have no such limits, while other companies will not cover evaluations at all.

If your insurance carrier is one of the rare ones that tells you that it will not pay for your child to be evaluated and/or treated for ADHD, ask if it pays for evaluation or treatment of other mental disorders. Specifically ask if it covers the disorders listed in the fifth edition of the *Diagnostic and Statistical Manual of Mental Disorders,* known professionally as the DSM-5, published by the American Psychiatric Association. If it does but won't cover your child's evaluation, try giving this explanation (diplomatically, of course): Your carrier may not be aware that ADHD has been recognized for more than 10 years as a disability by the Americans with Disabilities Act (ADA); by the Individuals with Disabilities Education Act (IDEA), which governs the provision of special education services to children in public schools; by the Social Security Administration; and by the Office of Civil Rights (OCR), which administers the laws that protect the disabled against discrimination based on their disability. If the company is paying for services for other mental disorders but not for ADHD, this is discriminatory against disabled people. Is the company aware that this policy could be construed as discriminating against those with ADHD because of their disability? The IDEA and the ADA consider ADHD a disability and protect children with ADHD from discrimination because of it. Indicate that you may need to contact the OCR about filing a complaint of discrimination against the company because of its policy not to cover services for ADHD. The company may change its mind; it may not have been aware of these legal developments. If the company does not provide coverage thereafter, you may wish to file such a complaint with your local branch of the OCR.

3. If you're in a managed care program, such as a health maintenance organization (HMO), preferred provider organization (PPO), or other managed care plan, you may end up having to pay for a professional of your choice if you're not satisfied with the expertise available within your program. Usually you will have to see a professional within your plan first. Should you wish to go outside your plan, your plan will then decide whether it will cover part or all of such expenses. If not, you'll have to pay the uncovered portion or even the entire bill.

Personnel at Your Child's School

If your child has already entered school, your local school district can be one of your greatest sources of professional help. Either before you make an appointment with another professional or while waiting for one, ask your local school district to perform an educational evaluation. The IDEA requires your child's public school district to provide a free evaluation if the child's school performance is being affected significantly by ADHD or other behavior or learning problems. Ask your child's school or central school district offices about your child's rights under this law and the state law that has been created to implement the federal law. This evaluation will be done by several school professionals who have expertise in the areas in which your child is having problems. Usually a school psychologist, social worker, your child's teacher, and the school principal or a member of the school's office of special education will be part of the team to evaluate your child. Often teachers with special training in learning or behavior disorders will serve on this team as well. Sometimes even occupational, physical, or speech–language therapists may also join the team if the child is having problems within their own area of expertise.

"I want him in special education. He needs help at school. The school says he doesn't qualify for such services. Is that true? How can I get him the help he needs at school?"

If this evaluation seems like an extra step to you, understand that no public school is likely to give your child special education services without it. In fact, you might as well request a school evaluation *before* going to an outside professional because it can take up to 6–9 months to get this evaluation and so that the psychological testing of your child's intelligence, learning abilities, and other areas of psychological development are done by the school at no cost to you. If you've already had this evaluation done, be sure to send the report to the professional who is to see your child *ahead of the appointment date* so that this person can digest its contents before seeing your child.

If you're unhappy with the school evaluation or the recommendation based on it, be sure to tell the chairperson of the evaluating team to see if the problems can be corrected. If not, you may wish to appeal the team's decision to the local school superintendent. Your school office can tell you your rights of appeal and the process you will have to follow. You can also request a second opinion or evaluation from an outside professional. Some school districts (the minority) will pay for such second opinions; be sure to ask.

Parents I have met have reported a tremendous range and variety of experiences in getting their children with ADHD evaluated for educational assistance. Some report dealing with sensitive school personnel who initiated an evaluation within a month or two, treated the parents as equals and as valued members of the evaluation team, made sure the parents understood their findings, and implemented reasonable recommendations quickly. Others report quite a different experience. With school budget problems and limited educational staff, it's no surprise that parents have sometimes found evaluations completed 6 months after they were requested, so that the children get no help until the next school year. School staff members have been harried, insensitive, condescending, disrespectful, and/or unwilling to describe the procedures, findings, and recommendations from the evaluation in terms a parent can comprehend. Add to this the fact that some school districts in this country are still trying to deny that ADHD is a real problem for children and are continuing to refuse to take any responsibility for helping such children, and that some school staff members may be completely ignorant or out of date in their understanding of ADHD, and it is small wonder some parents feel compelled to bring lawsuits against their school districts for violating the rights of children with ADHD to a free, *appropriate* public education.

Helpful Hints for an Effective School Evaluation

What can you do to make the school evaluation process a more positive and constructive experience?

1. Ask the central office of your child's school district for literature describing the procedures the school must follow in initiating an evaluation of a child for special education. This literature will explain the federal and state laws that govern the evaluation process, the rights you and your child have, the timetable the school system must adhere to in conducting an evaluation, and the appeal process. Most school districts have prepared such literature; be sure to take advantage of it.

2. Read *ADD and the Law* and *Learning Disabilities and the Law* by attorneys Peter and Patricia Latham (see "Suggested Reading and Videos" at the end of this book) for more information on your child's rights within the school system (and in other areas, such as employment and insurance). If your son or daughter is in college, you will want to read Michael Gordon and Shelby Keiser's book *Accommodations in Higher Education under the Americans with Disabilities Act* (again, see "Suggested Reading and Videos").

3. Speak with your child's teachers about their concerns about your child's school performance and take notes. This will prepare you to give specific information to any school administrators who question the purpose and focus of the evaluation.

4. Once the evaluation has begun, monitor the school system's adherence to the required timetable. If it looks as if the school is going to miss a deadline, ask about it immediately. Do not agree to sign a waiver unless the school has a very good reason for missing a deadline.

5. Throughout the evaluation, be cooperative but also firm in your conviction that your child needs assistance. For example, if unfinished class work is being sent home, say you wish the practice to stop; if your child is not completing class work at

school, the problem is at school, and that is where the solution to the problem is to be found. Don't let the school shift the burden of correcting the problem to you.

6. Attend the team meeting convened to review the results of all of the different professional evaluations with recorder in hand. State up front that you will find it easier to absorb everything if you can focus on listening without having to take notes. Nevertheless, take a few written notes during the meeting as well—many parents find it helps them relax and buys them some time to think. Always ask for clarification of terms; it is the job of these professionals to communicate results effectively and clearly to you.

7. Pay particular attention to the team's recommendations: Do they square with your impressions of what kind of assistance your child may need? Be sure to ask about timelines for implementing these recommendations. What is the school recommending? When would it begin? Who is to implement the recommendations? How will progress during the intervention be monitored? Before the meeting adjourns, set a date to reconvene after the recommendations have been in effect for a few months to discuss how your child is responding to the treatment programs.

8. Always begin this evaluation process by being as courteous, cooperative, and diplomatic as possible. Even if you have reason to be somewhat hostile, starting the evaluation process by making demands, confronting or challenging school officials, and insulting personnel may very well slow the process down and get you labeled as a troublemaker—a reputation that can hurt your effectiveness with the school system and may even spill over to affect your child's treatment at school. Bring any concerns to the attention of school administrators by having a frank discussion in which you are diplomatic, open to discussion, yet firm in your convictions that your child may need help.

9. If you are unhappy with the evaluation process, seek a second opinion. Have a clinical professional outside the school system, who is experienced in evaluating children with ADHD and learning disabilities, attend the school team meeting with you when the results of the evaluation are discussed. Let this professional advocate for your child's needs. In many cases, school personnel seem more inclined to respect the opinions of another professional than those of a parent.

10. If you are not satisfied with the results of the evaluation, file an appeal with the school administration following the guidelines set forth in the literature provided by the school district.

Moving On

Armed with as much information as you can gather about your local resources, you can choose what you feel is the best course of action for evaluation of your child. The next chapter will tell you what to expect from an evaluation by a psychologist or a physician and how a diagnosis will be made.

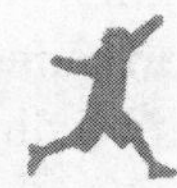

7 Preparing for the Evaluation

A thorough evaluation and an accurate diagnosis are the stepping-stones to successful management of your child's ADHD. Whether you are seeking a professional evaluation in place of or as a result of a school evaluation, try not to postpone taking action. Many professionals have long waiting lists, and you want to get in to see the appropriate person as soon as you can. While you're waiting for the appointment date, there's much you can do to ensure that the evaluation by a psychologist—as well as the medical checkup—answers all your concerns and serves your child's particular needs.

Preparing for a Psychological or Psychiatric Evaluation

Sit down and make up a list of answers to the following questions to help clarify your thoughts about your child's difficulties. Doing this task in advance can make the evaluation proceed more smoothly and quickly, perhaps even saving you money in the process. (Professionals usually charge by the hour or quarter hour for their time.)

1. What most concerns you now about your child? At the top of a sheet of paper, write headings such as "Home," "School," "Neighborhood," "Peers," and other areas where you see problems. Then, under each, list precisely what concerns you, sticking to the major problems that you feel occur more often or to a greater degree than they should for children at this age. Also write down those that concern you even if you're not sure they are deviant for your child's age, but note that fact next to each item of this sort. Save this list to take to your appointment.

2. On the back of that sheet of paper or on a new one, write down the headings "Health Problems," "Intelligence or Mental Development," "Motor Development and Coordination," "Problems with Senses," "Academic Learning Abilities," "Anxiety or Fears," "Depression," "Aggression toward Others," "Hyperactivity," "Poor

Attention," and "Antisocial Behavior." Then list anything that comes to mind that might indicate your child has a problem in these areas: chronic or recurring medical problems; problems with eyesight, hearing, and so forth; problems with reading, math, and so forth; lying, stealing, setting fires, or running away from home. You may already have listed some of these on the front of the paper, but it can help to reorganize them into these new categories for your child's professional evaluation.

3. Fill out the Home Situations Questionnaire, shown in Figure 1. Then, on another sheet of paper, list each situation for which you circled "Yes," and briefly write down what problem arises in that situation. For instance, if you said "Yes" to "When you are on the telephone," what does your child do at that time? Interrupt? Get into mischief out of your sight? Pick fights with siblings? Also jot down what you try to do to handle the situation. Make a photocopy of your completed questionnaire and take it and your descriptions of the problem situations to your appointment.

4. Understandably, parents sometimes hold back information that they find embarrassing to divulge to a stranger. Most often people are reticent about family problems that one or both parents believe are contributing to the child's problems: alcoholism or other substance abuse in the family, marital/couple conflict that spills over into mistreatment of the child, excessive discipline or physical punishment, or suspected sexual abuse, for example. No matter how difficult it is to talk about these problems, you must understand that withholding such information increases the possibility of mistakes in diagnosis, in the formulation of the important issues in the case, and in treatment planning. These matters have a direct bearing on a complete understanding of the case.

5. If at all possible, speak with or e-mail your child's teacher or teachers, and write down their major concerns about your child's school adjustment. Again, save this list to take to your appointment.

6. Now take one more sheet of paper and make a list of any problems you think are occurring in your family besides those concerning your child. Use the following headings if it will help: "Personal" (things that are troubling you about yourself), "Marital" or "Couple," "Money," "Relatives," "Job" (yours or your spouse's/partner's), "Other Children," and "Health" (yours or your spouse's/partner's). Take this list with you to your appointment.

These lists address the topics most likely to be covered in your interview with the professional. Keep them handy before your appointment and add items as you think of them. They should help to focus the evaluation quickly on the areas of greatest concern to you.

7. *Be sure to take along your child's baby book.* It will provide valuable information about the pregnancy and birth of your child, as well as the ages at which the child achieved important developmental milestones. If you don't have a baby book, write down any of the following information that you can recall: (a) any problems during

Home Situations Questionnaire

Child's name ______________________________ **Date** __________

Name of person completing this form ______________________________

Instructions: Does your child present any problems with compliance to instructions, commands, or rules for you in any of these situations? If so, please circle the word Yes and then circle a number beside that situation that describes how severe the problem is for you. If your child is not a problem in a situation, circle No and go on to the next situation on the form.

Situations	*Yes/No* (circle one)		*Mild*				*If Yes, how severe?* (circle one)				*Severe*
While playing alone	Yes	No	1	2	3	4	5	6	7	8	9
While playing with other children	Yes	No	1	2	3	4	5	6	7	8	9
At mealtimes	Yes	No	1	2	3	4	5	6	7	8	9
Getting dressed/undressed	Yes	No	1	2	3	4	5	6	7	8	9
Washing and bathing	Yes	No	1	2	3	4	5	6	7	8	9
While you are on the telephone	Yes	No	1	2	3	4	5	6	7	8	9
Watching television	Yes	No	1	2	3	4	5	6	7	8	9
When visitors are in your home	Yes	No	1	2	3	4	5	6	7	8	9
When you are visiting someone's home	Yes	No	1	2	3	4	5	6	7	8	9
In public places (restaurants, stores, church, etc.)	Yes	No	1	2	3	4	5	6	7	8	9
When father is home	Yes	No	1	2	3	4	5	6	7	8	9
When asked to do chores	Yes	No	1	2	3	4	5	6	7	8	9
When asked to do homework	Yes	No	1	2	3	4	5	6	7	8	9
At bedtime	Yes	No	1	2	3	4	5	6	7	8	9
While in the car	Yes	No	1	2	3	4	5	6	7	8	9
When with a babysitter	Yes	No	1	2	3	4	5	6	7	8	9

FIGURE 1. Questionnaire for identifying where compliance problems occur at home.

pregnancy with this child; (b) problems with the delivery; (c) your child's birth weight; (d) problems your child had shortly after birth; (e) any serious health, medical problems, or injuries your child has had since birth; and (f) any delays the child had in sitting, crawling, walking, learning to talk, or toilet training.

What to Expect

Probably the most important components of a comprehensive professional evaluation of a child with ADHD are these:

1. The clinical interview with the parents and child.
2. The medical examination (where necessary).
3. The scoring of behavior rating scales completed by the parents.
4. An interview with the child's teacher(s).
5. Completion of similar behavior rating scales about the child by the teacher(s).
6. Possibly IQ testing or testing of academic achievement skills, if this has not been performed by the school system.

Before any child can be diagnosed as having ADHD, a professional must collect a great deal of information about the child and family, sift through this information looking for the symptoms of ADHD, determine how serious the problem is likely to be, and rule out other disorders or problems. You can expect an evaluation to run an average of 2–3 hours—longer if your child also needs educational or psychological testing for learning or development problems.

When You Make the Appointment

When you call for an appointment, you'll be asked for basic information—your name and address, the child's sex and date of birth, child's school and grade placement, and so forth—and possibly your reasons for seeking an evaluation. You may also be asked to:

1. Give your permission for releases of information from previous evaluations.
2. Allow the professional to contact your child's treating physician for further information.
3. Provide the results of the most recent (if any) evaluation from your child's school.

4. Initiate a school evaluation, if this has not already been done.
5. Complete and return before your appointment a packet of behavior rating forms about your child.
6. Grant permission for your child's teacher(s) to complete similar forms.
7. Give permission for the professional to obtain information from any social service agencies working with your child.

You should agree to these requests in all cases, except possibly when you're seeking an unbiased second opinion because you strongly disagree with the first one obtained. In that case, you may want to ask the professional not to request the records from the first evaluation—and explain why—but never deny access to your child's teachers, even when you disagree with them. The information from teachers is too important to omit; just mention your disagreement beforehand.

In this initial phone meeting, beware of professionals who are willing to give specific treatment advice over the phone, who tell you that only they have the expertise to evaluate and treat your child, who ridicule other professionals in your community, who promise a cure, who tell you all they need for diagnosis is a hair or urine sample, and/or who will schedule an evaluation appointment that will take only a half hour or less. In all such cases, find another professional.

The Day of the Appointment

Several things will happen during your appointment: A psychologist will interview both you and your child and will perform tests if information is needed about the child's intelligence, language, academic skills, or other mental abilities. If a physician is conducting the evaluation, your child is not likely to receive any extensive psychological testing, and the interview with you may be much shorter (perhaps 30 minutes to an hour). Instead, your child may be given a more thorough physical exam and may be referred for a vision and hearing exam if one has not been done before or in the past few years.

The Interview with You

The interview with you is indispensable. Whenever possible, both parents should attend, since each has a unique perspective. If that's not feasible, the parent who can't be there can write down concerns and opinions that can be taken to the evaluation.

The interview with you serves several purposes: (1) It establishes a necessary rapport among you, the examiner, and your child. (2) It gives the professional your view of your child's apparent problems and narrows the focus of later stages of the evaluation. The more information you provide, the better appreciation the professional will have of your child's problems, the more quickly he or she can proceed, and the more accurate the diagnosis. Use the lists you have constructed so you don't forget anything you wanted to discuss. (3) It shows how the child's problems are affecting the family and gives the professional some sense of your own psychological integrity. (4) It can reveal information about your relationship with your child that could be important in pinpointing potential contributors to your child's problems. (5) But the most important purpose is to determine a diagnosis of your child's problem(s) and to provide you with reasonable treatment recommendations.

The examiner will take notes throughout the interview, including observations of you and how you are dealing with your child while at the clinic. A wise professional will know, however, that behavior in the office, particularly your child's behavior, is not likely to mirror typical behavior elsewhere. Research has shown that many children with ADHD behave normally during this evaluation. If this happens, don't accept any statement that it means your child is normal.

"The pediatrician says my daughter doesn't have ADHD. The day we took her for an appointment, the doctor spent 20 minutes examining her, and she behaved just fine. Why do you say she has ADHD when our doctor says she doesn't? Why do you disagree?"

Some professionals like to have the child present during the parental interview. This is fine as long as the subject of discussion will not upset your child or make you uncomfortable. Be sure to state your feelings on this matter. I typically prefer children of school age to stay in the waiting room while interviewing the parent(s) separately.

The interview should begin with an explanation of the procedures to be undertaken, the time it is expected to take, the estimated cost and manner of payment if not already discussed, and the fact that most of what you say will be confidential (many states' laws require professionals to report child neglect or abuse to the department of social services).

Information about Your Child

The interview will probably proceed to a discussion of your concerns about your child. Here is where your notes are helpful. The professional will ask for specific examples of behavior that concerns you, such as examples of your child's impulsive or inattentive behavior. You may also be asked how you are presently trying to manage your child's behavior problems and whether your spouse/partner is using a different approach. You will surely be asked when you first noticed your child's problems. This naturally leads to questions about any professional assistance you have already obtained. Some examiners like to ask parents what they believe has led their child to develop these problems. Feel free to give your opinion, but also don't hesitate to say you don't know.

If you completed behavior rating forms before the appointment and returned them, the professional may want to review some of your answers now, especially any that were unclear. Similarly, *you* may want to ask if the professional has any questions about your answers. You may also be asked about some answers on the forms that were sent to your child's teacher(s). If you are curious, ask to see a teacher's answers on these forms; it is your right to see them. Ask the professional to explain anything on these forms that is confusing to you.

The examiner will also talk with you about any developmental problems your child has. I customarily ask parents about the child's development so far in physical health, sensory and motor abilities, language, thinking, intellect, academic achievement, self-help skills like dressing and bathing, social behavior, emotional problems, and family relationships. Many professionals will also review with you a variety of behavior problems or symptoms of other psychiatric problems to see if your child also may be having these difficulties. Simply be truthful and indicate whether or not these other symptoms are present and to what degree.

The examiner may ask you about the symptoms of ADHD that were discussed in Chapter 1. If not, politely ask if the examiner typically uses the DSM-5 guidelines for diagnosing ADHD. Most professionals now use them. Ask the professional to review them with you, just to be sure all the criteria have been covered. I think a professional should also take care to ask you about any strengths and interests your child has. If yours does not, then mention some yourself. This information not only provides a more complete and balanced picture of your child, but gives helpful information to be used later in treatment.

At some point in the interview, the professional should conduct a careful review of your child's developmental, medical, and school histories. I always ask parents about their relationship with school staff. Knowing whether it's friendly, supportive, or filled with conflict, and whether communication has been open and reasonably clear or limited and hostile, greatly helps me in preparing for later contacts with the school staff if needed.

Information about You and Your Family

Professionals know that many families of children with ADHD are under more stress than other families and that the parents may be having more personal problems than most. Don't be offended if you're asked such personal questions. This information can be of great assistance in understanding your child's problems and developing more useful treatment recommendations for you. You will probably be asked about your own background, education, and occupation, as well as those of your spouse/partner. The examiner may ask if you, your spouse/partner, or your other children have had any psychiatric, learning, developmental, or chronic medical problems.

Before the interview is over, take a minute to review your notes. Share anything not yet covered or any other information you feel might be helpful. The vast majority of professionals will respect and appreciate your candor.

The Interview with Your Child

The professional will interview your child during the appointment, usually separately from you if your child is of school age, and make some informal observations of your child's appearance, behavior, and developmental skills. How much time he or she devotes to this interview will depend on your child's age and intelligence. Again, neither you nor the professional should place too much importance on the information obtained in this interview, since so many children behave atypically in a professional's office and most children with ADHD have only a very limited awareness of their own problems.

Mental health professionals usually ask children a lot of general questions dealing with these areas:

- Their awareness of why they are visiting a professional today—their own feelings and what their parents have told them.
- Their favorite hobbies, TV shows, sports, or pets, to create rapport.
- Where they go to school, who their teachers are, what subjects they take and like most, and the reasons for any specific difficulties.
- Whether they see themselves as having any behavior problems in the classroom and what types of discipline they get for misconduct.
- How they think they are accepted by other children at school.
- Their perceptions of any problems the parents have reported.
- What they would like to see changed or improved at home or at school.
- Whether they see themselves as having the symptoms of ADHD (as included in the DSM-5 criteria and/or in general terms).

Particularly with young children, some examiners find it helpful to let them play, draw, or simply wander about the office during the interview. Others may ask children to fill in the blanks in a series of incomplete sentences.

The Interview with the Teacher(s)

Few adults spend as much time with your child as a teacher does, so a teacher's opinions are a critical part of the evaluation. If the child has more than one teacher, at least the ones with whom the child spends the most time should be interviewed.

In person, by telephone, or these days even by e-mail, the professional will ask the teacher(s) about your child's current academic and behavioral problems, relationships with classmates, and behavior in various school situations (especially those involving work, as well as those with limited or no supervision, such as recess, lunch, in hallways, or on the bus). The professional should also find out what the teacher or teachers are currently doing to manage your child's problems and should go over any school evaluation done.

The Medical Examination

It is essential that children being evaluated for ADHD have a complete pediatric physical examination. Usually this has been done as part of annual school or summer camp physicals, but it may have to be repeated with more careful attention to medical problems that could be contributing to your child's current behavioral and school difficulties.

The Interview

The medical interview about your child will be similar to the psychologist's interview with you. However, the doctor will devote more time to reviewing the child's genetic background; pregnancy and birth events; developmental and medical history; and current health, nutritional status, and gross sensory–motor development.

The main distinction, however, is the attempt to distinguish ADHD from other possible medical conditions, particularly those that may be treatable. In rare cases, ADHD develops as a result of a clear medical problem, such as severe Reye syndrome, a near-drowning or severe smoke inhalation, serious head trauma, or recovery from a brain infection or disease. In other unusual cases, the ADHD may be associated with a high lead level in your child's body or with other metal or toxic poisonings. Any of these may require treatment in their own right separate from the ADHD. If your doctor strongly suspects that your child has a seizure disorder, additional tests such as an EEG or brain scan may be ordered for your child.

Besides searching for possible causes, the doctor will thoroughly evaluate any coexisting conditions that may require medical management, especially problems such as poor motor coordination, bed-wetting, soiling, and middle ear infections, for which children with ADHD are at higher risk. The doctor will also determine whether your child has any physical conditions that would contraindicate the use of medications to treat ADHD.

The physician's written recommendation will normally be required to document any need for physical or occupational therapy at school. For this and other reasons, the role of your child's physician in the evaluation of ADHD should not be underestimated. However, by itself it is usually inadequate to make a diagnosis of ADHD.

The Physical Exam

In the course of the child's physical examination, the doctor will follow up on any findings from the interview, looking for thyroid problems, lead poisoning, anemia, or other illnesses. The doctor may also do a brief neurological exam to screen for relatively gross neurological problems. Your child's height, weight, and head circumference will be measured and compared to standard charts for normal children. Hearing, vision, and blood pressure will also be screened.

Don't be surprised if your child's routine physical exam, height and weight, and routine neurological exam are all normal. Also, abnormalities in these areas are not necessarily signs of ADHD; the goal is to rule out the rare case of visual, hearing, or other deficits giving rise to some of the symptoms that may look like ADHD.

Laboratory Tests

Misled by research reports that lab measures have found differences between children with and without ADHD and by the fact that ADHD is a biologically based disorder, many parents ask for medical tests to confirm the diagnosis of ADHD. At present, there are no lab tests or measures that are of value in making a diagnosis of ADHD, so blood work, a urinalysis, chromosome studies, EEGs, averaged evoked responses, MRIs, computed tomography (CT) scans, SPECT scans (blood flow studies), or PET scans should not be used routinely in the evaluation of children with ADHD.

Certain limited tests may be required if your child is going to take a particular medication (see Chapter 19) but not the more common ones, such as Ritalin, Focalin, or Concerta (methylphenidate), Dexedrine (*d*-amphetamine), Adderall or Vyvanse (a combination of amphetamines), Strattera (atomoxetine), or Intuniv (guanfacine XR).

The Final Step: Making a Diagnosis

During the evaluation, the professional you have chosen has collected a wealth of information about your child and your family. The professional has probably already made a *differential diagnosis*—a preliminary step employing DSM-5 guidelines to differentiate what disorders your child may have from those your child does not seem to have. Now, using the behavior rating scales filled out before or during the appointment, as well as everything culled from the interviews and observations, the professional will make the best possible educated guess about which disorder(s) your child has. A diagnosis of ADHD most likely will be based at least in part on the DSM-5 criteria, but diagnosing psychiatric disorders in children is far from an exact science. The absence of entirely objective evaluating methods, and the reliance on the observations and opinions of parents and others, can introduce some uncertainty into the diagnostic process.

You should know that toward the end of 2011 the American Academy of Pediatrics issued guidelines that pediatricians are urged to follow in the evaluation of children for ADHD (*Pediatrics,* 2011, Vol. 128, No. 5, pp. 1007–1022). These guidelines are very consistent with the steps recommended earlier in this chapter for the proper evaluation of children for ADHD. The guidelines include strongly encouraging pediatricians to use the latest diagnostic criteria from DSM-5 and to obtain information directly from parents and teachers about the child's behavior and adjustment at home and school. The guidelines also suggest that the physician consider the use of well-developed behavior rating scales to be completed by parents and teachers. Noteworthy is that these guidelines also do not encourage the use of any medical, neurological, or laboratory-type tests as part of this diagnostic evaluation, since those tests are not validated for such use. If the evaluation of your child begins with your child's pediatrician, be aware that these guidelines now exist and, if necessary, make the pediatrician aware of them as well.

During the evaluation, the professional has also been formulating possible treatment recommendations, which will be presented to you along with the diagnosis. You and the professional together must then discuss which of these you will agree to have implemented. As an executive parent, you view the professional as your consultant. As a scientific parent, you weigh the information received against your own sense of your child and the other information you have gathered about ADHD, determine whether the conclusions and recommendations make sense, and then ask questions about anything that confuses or concerns you. Be sure to ask the professional to define any diagnosis rendered, because what the professional calls ADHD or ADD may not coincide with the way I am using those terms in this book (see the sidebar on pp. 150–151). If you're left with much doubt about the diagnosis, thank the professional and seek a second opinion.

As a principle-centered parent, you will go about the entire evaluation process with dignity and diplomacy, guided by Dr. Covey's seven principles (summarized in the Introduction) not only with your child but in your interactions with others.

Two Types of Attention Disorders Now Recognized by Clinical Scientists

Some children may have only problems with being inattentive and are not impulsive or hyperactive. Previously, they might have been diagnosed as ADHD–predominantly inattentive type based on the earlier version of the DSM, known as DSM-IV. However, many of these children actually appear to have a different attention disorder from that seen in ADHD. They are more often described as being more daydreamy or "spacey" than others, acting as if they are often in a mental "fog," staring more than others, seeming to be sleepy, and not very attentive to what is happening around them. Parents of these children tell us that these children are not only not hyperactive but are actually lethargic, sluggish, or slow-moving compared to other children. These children seem to wander through their daily lives only half-attending to events around them, acting like little absent-minded professors. As a result, they often miss a lot of the information in situations that other children are attending to, and so seem "out of it." They make more mistakes than other children in following oral or written instructions—but not because they go headlong or headstrong into their work and make impulsive mistakes, as children with ADHD do. Children with this type of inattention seem to have a problem with sifting through the information given in instructions and quickly identifying the important parts; their mental filter seems less able to sort out the relevant from the irrelevant. Unlike children with ADHD, they are likely to be quiet while working, yet mentally they are "not all there"—not fully processing the task and its instructions. Clinical scientists have named this condition *sluggish cognitive tempo* (SCT).

Research finds that children with this form of inattention differ from those with ADHD in having considerably fewer problems with defiance, aggression, impulsivity, and overactivity at home and school. These children also have a lot less trouble in their relationships with other children; if anything, they tend to be withdrawn, reticent, or even shy or socially anxious. On psychological tests, they have been found to perform much worse on tests involving perceptual–motor speed or hand–eye coordination and speed.

They also make more mistakes on a memory retrieval test. In particular, they have more trouble consistently recalling information they had learned as time passed. These problems were not seen in the children with ADHD. Other studies, including my own recently published large-scale study of both ADHD and SCT in U.S. children done in 2012, have found that they are also more likely to be diagnosed with depression or to have more anxiety symptoms than are typical children or even those with the more common combined type of ADHD. This large study also found that boys and girls did not differ in the prevalence of this disorder as they do with ADHD (boys are three times more likely to have ADHD). We also found that SCT symptoms developed somewhat later in childhood than

ADHD symptoms and did not decline with age. Both groups did equally poorly at school, but the children with SCT seem to have more trouble with the accuracy of their work, while those with ADHD have more problems with the quantity of work they do (productivity). Both groups were more prone to have learning disabilities but may differ in the pattern, with children with SCT possibly having a greater risk for math disorders. I also noted that SCT and ADHD could coexist in 35–49% of cases of the other disorder. When this occurred, the children were far more impaired and carried a far greater risk for other psychiatric and learning disorders than did children with either disorder alone. Research by Dr. José J. Bauermeister and colleagues at the University of Puerto Rico indicates that children with ADHD are far more demanding and stressful to raise than are children with SCT, and so create much more family conflict than in the families of children who have this other attention disorder.

Unfortunately, at present far less is known about treating SCT than about treating ADHD. The little research done has studied the stimulant medication methylphenidate (Ritalin) and shown that most children with SCT don't respond as well or as dramatically as those with ADHD. Where they did respond, it was to a lower dose, whereas moderate or higher doses appear to be more effective with ADHD. More telling was the finding that 30% or more of those with this type of inattention did not respond at all to stimulants, compared to fewer than 10% of those with ADHD. Children with ADHD also demonstrated a much greater therapeutic response to the medications than did those with this form of inattention. Children with SCT, in contrast, may be more responsive to behavior modification programs and social skills training programs than are children with ADHD.

There is still much research to be done on what types of psychological, educational, and medical treatments may be most useful for SCT. Don't expect most professionals to have heard of this second attention disorder unless they keep up with journal publications on ADHD. Also SCT is not listed in DSM-5 and so is not an officially recognized diagnosis as yet. It may be called ADHD with inattentive presentation, but that is not definite nor is SCT a type of ADHD. Much of what is written in this book does not apply to children with SCT, especially the theory of executive functioning and ADHD discussed in Chapter 2. SCT is far less likely to be associated with most of the problems with self-regulation and executive functioning seen in ADHD. Where there is some association, it is mainly with problems with self-organization and problem solving but not with time management, self-restraint, or emotional self-control.

8 Coping with the Diagnosis of ADHD

How You Are Likely to React

Having your child evaluated was a big step, and you invested your mental, physical, and emotional energies into doing it right. Now you've received a diagnosis: your child has ADHD. What next?

First, stop and try to acknowledge how you feel. From the several thousand parents I have counseled personally about ADHD, as well as the thousands of others I have heard from at my public speeches, I have come to realize that parents' emotional reactions to information about ADHD are an important part of their adjustment to their child's disorder. They also influence the quality of the investment they are able to make in helping and advocating for their child.

Denial or Relief?

Some parents may initially engage in *denial* of the label or diagnosis or the largely neurological basis of it. They hold desperately to their original view that nothing is so wrong that it cannot be righted by some diet, form of counseling, or simple behavior management methods. This reaction is likely to occur when the parents did not suspect that much was wrong with their child in the first place. Typically it is a day care worker, a preschool teacher, or even the parent of a playmate who broaches the possibility that a problem exists. When parents are the last to know that their child has ADHD, it is natural for them to deny or minimize the extent of the problem until they can reevaluate the information they are receiving and come to see the problems of their child on their own. If you find yourself resisting a diagnosis, the best way to erase your doubts is to seek a second opinion from someone you trust who knows about ADHD.

Other parents willingly accept the information they receive about ADHD, embracing its message as the answers they have desperately sought for so long. Finally they have a name for their concerns about their child and can pursue ways to help. These families welcome *relief* from the burden of uncertainty—and often of guilt as well. Knowing that ADHD has a biological basis allows them to let go of the previous sense that they personally created the problem.

Anger

For some parents a diagnosis of ADHD evokes *anger*—anger aimed at anyone who may have previously assured them that nothing was wrong; anger at those who blamed the problem on the parents' child-rearing methods or on family problems. All too often, practitioners in my field, relatives, and the media chastise, shame, or otherwise "bash" parents in their quest to lay blame for the disorder. When the parents finally realize they are not at fault, anger and resentment are not unreasonable reactions.

Grief

It is both natural and healthy to have a mild *grief* reaction to the information about your child's ADHD. Almost all parents, when confronted with the news that their child is disabled in some way, will grieve for this loss of normalcy. Some parents grieve over their child's future risks; others are reacting to the alterations the family must make to accommodate ADHD.

For most people, this grieving will pass as they reframe their views of their child and his problems. I have been told by others, however, that they never fully resolve this grief. They adapt to it and for a time seem to put it behind them as they confront the day-to-day responsibilities of child rearing and work. But when the child has been doing particularly well for a long period and then has a regression or a significant crisis, the feelings of mild sorrow return. This may happen to you as well. If so, talking with other parents who have children with ADHD can help, perhaps through your local parent support group or supportive Internet chat rooms or blogs. If the grief reaction persists, consider undertaking some short-term counseling with a professional who is knowledgeable about ADHD or therapy with parents of children with disabilities.

Acceptance

The natural and desired outcome of dealing with information on ADHD is *acceptance*—acceptance of what your child is and may become and, equally important, what your child is not and may never be. There is peace of mind at this stage, as if a cloud has been lifted, allowing the parents to see their child's problems and their own reactions to these problems more realistically. From this new perspective you can more clearly see that your child has a problem that she did not ask for, cannot help having, and needs your help in dealing with, including protection from those who will not understand. The child needs your advocacy to obtain her legal entitlements among the community and school services. This change in perspective can be profound and moving, both to the parents experiencing it and to anyone who has the privilege to witness it as I have.

If you've reached this stage, you may now thirst for knowledge about how best to help your child. Perhaps you are now motivated to enter a support group, counseling, or a formal child management training program that provides you with the skills and techniques that may help your child succeed. You will also find yourself seeking ways to modify the environment, not the child. For your child, an appropriate "prosthetic device" may be an organizing chart or a home point system instead of a wheelchair; access may mean a special seating arrangement rather than a ramp to a doorway. In both cases, the goal is to permit the child to succeed, given the circumstances.

Acceptance also means, however, recognizing that some things simply cannot be modified to permit children with ADHD to succeed maximally or adapt as well as do children without ADHD. Failure to accept some limitations for your child will instill intolerance, anger, and frustration in you, as well as put undue pressure on the child.

The bottom line is that your acceptance of your child's ADHD and all it may entail frees you to fulfill the role so crucial to your child's progress. More than other parents, you must actively support your child's self-esteem, perhaps via less traditional routes, whereas children without ADHD build their own paths through academic and social success. You need to exercise creativity to find successful outlets for your child, whether in organized sports, fine arts, hobbies, science, mechanical projects, or even nontraditional pursuits. Once you've truly accepted your child's ADHD, you can look beyond the child's limitations and see—as no one else can—his unique strengths and talents.

Understanding Treatment Options

As will become clear from Parts II–IV of this book, most children with ADHD are going to require a combination of behavioral (psychological), educational, and medication treatments to achieve the best results. Undoubtedly there exists a minority of cases in which the medications alone may be enough, but my own experience and that of many other career clinical scientists studying ADHD is that this will not be true for most. Some children simply do not respond to medications. And even among those who do respond, slightly less than half are not entirely normalized in their behavior or school performance or peer relationships when on their medication. And even in some cases where they may be normalized, the stimulant medications often cannot be used in the evenings with many children. So at these and other times, they are going to require some other forms of treatment to help in those situations. Furthermore, as explained in Chapter 4, many children with ADHD are likely to have additional psychological and learning disorders besides ADHD. Those additional disorders are not going to be addressed properly by the medications used for ADHD. Learning disabilities will not go away with medication treatment, nor will some of the social skills problems with the peer group, certain kinds of defiant and antisocial behaviors if they are present, or family conflicts if they are due to factors other than just the child's ADHD. Thus, for most children with ADHD, a treatment package of multiple interventions is likely to be the most useful.

Interestingly, however, the largest treatment study for ADHD done to date, called the Multimodal Treatment Study of ADHD (sponsored by NIMH), indicated that medication may be the most effective treatment option for children with ADHD. The study involved more than 570 children from five different sites across the United States and some sites in Canada. These children were given careful and thorough evaluations and then were randomly assigned to four different treatment groups: one receiving community referrals and then left to follow up on their own treatment; one receiving medication alone but very well managed; one receiving a substantial package of various psychosocial treatments but no medication; and one receiving both medication and psychosocial treatments. What this massive study initially found after 14 months of treatment is that medication, in proper dosages and with good monitoring, produces powerful effects on the symptoms and problems associated with ADHD. More than half of the medication-only cases were considered treatment successes or normalized, while this was true for only about a third of the psychosocial-treatment-only cases. Combining medication with a comprehensive psychosocial treatment package produced slightly more treatment responders (about 10–15% more), as well as some additional benefits for different subsets of children. The combination may also result in less need for medication or the need for a lower dose of medication. Psychosocial treatments alone can be effective but may not produce equivalent results to those achieved by medication. The study suggests that combined treatment is best.

Getting Educated about ADHD

It's fortunate that acceptance leads to a thirst for knowledge, because staying educated is the most fundamental ongoing task of the executive, scientific parent. In the thousands of cases of ADHD seen at the ADHD clinics at which I have worked over my 35 years of clinical practice, we have in fact learned that the single most important intervention we have provided is up-to-date information about the disorder. Here are a number of things you can do to get and stay educated about ADHD and the latest advances in treating it:

1. Read as many books about ADHD as you can. Some of the best, in my view, are listed at the end of this book ("Suggested Reading and Videos"). Remember, truth

is an assembled thing. The more you read and learn about ADHD, the closer to the truth about its nature, causes, and proper treatment you will come. You can obtain many of these books by ordering them through your local bookstore. The majority are also available through the ADD Warehouse (see "Suppliers" section in "Suggested Reading and Videos"). Or go to your local library, keeping in mind that smaller libraries rarely have current books. If a book was copyrighted more than 10 years ago, you should assume the information is not current enough. For current scientific articles and professional books on ADHD, check a local university library or medical center library. Look up the names of researchers mentioned in this book for reports on the latest scientific studies. Some school professionals or districts have also developed lending libraries on materials for parents; ask if your school district has anything on ADHD, ADD, or hyperactivity.

2. If like many people you have Internet access, then read the information at the websites *www.help4adhd.org* or *www.chadd.org* (Children and Adults with Attention-Deficit/Hyperactivity Disorder) in the United States and *www.caddac.ca* (Centre for ADHD Awareness, Canada) in Canada. There is also some useful information at websites of professional associations, such as *www.aacap.org* (American Academy of Child and Adolescent Psychiatry) and *www.aap.org* (American Academy of Pediatrics). These websites are explained in more detail at the end of this book under "Support Services for Parents." Be cautious in visiting other websites or just entering "ADHD" or "ADD" into your search engine, like Google, as you will get millions of hits and not know where to begin. There is a lot of misinformation on and outright propaganda against ADHD on the Internet, so approach it as if you were strolling through a Turkish bazaar with many websites simply trying to get your attention (and your money); consumer beware.

3. Watch commercially made videos on this subject. Some are listed at the end of the book, including seven of my own (available from The Guilford Press or the ADD Warehouse), but if the expense is prohibitive, see if your local school district has any you can borrow. Also check libraries and video rental stores, some of which are now setting aside shelf space for health, self-improvement, and psychology video programs. You can also find some useful videos, including a few of my own, on the Internet using the YouTube website, but again, be wary and even skeptical, as much of the information here is either just personal opinion or bias, or outright misrepresentation. Some videos of presentations by experts can also be found at the *www.caddac.ca* website noted above. I also have a website containing 10+ hours of presentations for parents and 25+ hours for professionals at *www.adhdlectures.com.*

4. Make an appointment with a local professional expert on the subject to get opinions and any educational materials available for loan. Be prepared to pay for the time he or she spends with you, or to have this billed to your health insurance program as a therapy session.

5. You can also join a local parent support group, such as CHADD or ADDA (see

"Support Services for Parents" at the end of this book), both of which publish informative newsletters and feature expert guest speakers at their frequent meetings. Your local group may also receive brochures and notices on one-day seminars and workshops held in your area. Although such workshops are often aimed at professional audiences, parents may be permitted to attend. Ask any professional you're working with to let you know about these events too.

6. The national arms of these parent support associations are also great resources. Both CHADD and ADDA hold 2- to 4-day annual conventions, where you can hear numerous speakers on most aspects of raising a child with ADHD. Call the national organizations to find out when and where such conferences are held. It can be tremendously inspiring and reassuring to attend a 3-day conference with hundreds of other parents of children with ADHD, all striving to learn more about caring for and raising these children.

Throughout this process of self-education, remember that your child is struggling with a developmental disorder and that you're undertaking this somewhat monumental task to help the child surmount as many of the problems this disability poses as you can. Bolstered by the empathy that naturally flows from acceptance, and armed with all the knowledge you can amass, you are prepared to help your child as no one else can. The next chapter will give you some fundamental principles to follow in that endeavor.

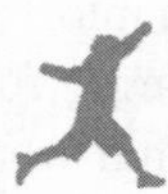

9 Fourteen Guiding Principles for Raising a Child with ADHD

Part I (Chapters 1–5) explained that ADHD is a developmental disorder of self-control—or what some professionals call the *executive functions* critical to planning, organizing, and carrying out complex human behavior over long periods of time. That is, in a child with ADHD, the "executive" in the brain that is supposed to be organizing and controlling behavior, helping the child plan for the future and follow through on those plans, is doing a very poor job. The child is not suffering from a lack of skill or knowledge in many cases, so showing the child how to do something to correct her problems will not be of much help. Instead you will find it more effective to combine such teaching or skills or knowledge with the following: give clear instructions, rearrange the work so it's more interesting and motivating, break it down into shorter quotas with frequent short breaks, rearrange the setting to be less distracting and to help focus the child's attention on what is important to do in that situation, redirect the child's behavior toward future goals versus immediate gratification, and provide immediate rewards for a completed task or adherence to rules. In short, we want to help children with ADHD "show what they know" in situations that were previously a problem for them.

Sound simple? It *is* relatively simple—in theory. In practice it's not always easy to implement. Over 35 years of clinical experience and teaching, I've found that parents benefit greatly from 14 general principles distilled from our current understanding of ADHD. As touchstones in the daily behavior management of children with ADHD, these principles have served parents well in designing both home and classroom management programs for these children. Brief illustrations of some of the principles are given here; specific techniques are detailed in Chapter 11.

Remember that principle-centered parenting of a child with ADHD means (1) pausing before reacting to the present misconduct of the child, (2) using this delay to reflect on the principles contained in this book, and (3) choosing a response to the child that is consistent with these principles. To keep you grounded in this approach to rearing your child, I suggest you photocopy the list of principles provided at the end of this chapter (p. 168) and tape it to both your bathroom mirror and your refrigerator door. You can also put a copy on a wall in your workspace if you work outside the home. Glancing at these 14 guiding principles when you wake up, and seeing them throughout the day, will give you a gentle reminder of what type of parent you are striving to be with your child with ADHD.

1. Give Your Child More Immediate Feedback and Consequences

As Dr. Virginia Douglas, a renowned Canadian psychologist and expert on ADHD, and others noted long ago, children with ADHD seem much more under the control of the moment than normal children do. Either you become part of that moment, or you will have little influence over your child with ADHD.

As already explained, when confronted by a job that they find tedious, boring, or unrewarding, children with ADHD will feel the urge to find something else to do. If you want them to stay at a task, you'll have to arrange for positive feedback and consequences that occur throughout the task that will make the task more rewarding, as well as mild negative consequences for shifting off-task. Similarly, when you're attempting to change negative behaviors, you must provide quick rewards and feedback for behaving well and swift negative consequences for acting inappropriately.

Positive feedback can be given in the form of praise or compliments, as long as you state expressly and specifically what the child did that was positive. But don't expect that to always be enough. You can also use forms of physical affection, but don't overdo it as children may see this as being insincere. In many instances you will have to use rewards such as extra privileges, or systems by which the child earns tokens or points toward privileges, because your praise will not be enough to motivate the child to stick with the assigned task. Whatever type of feedback you give, however, the more immediately it can be provided, the more effective it will be at changing future behavior.

For example, if a child with ADHD normally has problems playing nicely with a younger sibling, the most effective reinforcement of cooperative play would be for you to be on the alert for any instances of cooperation, sharing, and kindness shown by the child with ADHD and then give immediate praise (and tokens) when you spot it. Likewise, the child should receive immediate and mildly negative feedback and consequences after bullying the younger child. You tell the child exactly what he has just done wrong (rather than yelling) and why it is not acceptable; then you remove a privilege the child had access to that day, or some earned tokens in a token program (see Chapter 11).

2. Give Your Child More Frequent Feedback

Children with ADHD need feedback and consequences that are not just swift but also frequent. Immediate consequences or feedback can be helpful even when given occasionally, but they are more beneficial when given often. Admittedly, going too far with this can get irritating and intrusive to your child and tiring for you, but it is necessary to do this as much as your time, schedule, and energy permit—especially when you're trying to change some form of significant misbehavior. For instance, rather than waiting to praise a child who has considerable trouble finishing homework when all of the homework is finally done, or punishing the child for not finishing after several hours when it should have taken 20 minutes, instruct the child that she can now earn points for completing each math problem, with the points adding up toward purchasing a privilege. A reasonable time limit—say, 20 minutes—is also set for the whole assignment, and when the time expires the child is fined (loses) one point for each problem not done. During the work period you praise the child frequently for remaining on-task and provide words of encouragement to keep working hard at the same time you're tallying points.

Often parents get very busy with their own household responsibilities and forget to check frequently on the child. One way to remind yourself is to place small stickers with smiley faces on them around the house in locations where you frequently look—in the corner of bathroom mirrors, on the edge of the face of a kitchen clock, and so on. Whenever you spot a sticker, comment to your child on what you like that the child is doing at that very moment—even if it's just sitting quietly watching TV. You can also set a cooking timer or watch for various brief intervals or use the device called a MotivAider, which is worn on a belt or in a pocket and vibrates at the programmed intervals. This device is available on the Internet (enter the name in your search engine) or from the ADD Warehouse (see "Suppliers" section in "Suggested Reading and Videos" at the end of the book).

3. Use Larger and More Powerful Consequences

Your child with ADHD will require more salient or powerful consequences than other children to encourage him to perform work, follow rules, or behave well. These can include physical affection, privileges, special snacks or treats, tokens or points, material rewards like small toys or collectible items, and even occasionally money.

This may seem to violate the common wisdom that children should not be materially rewarded too often because such rewards may replace intrinsic rewards such as the pleasure of reading, the desire to please parents and friends, the pride of mastering a job or new activity, or the esteem of peers for playing a game well. But these forms of reinforcement or reward are much less likely to influence children with ADHD to behave well. They also do not consistently motivate these children to start working, to inhibit their urges to do inappropriate things, and to persist in their work. The disorder may also be associated with a biologically based deficit in the capacity for self-motivation, one of the executive functions, which requires parents to augment their praise or these other social or symbolic rewards with more powerful consequences than are needed for other children to sustain persistence toward a task. The nature of your child's disability dictates that you will likely have to use larger, more significant, and sometimes more material consequences to develop and maintain your child's positive behaviors.

4. Use Incentives before Punishment

It is common for parents to resort to punishment when a child misbehaves or disobeys. This may be all right for a child without ADHD, who misbehaves only occasionally and thus receives a small amount of punishment. It is not all right for a child with ADHD, who is likely to misbehave much more often and could receive a great deal of negative consequences. Research shows that children with ADHD are all ready being punished substantially more often than typical children and so starting your behavior-change plan with even more punishment is unlikely to work. Punishment, when used alone or in the relative absence of ongoing rewards and positive feedback, is not very effective at changing behavior. It usually leads to resentment and hostility in your child, and eventually to the child's avoidance of you. Sometimes it can even lead to efforts at what psychologists call *countercontrol:* your child tries to find ways to strike back, retaliate, or get even with you for the excessive punishment.

It is critical that you avoid this all-too-common drift toward using punishment first. Frequently remind yourself of this rule: *Positives before negatives*. It might help to remember that your child receives more than enough reprimands, punishments, and rejection from others who do not understand the child's disability. Do they really need just more of the same from you to improve her behavior? Not likely. Starting your plan with rewards and incentives is more likely to teach what you expect your child to do rather than just what not to do.

The rule of using positives before negatives is simple: when you want to change an undesirable behavior, first decide what positive behavior you want to replace it with. This will instinctively lead you to start watching for that positive behavior or teaching it if you think your child is unclear about what you expect. When that behavior occurs, you will be more likely to praise and reward it.

Only after this new behavior has been rewarded consistently for at least a few days to a week should you begin punishing the undesired opposite behavior. Even then, try to use only mild punishment such as the loss of a privilege or special activity or a brief time-out, and keep the punishments in balance with the rewards: only one punishment for every two or three instances of praise and reward. Punish consistently but selectively, only for the occurrence of this particular negative behavior. *Do not punish your child for everything else she is doing wrong.*

Let's look at the example of a child who frequently interrupts, intrudes, and blurts out comments at the dinner table. You speak with the child just before the next family mealtime about what you would like to see the child do more of at the table: try not to talk so much, wait until others are finished before talking, and talk only after finishing chewing food. You explain that the child can earn points for following these rules. Throughout the meal, you mark points on a small card and make sure the child sees this occurring, at the same time giving some nonverbal cue such as a wink that lets the child know you appreciate how hard the child struggles to adhere to these rules. You ignore rule violations for a week or so and then let the child know just before the next meal that from now on breaking a rule means losing a point. Remember that a fine or penalty should be imposed no more than once for every two or three rewards you dispense.

5. Externalize Time and Bridge Time Where Necessary

As my theory of ADHD makes plain, children with ADHD are delayed in their development of the ability to use an internal sense of time and of the future to guide their current behavior. Because they do not have the same capacity to sense and use time as normal children, they cannot respond to demands that involve timelines and preparation for the future as well as others can. They need some external reference to the time period allowed for an assigned task. Because they seem to live in the moment or "the now," they are less sensitive to mental information about time but are more sensitive to things that are occurring around them in that "now." They are more likely to be guided by time when you provide external reminders about time and the time interval assigned for a task. For instance, if your child is given 20 minutes to clean up his room, you will need to set a cooking timer for 20 minutes, place it where it will be visible in the child's room, and draw his attention to it. You can also use the Large Time Timer, a 1-foot-high clock that you can set for a time interval that is represented by a red disc. As time passes, the disc shrinks in size until time is up when a signal alerts the child. You can get this by just entering Large Time Timer into your Internet search engine, like Google, or at the ADD Warehouse *(www.addwarehouse.com)*. For older children or teens, you can try using a watch with a built-in timer and alarm, the MotivAider discussed above, the WatchMinder wrist watch (check the Internet for it or, again, go to *www.addwarehouse.com*), or just a recorder on which you have recorded your voice that counts backward for a specified time interval, perhaps indicating when each minute has elapsed ("10 minutes until time is up, 9 minutes until time is up," etc.). Use any means you can to externalize the time interval and to give the child a more accurate way of marking time during the work period.

For tasks that involve much longer time intervals, like book reports or science projects assigned to your child as homework, you will need to *bridge* time—that is, break the assignment into small daily steps so that a little piece of the task is done every day. By bridging time, you are building little bricks in the bridge across the gap in time between when the work was assigned and when it may be due (a few weeks or even a few months from now). Without these methods, the child will likely leave the work to be done until the very last minute, which often makes it impossible to do a good job.

6. Externalize the Important Information at the Point of Performance

Because working memory, or the ability to keep in mind information necessary to complete a task, is impaired significantly in children with ADHD, I have found it very helpful to place important information in a physical form at the point where the work has to be done. I call this point where the work is being done the *point of performance*—a phrase that Dr. Sam Goldstein invented to refer to the critical place and time for performing a behavior or a task in the natural setting, like home or school. If your child has homework to do at the kitchen table (where she can be supervised during dinner preparation, for example), place before her on the table a card listing important rules and reminders, such as "Stay on task, don't space out, and ask for help if you need it" or "Read directions carefully, do all the work, and when finished go back and double-check all your answers for completeness and accuracy." These reminders should be tailored to address the problems that each child has at that point of performance. If your child usually has trouble when a friend comes to the house to play, take her aside right before the friend is to arrive and review the social rules she needs to follow, such as "Share your toys, control your temper, take turns in games, and ask your friend about herself and her interests." You could even write these down on a card and review them with your child in private a few times while the friend is also at the house. Again, the more you can make important information available at points of performance, the more likely the child will be to remember that information and use it to guide her behavior.

7. Externalize the Source of Motivation at the Point of Performance

As my theory suggests, children with ADHD have trouble not only with using their internal timer and mental rules but also with self-motivation. They are not able to muster the internal motivation frequently needed to stay with work that is otherwise boring, tedious, effortful, or protracted. This deficit in intrinsic motivation can be overcome to a large extent by giving the child an external motivation boost such as an incentive, reward, or reinforcer to behave himself, restrict his activity, and follow rules—whatever is difficult for the child at that point of performance. As I discussed earlier about being a principle-centered parent, Dr. Stephen R. Covey refers to this sort of thing as creating a win/win situation in his seven habits of highly effective people (see the Introduction). This incentive can be an offer to let the child have something he wants when the work is done (a special snack or treat), to have a privilege he enjoys (extra TV time or time on video games or social networking devices), or to earn some tokens or points that he can save up toward a later privilege.

8. Make Thinking and Problem Solving More Manual or Physical

Children with ADHD do not seem to be able to manipulate or play around with mental information as well as others do when they must stop and think about a situation or problem. They respond impulsively, without giving due regard to their options. I think it may be helpful, therefore, to find ways to represent a problem and its alternative solutions in a more physical way. For instance, if your child has to write a short essay for school and doesn't seem to be responding well to this assignment, have her use a word processor and simply write down everything that comes to mind over a short period of time. This way every thought gets captured rather than being lost to forgetfulness, and the child can then expand on and play around with the ideas in a physical form instead of a mental one. The same thing can be done using index cards or even by drawing little pictures or symbols on a blank sheet of paper, where each represents some idea that has to be kept in mind to solve the problem.

This may be the most difficult type of information to externalize, but it seems particularly effective with schoolwork. So whenever problem solving of any type must be done, see if you can think of some way to make the problem and the parts of possible solutions physical so that your child can touch them, manipulate the pieces, move them around, and come up with new arrangements of the pieces of information that might help him solve the problem. This is just like using the form board and paper furniture pieces that designers often use in furniture stores to help you visualize various room arrangements of furniture you are thinking of buying. By making it manual and visible, you can better see the options to a problem and what is likely to work to solve it. The two discoverers of DNA, Drs. Francis Watson and James Crick, appear to have done just this when they puzzled over the structure of DNA. They put down on scraps of paper the various parts known to be involved in DNA, and then just kept playfully moving them around in different arrangements until, quite by accident, the correct arrangement became apparent.

9. Strive for Consistency

You must use the same strategies for managing your child's behavior every time. Applying consistency means four important things: (a) being consistent over time,

(b) being persistent and not giving up too soon when you are just starting a behavior change program, (c) responding in the same fashion even when the setting changes, and (d) making sure that both parents are using the same methods. Being unpredictable or capricious in your enforcement of the rules is a common invitation to failure. So is losing hope when your new method of management fails to yield dramatic, immediate results. Try a behavior change program for at least 1–2 weeks before deciding it isn't working. Don't fall prey to the trap that snares many parents: responding to behaviors one way at home but an entirely different way in public places. Finally, try to maintain a united parental front as much as you can, granted the inevitable differences in parenting styles.

10. Act, Don't Yak!

Dr. Sam Goldstein, a psychologist and expert on clinical work with ADHD (see the sixth principle, above), said it beautifully when he advised parents to stop talking and use consequences: *Act, don't yak!* As said at the beginning of this chapter, your child does not lack intelligence, skill, reasoning, or information, so simply talking to the child won't change the underlying neurological problem that makes her so uninhibited. Your child is much more sensitive to the consequences and feedback you use and much less sensitive to your reasoning than is a child without ADHD. So act quickly and act frequently and your child will behave better for you. Keep talking and all you will get is aggravation, not compliance.

11. Plan Ahead for Problem Situations

I'm sure you're familiar with the scenario: You're in a store and your child with ADHD begins to tear open packages, pull things off shelves, and generally create havoc, despite your repeated threats and commands. You become flustered and frustrated, unable to think quickly and clearly, so a solution eludes you. Your dismay is intensified by the disdainful glares of salespeople and other shoppers, and you try to skulk out of the shop, pulling your screaming child behind you.

I am often struck by parents' ability, when pressed, to predict where their children are likely to misbehave. So I am surprised by how few seem to put this information to good use. Why not use it in preparing for such problems to arise again? You can save yourself much anguish if you learn to anticipate problem situations, consider ahead of time how best to deal with them, develop a plan of action before entering that problem situation, share the plan with your child beforehand, and then follow through on your plan should a problem arise. People may find it hard to believe that even just sharing the plan with the child before entering a potential problem setting greatly reduces the odds that behavior problems will arise. But it works!

Try these five simple steps before entering any problem setting:

Step 1: *Stop* just before entering the site of a potential problem, such as a store, restaurant, church, or friend's home.

Step 2: *Review with your child two or three rules* that the child often has trouble following in that situation. For a store the rules could be "Stay next to me, don't ask for anything, and do as I say." No long-winded explanations, just a brief statement of the rules. Then ask the child to repeat these simple rules back.

Step 3: *Set up the reward or incentive*—selecting a snack at the checkout counter or stopping for a frozen yogurt on the way home, for example—that your child can earn by obeying the rules.

Step 4: *Explain the punishment* that may have to be used, such as a loss of points or a privilege.

Step 5: *Follow your plan* as you enter the situation and remember to give your child immediate and frequent feedback while there. If you must, punish your child swiftly for any acts that violate the rules.

12. Keep a Disability Perspective

At times, when faced with a difficult-to-manage child with ADHD, parents may lose all perspective on the immediate problem. They may become enraged, angered, embarrassed, or at the very least frustrated when their initial attempts at management do not work. They may even stoop to the level of the child and argue about the issue as another child might do. You must remember at all times that *you are the adult;* you are this disabled child's teacher, coach, and shepherd. If either of you is to keep your wits about you, it clearly has to be you.

One way to keep your cool in trying circumstances is to try to maintain some psychological distance from your child's problems. Look away from the child, count to 10, think of another place you would rather be (the beach), and try to reevaluate the situation more rationally. You can even pretend you are a stranger so you can view the situation for what it really represents—a parent's routine attempt to deal with a child with behavioral disabilities. If you can do this, you are likely to react to your child more reasonably, fairly, and rationally than if you let your child's problems upset you and respond impulsively in kind.

This is hard, so you may have to remind yourself of your child's disability each day—perhaps even several times a day, and especially when you are trying to deal with disruptive behavior.

13. Don't Personalize Your Child's Problems or Disorder

Don't allow your own sense of self-worth and personal dignity to become wrapped up in whether or not you "win" an argument or encounter with your child. No one is keeping score here. Stay calm if possible, maintain a sense of humor about the problem, and by all means try to follow the other principles listed here when you respond to your child. Sometimes this may even mean removing yourself from the situation for a moment by going to a different room to gather your wits and regain control over your feelings. Don't conclude that you're a bad parent when a situation goes wrong or does not turn out as you wanted. All parents fail at managing their children occasionally, and that doesn't make them bad parents. What is more important is your desire to strive to get it right or done better the next time, which leads to my last principle.

14. Practice Forgiveness

Practicing forgiveness is the most important principle, but often the most difficult to implement consistently in daily life. It means three things. First, each day, after problems have occurred and been settled, practice letting go of your anger, frustration, or disappointment. Try just 3 minutes of meditation called mindfulness in which you sit for a moment, close your eyes, focus on your breathing or heart rate, clear your mind of all thoughts, and let any bad thoughts go out of your mind. Conclude this brief respite by simply saying in your mind about your child "I love you and I forgive you." You can also try practicing forgiveness at the end of the day after your child is put to bed or before you retire for the night. Take just a moment to review the day and forgive your child for any transgressions. Let go of the anger, resentment, disappointment, or other personally destructive emotions that have arisen that day because of your child's misconduct or disruptions. The child cannot always control what he does and deserves to be forgiven.

Do not misunderstand this essential point. It does not mean that your child should not be held accountable for misdeeds. It means that you should let go of any bitterness over them.

Second, concentrate on forgiving others who may have misunderstood your child's inappropriate behavior that day and acted in ways offensive to you and your child, or simply dismissed your child as lazy or morally defective. You know better; don't buy into what others think about your child. Take any corrective action that's needed and continue to advocate for your child, but let go of the hurt, anger, humiliation and resentment such instances may have inflicted on you.

Finally, you must learn to practice forgiving yourself for your own mistakes in the management of your child that day. Children with ADHD have the capacity to bring out the worst in parents, which frequently results in parents feeling terribly guilty over their own errors. Without giving yourself license to make the same errors repeatedly without consequence, let go of the self-deprecation, shame, sadness, humiliation, resentment, or anger that accompanies such acts of self-evaluation. Replace them with a frank evaluation of your performance as a parent that day, identifying which areas to improve and making a personal commitment to strive to get it right the next day.

You will find this principle the hardest to adhere to, but the most fundamental to the art of effective and peaceful management of your child with ADHD.

14 Best Principles for Managing ADHD

1. Give Your Child More Immediate Feedback and Consequences
2. Give Your Child More Frequent Feedback
3. Use Larger and More Powerful Consequences
4. Use Incentives before Punishment
5. Externalize Time and Bridge Time Where Necessary
6. Externalize the Important Information at the Point of Performance
7. Externalize the Source of Motivation at the Point of Performance
8. Make Thinking and Problem Solving More Manual or Physical
9. Strive for Consistency
10. Act, Don't Yak!
11. Plan Ahead for Problem Situations
12. Keep a Disability Perspective
13. Don't Personalize Your Child's Problems or Disorder
14. Practice Forgiveness

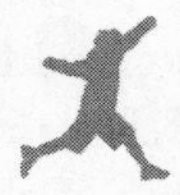

10 Just for Parents

HOW TO TAKE CARE OF YOURSELF

Undoubtedly you already know how stressful it can be to raise a child with ADHD. These children require a lot more monitoring and supervision than other children as they launch headlong into life with all its hazards. They can be demanding, defiant, loud, selfish, and aggressive; even their more benign incessant talking takes its toll. One recent study showed that parents of children with ADHD, especially those of preschool/kindergarten age, suffer higher levels of stress, depression, and self-blame than parents of children without ADHD. Another study showed, in fact, that parents of children with ADHD endure the same stress levels as parents of children with severe developmental disabilities, such as mental retardation and autism. To make matters worse, many parents also end up socially isolated as relatives, friends, and neighbors try to avoid contact with the family.

As I've seen all too often, this pattern can carry parents along on a downward spiral that leaves them drained and exhausted, demoralized and in despair. Taking care of their child has left them nothing for themselves, and ultimately this leaves them with no resources to care for the child either. Obviously, that's a situation that serves no one.

I can't pretend to give you a panacea for all of the ills that can strike a family struggling with ADHD. A certain amount of stress is inevitable. It does not, however, have to destroy you or anyone else in your family. So this chapter is just for you: some specific tips and general suggestions for preventing stressful events, minimizing the impact of the unavoidable ones, and giving yourself the break that you richly deserve.

Heading Off Stressful Events

The first thing you need to do to reduce the number of stressful events that you have to cope with is identify the exact sources of your stress. Many parents I've worked with seem to focus on their emotional reactions to stress, rather than on the sources of that stress. They in fact mistake one for the other and believe they need to eliminate the feelings of tension, irritability, depression and sadness, the fatigue, and the headaches, rather than the events that are precipitating them. Granted, there are stressful events that can't be avoided—more of them for you than for parents of children without ADHD. For these you will have to resort to stress reduction techniques such as formal relaxation methods, meditation, exercise, perhaps even medication in extreme cases. But in other cases—and you might be surprised by how many—you can identify and avoid or at least reduce the source of the stress and head it off. Try this simple method:

1. When you have some quiet time, sit down with paper and pencil and think back over the times in the last few weeks when you felt stress reactions: irritability, anger, hostility, anxiety, or depression. Then list the stressors—not how you felt, but the events that immediately preceded each stress reaction. What was it about that situation that you think may have precipitated your stress response? What did your child or someone else do that elicited this negative reaction from you? What did others do to your child? What might your spouse have done? What event came up that made you feel this way? Leave a few blank lines after each stressor you identify.

2. Now look closely at the first event. What could you have done to avoid or eliminate that event or problem? Did your reaction worsen the situation? Would any of Dr. Covey's seven principles (see the Introduction) have helped you eliminate the stressor? Or would any of the 14 principles for raising a child with ADHD (see Chapter 9) have helped you avoid the situation? Can you see how any of these principles might help you eliminate or avoid this stressor the next time around? Or can you simply plan to avoid the stressful event or person altogether? Write down at least one coping method after each of the stress events listed.

3. Now focus on one (or at most two) of these stressors and resolve either to avoid the stressor in the future or, if it is unavoidable, to use your coping method the next time the event arises. Close your eyes and visualize yourself responding differently and more effectively in just that situation.

4. Remind yourself of your plan by posting small notes to yourself around your home and work space.

5. Take a few minutes each day to practice visualizing your use of this new action plan. This practice will fortify your confidence that you can in fact head off the source of stress when it threatens to rise again.

6. Once your confidence has been built up or you have actually tried the new plan, move on to another stressor or two. Work on only one or two stressors at a time until you've mastered or eliminated them; then move on to one or two more. Success here comes in small steps as you deal with just one or two stressors at a time, not by trying to deal with all of them at once.

Coping with the Inevitable

Because stress seems to be a part of life for everyone these days, many effective techniques have been devised for reducing its negative impact. Any professional you're working with can steer you to sources of more information on the subject, but so can the Internet, your local librarian, or a bookseller. You can even find audio recordings and videos that will teach some of the best-known methods. Space limitations make it impossible to go into depth here, so only a few brief suggestions follow.

1. Delay Your Response

Most of us respond quickly and impulsively to a stressful event. When we're emotionally aroused—angry or anxious—we get physically aroused as well: our pulse quickens, we may feel flushed, and adrenaline readies us for "fight or flight." Unfortunately, none of this contributes to mental sharpness. In fact, it's those impulsive responses that we usually end up regretting. So sometimes the best thing to do is nothing. If the only way to delay your response is to get away, just leave the room for a brief time or send your child away with a calm "I'll discuss this with you in a few minutes."

When you're confronting a stressful encounter with your child, try simply waiting to let your mind play on the situation and its possibilities. This doesn't mean filling your mind with thoughts like "Oh, what will I do? What will I do?" or "I know I can't handle this" or "This won't work, I have no options, and I don't know what to do." Rather, try to remain calm and let your mind engage the problem. That's the wonderful thing about the human mind: the only thing you have to do to help it come up with ideas is not interfere with its natural problem-solving ability. Just give it a little time.

2. Practice Relaxation or Meditation

Many people use relaxation techniques on a regular basis to lower their overall stress level. Because these techniques can have a considerable preventive effect, they'll serve you well when you're facing an upcoming stress event that can't be avoided. For example, say the school has called to say your child is being sent home for starting a fight with another child and you must meet with the principal the next day. Stress is likely to build before the meeting as you ponder the possible repercussions. Practicing techniques like progressive muscle relaxation can keep you from blowing the situation way out of proportion. There are many books that sum up this method and others. Progressive muscle relaxation involves deep breathing and relaxing of each muscle group in turn, followed by mental imagery of yourself in a relaxing, beautiful place. It's easy to learn but is most effective when you've had some practice, so anticipate stress and start practicing ahead of time.

3. Broaden Your Focus

Another way to avoid blowing things out of proportion is to broaden your focus when you are involved in a stressful situation. Try to avoid zeroing in on the small details and instead focus on the entire situation from the perspective of your own or your child's lifetime. This can often help you realize that the stressful event is not as important as you are making it out to be, that it can be managed, and that even if it does not go well, it is not as big a deal as you may think. At the school meeting in our earlier example, you could listen to the details of what the principal is saying while concentrating on the fact that this is just one school meeting, that the opinions expressed are not final and will not cause havoc in your life or your child's, and that as an executive parent you are ultimately in charge of this meeting and of what happens to your child.

4. Begin with the End in Mind

Before and throughout a stressful situation, visualize how you want the situation to turn out for your child. Keeping your positive goals in mind can lessen the impact of negative remarks, decrease the intensity of your own reactions, and thus avoid heightening the conflict and worsening its outcome.

Practicing Personal Renewal

Raising a child with ADHD places huge demands on the mind, body, heart, and spirit. To replenish yourself emotionally, feel more in control of your life, and better equip yourself to handle unexpected stressful events, consider the following suggestions. You've heard many of them before, but there's bound to be something new as well. You deserve to take as good care of yourself as you do your child, and that means setting aside some time for yourself. If you're tempted to protest that you have no time, see the suggestions in the sidebar (pp. 173–174).

1. Take a Long Weekend Away

Sometimes the only way to renew your energies is to get away. Don't hesitate to do this. Go by yourself and have your spouse/partner look after your child. Visit a friend, go to a spa, loll on the beach with a good book, or do something that appeals uniquely to you. Recharging your emotional batteries and catching up on your sleep are well worth the trouble of arranging this getaway. If there's someone you trust to

One Key to Survival: Time Management

Time management does not come naturally to most people because it is not really time management at all. Time cannot be manipulated or managed; it just is and seems to flow along. Time management is self-management to the passage of time, a skill to be acquired. It takes practice and effort, but its rewards can be enormous—especially in families affected by ADHD, where parents have so many demands on them.

There are many excellent books in libraries and bookstores that can give full details on how to manage your time effectively. Most of them begin by explaining that your first step must be to set specific, well-defined, reasonable goals for both the long and short terms. When you do this you end up with a plan for each day, each week, each month—a plan that you can follow realistically, giving you the sense of satisfaction that you have achieved what you set out to do. A child with ADHD, by nature disorganized and disruptive, can make you feel as if your life has no order whatsoever, so getting this sense of accomplishment is particularly important to you.

Experts on time management divide time use into five categories: important and urgent, important but not urgent, urgent but not important, neither urgent nor important (busy work), and wasted time. Knowing the difference can help you identify where your work usually falls, and can perhaps show you how to alter the nature of your current home or job activities to achieve your goals.

1. *Important and urgent.* Tasks that must be done immediately or in the very near future. Because they are urgent and important, they often get done. Usually this is not where time gets wasted.

2. *Important but not urgent.* It is here that effective parents can be readily distinguished from ineffective ones. These are tasks that you or others consider important for you to do, but they are not urgent. Most of the time you simply never get around to doing them. Time management can help elevate these personal priorities to a more urgent status so that you do get them done. Taking time for personal renewal, for exercise, for connecting with close friends, or for your intimate relationship with your partner often falls into this category and gets neglected to your longer term detriment.

3. *Urgent but not important.* Often minor or trivial stuff that others make urgent with their deadlines but that, if thought about, are of only modest importance. Yet because they are urgent (immediate) you may give more attention to these than to your more important but less urgent goals. Returning e-mails, text messages, postings on Facebook, and answering requests through the mail can fall into this category because we feel as if we must respond to them as quickly as we can or as requested by others. The vast majority, however, are not important.

***One Key to Survival: Time Management** (cont.)*

4. *Busy work*. This can involve tasks of marginal importance, such as housework, returning unsolicited telephone calls, running errands, reviewing junk mail, yard work, and the like. You may do them before the important ones because they are brief and diversionary or give you a feeling of productivity, but they rarely contribute to your real goals for yourself or your child with ADHD.

5. *Wasted time*. Whether it's watching lousy TV shows or 24-hour cable news networks, sitting through a bad movie, or attending an unnecessary committee meeting, this type of activity usually makes you feel you could have spent the time better doing something else. Most people think this is the cause of their poor time management, but usually, experts say, the real cause is allocating too much time to categories 3 and 4 and not enough to category 2. Take a look at how you spend your time. Could this be true of you?

Watch out for the real time wasters too: indecision, blaming others for your lack of time, pursuing perfection instead of excellence, getting off-track because of distracting stimuli, trivial social networking (e-mail, instant messaging, texting, Facebook posting, etc.), and letting those little tidbits of time spent waiting go unfilled.

care for your child, try to get away with your spouse/partner now and then as well—adult relationships need renewal too.

2. Find a Hobby or Social Activity

The last thing that a child with ADHD needs is a martyr for a parent—someone who has sacrificed all personal pleasures and recreational time for the sake of spending time with the child. That parent will be weary, exhausted, stressed, and often ill-tempered or irritable. You owe it to yourself and to your child to find something that will provide a sense of personal gratification and fulfillment on a regular basis.

One parent I know was an amateur winemaker and formed a small club of fellow enthusiasts who met periodically to make new wines, study winemaking, and travel to wine tastings. Others have joined bowling leagues, choral groups, quilting groups, running clubs, instrumental music groups, book clubs, or sports teams. There are also informal get-togethers like coffee klatches and potluck suppers. Then there are the private hobbies like woodworking, fly tying, model building, antique collecting, researching your family's genealogy, painting, sewing, quilting, or crocheting, reading . . . the list is endless. The point is that as long as you enjoy it, pursuing a personal interest can give you the same sense of renewal as going on a short trip.

3. Become Active in a Support Group

Maybe the last thing you want to do when you need to be reinvigorated is meet with a group of people who have the same problems you do, but attending support group meetings regularly has multiple benefits. True, parent groups are a great source of information and advice, but they also provide the release of commiseration, and many parents end up making real friends there. Some groups even have babysitting cooperatives; see if your local chapter is willing to support one.

4. Seek the Comfort of Close Friends

Don't forget to renew your friendships with those you've been close to for years. Most of us let these relationships get away from us when we're busy, but we all need the "sure refuge" that Aristotle called true friends. Unburdening yourself to a close friend has tremendous therapeutic value; someone who knows and cares for you well can provide not only a shoulder to lean on, but also a new perspective on your problems.

5. Practice Shared Parenting

If taking any of these suggestions sounds like pampering yourself and you think you have no time for that, you may need to talk to your spouse/partner about redistributing some of the load of parenting your child with ADHD. Often a disproportionate share of this load falls on the mother, and even if this isn't the case in your home, you can probably benefit from agreeing that each of you will take full responsibility for the child every other day (or, if one or both of you work away from home, every other evening). This gives you predictable times for pursuing personal interests, as well as just giving you time to take a deep breath and have a little time off.

6. Practice Becoming Aware of Moments

Many of the world's great religious teachers and philosophers have advised us to focus our mind on the natural beauty, joy, peace, and wonder in the world around us at any point in time. Yet we become so wrapped up in preparing for upcoming events that we often miss the wonder of this very moment. My former colleague Dr. Jon Kabat-Zinn has written a book that I highly recommend, *Wherever You Go, There You Are*. A principal theme of this book is that concentrating on the moment—its sensory richness and textures and its scope, both broad and minute—repays our investment of time a hundredfold in the renewal of our personal energy, mental perspective, and emotional balance and control. It can greatly diminish the sense of stress, time, and urgency that parents of children with ADHD feel daily.

This method is often called "mindfulness meditation." As mentioned earlier, this involves stopping what you are doing, closing your eyes, using a focal point for your attention, such as your breathing, and then letting all other thoughts go out of your mind as you concentrate on this focal point. If any thoughts enter your mind, then just note their occurrence and let them pass on but don't prolong them or engage them in any mental conversation with yourself. Then open your eyes and just try to focus only on the sensory information you are receiving at that moment or on your breathing, what some might call the texture of that moment in experience, with no regard to any thoughts, what has just passed, or what may be coming up next.

7. Identify and Alter Stressful Thinking Patterns

Emotionally at least, in large part, you are what you think. You've probably noticed that while you feel and act humiliated by, say, the tantrums your child with ADHD throws in stores, other parents seem to go about managing their children's similar misbehavior matter-of-factly, without alarm or distress. Well, you may reason, maybe they can be calm because their children don't act this way every time they go into a store, while yours does.

Not necessarily. Many years ago a famous psychologist, Dr. Albert Ellis, developed a theory that we determine how we will feel in a given situation by *what we are thinking* about those events or people. When we think negative, distressing, and self-critical thoughts, we fan the flames of our negative emotions. But if we identify these negative thought patterns and change them to constructive, positive, self-empowering ones, we can actually diminish or even eliminate the negative emotional reactions.

So when your child throws a tantrum in a store, you may think:

> "How can my child embarrass me like this? Everyone must be watching. What are they thinking of me? They must think I'm a terrible parent because I can't manage my child properly. I knew I should have stayed home. How dare this child humiliate me like this? Now I can never come back here again. Why am I such a lousy parent?"

The other parents you've seen behaving so calmly in the same situation may be thinking:

> "I am not going to give in to my child's attempt at extortion. He knows the rules, and I told him before we got here that we were not buying any toys or candy on this trip. I am this child's teacher, and he may have to learn the hard way that I will not be intimidated by these tantrums. In a few minutes he will calm down. It's unfortunate that he has to embarrass himself like this and disturb other people's

shopping. I've seen many parents have to discipline their children for these kinds of outbursts. In fact, many children occasionally act this way in stores. But to give in to him now would teach him the wrong lesson."

You can learn to identify negative thought patterns by keeping a small notebook with you and writing in it what you were saying or thinking to yourself when an event that triggered a stressful or emotionally upsetting reaction occurred. Once you've begun to identify your negative or distressing thought patterns, try substituting more positive, upbeat, constructive, and forgiving ones the next time you sense that same stressor occurring.

8. Exercise Regularly

OK, we've all heard this advice before, but where stressful lives are concerned it's *very* important to heed it, so it's worth saying again: regular exercise lessens stress, builds stamina, refuels our energy for self-control, and makes us generally more able to meet the demands of the day. If you don't think you can spare the time, try combining it with another self-renewal activity: ask a friend to become a cycling partner, put together a regular foursome for golf (and walk, don't ride, the course), or plan regular hiking weekends with old friends (and see the sidebar on time management). But keep in mind that you'll benefit from as little as 20–30 minutes of light exercise three times a week, according to the fitness experts.

9. Avoid Chemical Substances

Again, you've heard it before: alcohol, caffeine, and nicotine can take a lot more out of you than they give back. We all know the hazards of smoking by now, but alcohol and caffeine consumption seem to be more matters of quantity. Quite simply, moderation is essential if you're to preserve your energies. Alcohol is a sedative; when used chronically to excess, it can result in fatigue, irritability, low frustration tolerance, and a withdrawal from responsibilities. Nicotine and caffeine are both stimulants; they can increase heart rate, blood pressure, breathing rate, brain activity, muscle tension, restlessness, and perceived stress or nervousness in a situation. The last thing you need is to overreact, I'm sure you'll agree. So take a minute to evaluate your habits and whether they're serving you well.

Part III

Managing Life with ADHD: How to Cope at Home and at School

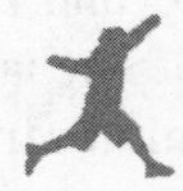

11 Eight Steps to Better Behavior

When a child has ADHD, a family often finds that the home is more a battlefield than a haven or a sanctuary. The child violates household rules, neglects chores, resists homework, and generally disturbs the peace. There is no cure for ADHD, but there are some sound principles by which you can work with your child to improve behavior, social relationships, and general adjustment at home. This chapter presents the management principles that I have taught at the ADHD clinics with which I have been affiliated over my career. More than 75% of the families who come to our clinic find the principles help them to significantly improve their children's behavior and their overall relationship with their children.

The tactics described here are designed expressly to reduce stubborn, defiant, or oppositional behavior while they increase a child's cooperativeness. The result in the great majority of cases is that the child becomes more successful at meeting daily demands for working and living within the larger family unit and acquires a wide range of positive behaviors that contribute to greater success in school, in the community, and in society at large.

Here's what you can expect to achieve by diligently applying these principles:

1. To strengthen the parent–child relationship through mutual respect, cooperation, and appreciation; to make that relationship more loving and friendly.

2. To reduce the daily conflict, hassles, arguments, and even temper outbursts—yours as well as your child's—that may now permeate your daily interactions.

3. To improve your child's range of appropriate and socially acceptable behaviors, while you decrease the child's reliance on antisocial and unacceptable social behaviors.

4. To prepare your child to be socialized. The variety of child behavior problems

> for which this treatment program can be applied extends well beyond the home—to all situations where parents must expect their children to behave in prosocial (effective and socially supportive) ways, must trust them to carry out family and social responsibilities, and must foster positive and cooperative social interactions between this child and other children and adults.

When young children learn to comply with parental requests and rules, they are acquiring a basic attitude of social cooperation and an openness to learning from adults that is absolutely critical to continuing social development and later adult social adjustment. And you will have fulfilled one of the most fundamental roles of a parent in society: the preparation of a child to be socialized within that family's larger social community. Make no mistake about the importance of this parental responsibility. The psychological research is crystal-clear on this point: the young child who learns that disobedience, resistance to parental requests, stubbornness, tantrums, and aggressive behavior are successful means of escaping from adult requests and the imposition of social responsibilities is at high risk for later antisocial and criminal activity, school failure, peer and community rejection, and early substance abuse. This program is designed to address that risk directly and to improve your child's openness to being socialized by you and other important adults and to cooperating with you, peers, and the larger social community. This spirit of social cooperation and openness to the rules and wisdom of society is critical to the eventual adult adjustment of any child.

Is This Program for You?

This program can help you manage the behavior of a child with ADHD who:

- Is between 2 and 10 years old.
- Has generally normal language development.
- Is not seriously oppositional or defiant (see sidebar, pp. 183–184).
- Is not likely to try to assault you or become seriously destructive when you try to set limits on the child's behavior.

Do not attempt this program if:

- Your child's language development is below that of the average 2-year-old.
- Your child is age 13 or older (the program described in Chapter 14 may be more appropriate).

How Defiant Is Your Child?

Circle any of the following items that you believe your child displays *to a degree that is excessive or inappropriate for the child's age group* and that has been present for at least 6 months.

1. Often loses control of temper.
2. Often disputes or argues with adults.
3. Often actively rebels against or refuses adults' rules or requests.
4. Often deliberately does things that annoy other people.
5. Often blames others for own misdeeds.
6. Often is easily irked or annoyed by others.
7. Often is resentful and angry.
8. Often is spiteful or revengeful.

If you circled at least four of these items, your child has a significant degree of defiant or oppositional behavior and may have oppositional defiant disorder. You may want to consider having a mental health professional assist you with this program. Certainly if you circled six or more, you will probably run into a great deal of resistance from your child and should not attempt this program without professional help. Whether your child has more or fewer than four of the behavior problems listed above, circle any of the following items that your child has shown during the past 12 months. (This list, of course, applies to children up to age 18 years.)

1. Often intimidates, harasses, or threatens others.
2. Often begins physical fights with others (not including fights with siblings).
3. Uses a weapon that can cause serious physical injury to others (for example, a bat, brick, broken bottle, knife, gun).
4. Is physically cruel to people (for example, ties up and abandons a victim, systematically cuts or burns a victim).
5. Steals, with confrontation with a victim (for example, mugging, purse snatching, extortion, or armed robbery).
6. Forces someone into sexual activity.
7. Often lies or breaks promises to obtain items or favors, or to avoid debts or obligations (that is, "cons" other people).

How Defiant Is Your Child? *(cont.)*

8. Steals items of significant value, without confrontation with the victim (for example, shoplifting, burglary, or forgery).
9. Often stays out after dark without permission, beginning before 13 years of age.
10. Is physically cruel to animals.
11. Deliberately destroys others' property (other than by setting fires).
12. Deliberately sets fires, with the purpose of causing serious damage.
13. Runs away from home overnight at least twice while living in parents' or parent surrogates' home (or once without coming back for a prolonged period).
14. Is often truant from school, beginning before 13 years of age.
15. Breaks into someone else's home, building, or car.

If your child has shown three or more of these problems within the past year, seek the assistance of a professional with this program. Your child may have conduct disorder, a serious pattern of antisocial behavior and violation of the rights of others. Families with children who show such behavior problems are in need of more professional help than can be provided by this book.

To find professional help, ask whether the mental health or medical professional you are already working with is familiar with *behavioral parent training or child management programs*. If not, ask for a referral to a professional who teaches such programs. Or contact your local ADHD parent support association or school psychologist for the names of professionals they know who employ such training programs in their practice. A full program as it should be conducted by a professional is detailed in my book *Defiant Children: A Clinician's Manual for Parent Training* (see "Suggested Reading and Videos"). Ideally, you should find someone who has used this particular program.

Try this program only with professional assistance if your child:

- Has been diagnosed as having a pervasive developmental disorder (such as autism), a psychotic disorder (such as schizophrenia), or severe depression.
- Is seriously defiant (see the sidebar). A final word of caution: If you are not ready to change your own behavior to help your child, this program is not for you. For some parents the principles demand significant changes in parent–child interaction, and if you're not prepared to comply fully with the program, it is bound to fail.

How to Use This Program

This program is explained in detail in my book *Your Defiant Child: 8 Steps to Better Behavior.* You may want to read that book before attempting to use these methods with your child, as this chapter provides just an overview of the program. The program will take the average parent about 8 weeks to complete. (The eight steps of the program are given in the sidebar at the bottom of this page.) You should plan on spending at least a week at each step before moving on. Do not go on to the next step until you feel comfortable with the step you have practiced that week. Your child has taken months—even years—to develop the current behavior pattern with you, so don't expect it to change quickly. Each step of this program builds on the previous one, so you must apply them in the order given. And *never* skip over the first three steps and go straight to the methods that involve discipline or punishment. To be effective, these later steps on discipline *must* be preceded by the earlier steps. Remember the rule you learned in Chapter 9: *Rewards before punishment*.

Step 1: Learn to Give Positive Attention to Your Child

Purpose and Goals

The attention you give a child is a very powerful reward or consequence. This is why your children seek you out, strive to get your attention, and bask in the glow of any positive attention you give them. This attention need not be positive, however, to be desirable to a child. In the absence of positive attention, negative attention—reprimands, criticism, or yelling—may seem worth seeking out, because any attention

Eight Steps to Better Behavior

Step 1: Learn to pay positive attention to your child.

Step 2: Use your powerful attention to gain compliance.

Step 3: Give more effective commands.

Step 4: Teach your child not to interrupt your activities.

Step 5: Set up a home token system.

Step 6: Learn to punish misbehavior constructively.

Step 7: Expand your use of time-out.

Step 8: Learn to manage your child in public places.

is better than none. A child who gets scolded for interrupting a phone call may obey the command to stop that time, but will surely be more likely to interrupt the next time.

Even positive attention is often flawed. When parents combine praise and criticism in backhanded compliments such as "You did a nice job cleaning up your room, but why can't you do that every day without being told?" they greatly reduce the power of their attention to reinforce children's positive behavior.

Learning *when* to give your child your attention and when to withhold it are important goals of this program. Also important is *how* you pay attention to your child when you do so, the subject of this first step of the program. We will come back to this in the second step as well.

If you don't believe that how and when you pay attention to your child has a powerful influence on the child's compliance and other aspects of behavior, do the exercise in the sidebar on the facing page. The goal of this step of the program is to help you become a parent with the characteristics of the best job supervisor you've ever had. The purpose is to change *your* behavior. Changes in your child should follow slowly, naturally, and eventually from changing yourself.

Instructions

This first step of the program involves learning how to pay attention to your child's desirable behavior during playtime. If your child is below 9 years of age, select a 20-minute period each day as your "special time" with your child—after other children are off to school in the morning if you have a preschool child, or after school or dinner for school-age children. No other children are to be involved! If your child is 9 years or older, you don't have to choose a standard time. Instead, choose a time each day as it arises when your child seems to be enjoying a play activity alone. Then stop what you're doing and begin to join in the child's play, following the instructions given here.

If you've set up a standard time, simply say "It's now our special time to play together. What would you like to do?" The child chooses the play activity, within reason (TV, a nonactivity, is out). If you have not set up a standard time, simply ask if you can join in.

In either case, don't take control of the play or direct it. Relax and casually watch what your child is doing for a few minutes before joining in. Obviously, you should not try to have this special playtime when you're upset, very busy, or planning to leave the house soon for some errand or trip. Your mind will be preoccupied by these matters, and the quality of your attention will be quite poor.

After watching your child's play, begin to describe out loud what your child is doing to show your interest. In other words, occasionally narrate your child's play. Try to keep what you say exciting and action-oriented, not dull and in a monotone. Young children really enjoy this. With older children, you should still comment, but less so.

Are You the Best or Worst Supervisor You Can Imagine?

1. Divide a sheet of paper into two columns and write "Worst Supervisor" over the left column and "Best Supervisor" over the right column.

2. Now recall the worst person you've ever worked for and think about how that person treated you. What did the supervisor say or do that made you dislike that style of management or interaction? This is a person you would not like to work for again if you could avoid doing so. Why? List in the left column at least five different negative characteristics. Parents usually give statements such as "Doesn't appreciate what I do," "Doesn't seem to listen to my point of view," "Dishonest," "Too bossy or overcontrolling," "Interrupts my work without apologizing," "Acts like I am his slave," "A real dictator," "Hot-tempered," "Very critical of others."

3. Next, think of the best person you've ever worked for—someone you'd enjoy working for again. If that person had asked you to do some extra work beyond the call of duty, you would have gladly volunteered to help out. Why? List in the right column five positive characteristics. Parents often give me answers such as "Honest," "Appreciated my work, even the little things," "Took an interest in me and my opinions," "Encouraged my efforts to improve my work," "Respected my time and my work," "Very positive and upbeat about herself and our work together."

4. Now look at the information in the two columns and honestly decide in which column your child would place you.

More than 90% of the parents I have worked with in various clinics are shocked to find that they are more likely to be acting like the "Worst Supervisor" with their children than the "Best Supervisor." *The way you give attention to your children when you supervise them can create the same feelings in them as it has in you.*

Ask no questions and give no commands! This is critical. Questioning is disruptive and should be limited to trying to clarify when you're uncertain of what your child is doing. Remember that this is your child's special time to relax and enjoy your company, not a time to teach or take over the child's play.

Occasionally, provide your child with statements of praise, approval, or positive feedback. Be accurate and honest, not excessively flattering. For instance, "I like it when we play quietly like this," "I really enjoy our special time together," and "Look at how nicely you have made that" are all positive, appropriate comments. If you find yourself at a loss for words, try some of these responses:

Nonverbal signs of approval

Hug

Pat on the head or shoulder

Affectionate rubbing of hair

Placing arm around the child

Smiling

A light kiss

Giving a thumbs-up sign

A wink

Verbal signs of approval

"I like it when you . . . "

"It's nice when you . . . "

"You sure are a big boy/girl for . . . "

"That was terrific the way you . . . "

"Great job!"

"Nice going!"

"Terrific!"

"Super!"

"Fantastic!"

"My, you sure act grown up when you . . . "

"You know, 6 months ago you couldn't do that as well as you can now—you're really growing up fast!"

"Beautiful!"

"Wow!"

"Wait until I tell Mom/Dad [other parent] how nicely you . . . "

"What a nice thing to do!"

"You did that all by yourself—way to go!"

"Just for behaving so well, you and I will . . . "

"I am very proud of you when you . . . "

"I always enjoy it when we . . . like this."

If your child begins to misbehave, simply turn away and look elsewhere for a few moments. If the misbehavior continues, tell your child the special playtime is over and leave the room. Tell your child you will play later when he can behave nicely. If the child becomes extremely disruptive or abusive during play, discipline the child as you might normally do.

Each parent is to spend 20 minutes with the child in this special playtime. During the first week, try to do this every day or at least five times. After the first week, continue this special playtime indefinitely at least three or four times a week.

Don't worry if you give too many commands, ask too many questions, or make too few positive comments at first. Just try harder to improve your attending skills the next time. You may want to spend this kind of special playtime with the other children in your family once you have improved your skills with the child who has ADHD.

If your practicing with your child goes reasonably well, you will probably find that your child enjoys your company. Your child may even ask you to stay and play longer after your "special time" is up. On rare occasions, you may even find that your child starts to compliment you for the things that you do well or do for the child.

If you still don't feel comfortable acting this way with your child, spend another week practicing your new attending skills before going on to step 2. You're ready to move on to the next step when you find you can observe and play with your child while commenting on her activities, without taking control of the play and directing it and asking lots of unnecessary questions. You should also find it relatively easy to give praise and positive feedback to your child for the good things you notice about the child's play and interactions with you. If you spend most of the playtime not saying anything to your child, then you need to practice this week's exercises for another week or so. For steps 1 to 4, you will know that you are ready by how your own behavior is changing, not by how well your child is improving. You should not expect much change from your child during these four steps.

Hints

1. Always show your approval immediately. *Don't wait!*
2. Always be specific about what you like.
3. Never give a backhanded compliment.

Step 2: Use Your Powerful Attention to Gain Compliance

Purpose and Goals

You are now going to take the style of paying attention you practiced during play and extend it to when your child is obeying you or complying with your instructions. It's the same style, just a different focus of your attention and comments. Your goal is to improve the manner in which you supervise work, in the hope that it will increase your child's willingness to work for you (obey) and improve how hard he works.

Instructions

When you give a command, give the child immediate feedback for how well she is doing. Don't just walk away; stay and pay attention and comment positively on your child's compliance (see the list of verbal signs of approval above).

Don't give any more commands or ask any questions while your child is working or obeying. Too often parents give multiple commands or ask unnecessary questions, which distracts the child from the task assigned.

Once you have noted your child's compliance, you can leave for a few moments if you must, but be sure to return frequently to pay attention and praise your child's compliance.

Should you find that your child has done a job or chore without being told to do so, provide especially positive praise, perhaps even a small privilege to help your child remember and follow household rules and jobs without always being told to do so. Even children with ADHD, despite their disability, can improve in their ability to recall and follow rules and instructions, and one way to help them is to reward them when they do so spontaneously.

This week, begin to use positive attention to your child for virtually every command you give. In addition, choose two or three commands your child follows inconsistently and make a special effort to praise and attend to your child whenever he begins to comply with these particular commands. In short, "Catch 'em being good!"

Setting Up Compliance Training Periods

It is very important during the next 1 or 2 weeks that you take a few minutes now and then to train compliance in your child. Select a time when your child is not very busy and ask her to do very brief favors for you, such as "Hand me a pencil" or "Can you reach that towel for me?" We call these *fetch* commands, and they should require only a very brief and simple effort from your child. Give about five or six of these, but only one at a time during these few minutes. As your child follows each one, be sure to provide specific praise, such as "I like it when you listen to me," "It is really nice when you do as I ask," or "Thanks for doing what I asked." Then let your child go on to do something else.

Try to do this several times a day. Because the requests are very simple and brief, most children (even children with behavior problems) will do them. This provides an excellent opportunity to "catch your child being good" and to praise his compliance. If your child does not obey one of the commands, skip it and make another brief request. Your goal at this point is not to confront or discipline noncompliance, but to catch, attend to, and reward compliance. By doing so, you increase the likelihood that your child will comply with your other, necessary instructions.

You will know that you're ready to move on to the next step when you feel comfortable pointing out the small things that your child is doing well for you and when your child is complying with most or all of your requests during your compliance training periods and you find it quite easy to praise compliance with each one.

After a week of practicing this, many parents tell me they begin to see a noticeable though not dramatic difference in their children's behavior toward them.

Step 3: Give More Effective Commands

Purpose and Goals

The purpose of the third step is to improve the manner in which you ask your child to do work for you or obey your instructions. In my work with children who have behavior problems, I've noticed that if parents simply change the way they give commands to their children, they can often achieve significant improvements in the children's compliance.

Instructions

When you're about to give a command or instruction to your child, be sure to do the following.

Make Sure You Mean It!

Never give a command that you don't intend to follow through on. You should plan on backing up any request with appropriate consequences to show that you mean what you say. It's better to focus on a few commands that you mean than to spew out hundreds and follow up on less than half of them.

Do Not Present the Command as a Question or Favor

State the command simply, directly, and in a business-like tone of voice. Don't say "Why don't we pick up the toys now?" or "It's time for dinner. Wash your hands, OK?" These are command–questions or command–favors. The inflection at the end of the statement asks for your child's assent, which is far less effective than a more direct statement such as "Pick up the toys now" or "It's dinnertime; wash your hands." You don't have to yell or scream; just be firm and direct, sort of like Clint Eastwood might say it—with conviction, and all business.

Don't Give Too Many Commands at Once

Most children are able to follow only one or two instructions at a time. For now, try giving only one specific instruction at a time. If a task you want your child to do is complicated, break it down into smaller steps and give only one step at a time.

Make Sure Your Child Is Paying Attention to You

Be sure to make eye contact with your child. If necessary, gently turn the child's face toward yours to ensure that she is listening and watching.

Reduce All Distractions before Giving the Command

A very common mistake that parents make is to try to give instructions while the child is engaged in watching TV, listening to a music player, playing a video game, or social networking on a smart phone or a computer. Parents cannot expect children to attend to them when something more entertaining is going on. Either turn off these distractions yourself or tell the child to turn them off before giving the command.

Ask the Child to Repeat the Command

Asking the child to repeat the command is useful when you're not sure your child has heard or understood the command. Also, repeating a command seems to increase the likelihood that a child with a short attention span will follow through.

Make Up Chore Cards

If your child is old enough to have chores and to read, you may find it useful to make up a chore card for each job. Simply list on an index card the steps involved in doing that chore correctly. Then when you want your child to do the chore, simply hand the child the card and state that this is what you want done. These cards can greatly reduce arguing over whether a child has done a job properly.

Set Deadlines

You might also indicate on the cards how much time each chore should take and then set your kitchen timer so the child knows exactly when it is to be done. Whether you use the chore cards or not, give your child a specific deadline in the immediate future. Don't say "Sometime today you will have to take out the trash" or "Before noon you must clean up your room." Instead, wait until the time for the work to be done and then say, "It is now time to take out the trash. You have 10 minutes to get the job done. I am setting the stove timer for 10 minutes. See if you can beat the clock." To be more than fair, 5–10 minutes before the task is to be started, you can always go to your child and give him a warning that in 5 (or 10) minutes you will return to have him start the job.

Practice giving effective commands for the next week, continuing to do the exercises from the previous two steps as well. You will have a sense that you're ready to move on when you give most of your work requests or commands in a neutral, imperative form rather than as a favor or question. You should also notice that your commands are simpler in form. Before moving on to the next step, ask yourself if you've reviewed your child's routine chores to see if a chore card with an assigned time limit was necessary to help with any of them. Also, do you now set a time limit with most tasks assigned? Giving explicit commands, keeping them relatively simple, and setting time limits for completion are three main indications that you're ready to go on to the next step.

Step 4: Teach Your Child Not to Interrupt Your Activities

Purpose and Goals

Many parents of children with behavior problems complain that they are unable to talk on the phone, cook dinner, or visit with a neighbor without their children interrupting. The fourth step will help you teach your child to play independently of you when you are occupied. Many parents provide a lot of attention to a child who is interrupting and almost no attention when the child stays away, plays independently, and does not interrupt. No wonder kids interrupt parents so much!

Instructions

When you're about to become occupied with some activity, such as a phone call, give your child a direct two-part command—one part that tells the child what to do while you're busy and another that specifically tells the child not to interrupt or bother you. For instance, you can say, "I have to talk on the telephone, so I want you to stay in this room and watch TV. Don't bother me." The task you give a child should *not* be a chore, but some interesting activity such as coloring, playing with a toy, watching a favorite children's TV program, or cutting out pictures. Then stop what you're doing after a moment, go to your child, and praise him for staying away and not interrupting. Remind the child to stay with the assigned task and not to bother you, then return to what you were doing. Wait a few moments longer before returning to your child and again praising him for not bothering you. Return to your activity, wait a little longer, and again praise your child. Over time you will gradually be able to reduce how often you praise your child while increasing the length of time you can stay at your own task. Initially you'll have to interrupt yourself to praise your child very frequently, say every minute or two. After a few times like this, wait 3 minutes before praising your child. Then wait 5 minutes, and so on. Each time, return to what you're working on for a slightly longer time before going back to praise your child. The same approach applies to teaching anything new to your child: start with very frequent attention and praise, and then gradually reduce how often you compliment the new behavior.

If it sounds as if your child is about to leave the activity and come to bother you, immediately stop what you're doing, go to your child, praise her for not interrupting, and redirect the child to stay with the task.

As soon as you finish what you're doing, give the child special praise for letting you complete your task. You may even periodically give your child a small privilege or reward for having left you alone while you worked on your project.

This week, choose one or two activities—preparing a meal, talking to an adult, writing a letter, accomplishing any special project, using the telephone, reading, watching TV, doing paperwork, talking at the dinner table, visiting others' homes, housecleaning—with which to practice. If you choose talking on the phone, you might want to have someone call you once or twice a day simply as practice. That way, when important calls do come in, you have already trained your child so you can handle these calls with less interruption.

After a week of practice, ask yourself how easy you now find it to stop what you're doing to praise your child for leaving you alone and how often you remember to give your child something to do when you don't want to be interrupted. If these practices are becoming part of your typical interactions with your child, you are ready to move on.

Step 5: Set Up a Home Token System

Purpose and Goals

Children with behavior problems often need a more powerful program than praise to motivate them to do chores, follow rules, or obey commands. One way to pair compliance with powerful rewards is a home poker chip program (for children 4–8 years old) or a home point system (for 9-year-old and older children). Although you'll probably see quick results, the positive changes in your child's behavior are not likely to last if you stop using the program too soon, so plan on sticking with this program for about 2 months.

Instructions for a Chip Program

Find a set of plastic poker chips, then sit down with your child and start your reward program with a very positive tone. Say that you feel your child has not been rewarded enough for doing nice things at home and you want to set up a program so she can earn privileges for behaving properly. For a 4- or 5-year-old, explain that each chip, regardless of color, is worth one chip. For a 6- to 8-year-old, assign different denominations to the colors: white = 1 chip, blue = 5 chips, and red = 10 chips. Then tape a chip of each color to a small piece of cardboard, label them with their points, and post the card where your child can easily refer to it.

You and your child should then make a bank—from a shoe box, a coffee can (with a dull rim), a plastic jar, or some other container—for storing the chips earned. Have some fun decorating it with your child.

Now compile a list of the privileges the child will earn with the poker chips. These should include not only occasional special privileges (going to movies, roller skating, buying a toy), but also the everyday privileges your child takes for granted (TV, video games, the Internet, using a cell phone, playing with special toys already in the home, riding a bike, going over to a friend's home, etc.). Be sure to list at least 10, preferably 15. They don't have to cost money; you can include any activity around the house that your child seems to enjoy.

Now make up a list of the jobs and chores you often ask your child to do: setting the table for a meal, clearing the table after a meal, cleaning a bedroom, making a bed, emptying wastebaskets, doing homework, and other typical household chores. Also you should list self-help tasks that cause conflict, like getting dressed for school, getting ready for bed, washing and bathing, and brushing teeth.

Next, decide how much each job or chore is worth in chips. For a 4- to 6-year-old, assign from one to three chips for most tasks and perhaps five for really big jobs. For a 6- to 8-year-old, use a range of 1 to 10 chips and perhaps give a larger amount for big jobs. Remember, the harder the job, the more chips you will pay.

Now calculate how many chips you think your child will earn in a typical day if he does most of the tasks you usually assign; write this number on a scratch pad. We generally suggest that two-thirds of the child's daily chips be spent on common privileges and one-third be saved toward the purchase of special longer term rewards. If your child can earn about 30 chips a day for doing daily work, for example, 20 should be spent on everyday privileges. The easiest way to do this is to start assigning a price to each daily privilege and then add them up to see if they total about two-thirds of the child's daily earnings. If the total is higher, go back and reduce the price of the privileges until they do add up to about two-thirds. Don't worry about exact numbers; just use your judgment and be fair.

Now go back and assign a price to the special privileges. Ask yourself how often you think your child should have access to these, then multiply the number of days you feel your child should wait to have each long-term privilege by the number of chips saved (one-third of the daily income). If your child earns 30 chips a day, and you wish your child to be able to rent a video game every 2 weeks, the price of that privilege should be 14 days × 10 chips, or 140 chips. Do this for each long-term privilege, again not worrying about precise amounts. An example of a home chip program is provided in Table 3.

Be sure to tell your child that she will have a chance to earn bonus chips when chores are done with a good attitude. That is, if the chore is done promptly and pleasantly, you will give your child extra chips. Be sure to also say that you like her positive work attitude. You should not give these chips all the time.

Be sure to tell the child that chips will be given only for jobs done on the first request. If you have to repeat a command, the child will not receive any chips.

Finally, be sure to go out of your way this week to give chips away for any small appropriate behavior even if it is not on your list of chores. Remember, you can reward a child even for good behaviors that are not on that list. Be alert for opportunities to reward the child.

Do not take chips away this week for misbehavior!

Once your child has earned the chips, he has the right to spend them. There will, of course, be times such as bedtime when it just is not reasonable or convenient for your child to have that privilege at that time, but he should be able to ask you when he can have this reward so you can schedule it at the next convenient time.

Instructions for a Home Point System

Set up a notebook like a checkbook with five columns—one each for the date, the item, deposits, withdrawals, and the running balance. When your child is rewarded

TABLE 3. Sample of a Home Chip Program Job and Privilege List for a 6- to 8-Year-Old

Job	*Payment*	*Reward*	*Cost*
Get dressed	5	Watch TV (30 minutes)	4
Wash hands/face	2	Play video games (30 minutes)	5
Brush teeth	2	Play outside in yard	2
Make bed	5	Ride bike	2
Put dirty clothes away	2	Use a special toy	4
Pick up toys	3	Go out for fast food	200
Take dirty dishes to sink after eating	1	Rent a video game or movie	300
Homework (per 15 minutes)	5	Go bowling/miniature golf or roller/ice skating	400
Give dog fresh water	1	Stay up past bedtime (30 minutes)	50
Take bath/shower	5	Have a friend over to play	40
Hang up coat	1	Have a friend sleep over	150
No fights with sibling		Go to a video arcade	300
Breakfast to lunch	3	Get my allowance ($2/week)	100
Lunch to dinner	3	Choose a special dessert	20
Dinner to bedtime	3	Go play at a friend's home	50
Use nice voice with Mom/Dad when asking for something	1		
Get pajamas on	3		
Come when called	2		
Tell the truth when asked about a problem	3		
Positive attitude	Bonus		

Note. I estimated that this child would earn about 50 chips each day for doing just the daily routine tasks on a typical school day. I then made sure that 25–30 of these chips would be needed to buy the daily privileges of television (1 hour), video games (1 hour), playing outside, riding a bike, and playing with a special toy that Mom and Dad control access to (such as a remote control car, a racecar set and track, a train set, an army battle station with troops, a doll with clothes and accessories, a personal MP3 player or iPod, in-line skates, skateboard). The remaining privileges were priced by determining how often the child should have access to that reward—that is, how many days of waiting and saving.

with points, write in the job under "item" and enter the amount as a "deposit." Add it to the child's balance. When she buys a privilege, note the privilege under "item," place this amount in the withdrawal column and deduct this amount from the "balance." Only parents are to write in the notebook. The child may look at the book any time she likes but may not make entries.

The program works just like the chip system, except that you record points in the book instead of giving poker chips and use larger numbers for the value of each job. We generally use a range of 5–25 points for most daily jobs and up to 200 points for very big jobs. A good rule of thumb is to give about 25 points for every 15 minutes of effort that a job might require for her to complete.

Hints

1. Review the list of rewards and jobs every few weeks or so and add new ones as you deem necessary. Check with your child for new rewards she may want on the list.
2. You can reward your child with chips or points for almost any form of good behavior. They can even be used in conjunction with step 4 to reward your child for not interrupting your work.
3. Do not give the chips or points away before the child has done what he was told to do, but be as quick as possible in rewarding the child for compliance. Don't wait to reward!
4. Both parents should use the chip or point system to make it as effective as possible.
5. When you give points or chips for good behavior, smile and tell your child what you like that she has done.

Try this program for at least 1 week before moving on to the next step. You'll know that you're ready to move on when your child is doing most of the assigned jobs or chores, your child seems to be enjoying the program, and you find it fairly easy to remember to give out the chips/points. Do not move on to the next step until you believe this program has become routine. Some parents find that this takes 2 weeks.

Step 6: Learn to Punish Misbehavior Constructively

Purpose and Goals

The sixth step is the most critical part of the program. Using this method of discipline with children when they misbehave or fail to comply with a command requires great skill. The goal is to decrease your child's defiant behavior, refusals to obey, or other misbehavior.

"If ADHD is causing my child to disobey," you may ask, "how can any method of discipline help?" ADHD does *not* directly cause children to refuse or defy your requests. It does, however, cause them problems with complying if the task assigned is lengthy, boring, repetitive, or otherwise tedious. It also causes them to be distracted more during the task. Refusing to obey initially with a request is not ADHD behavior. It is defiant behavior and can be greatly reduced by using this program.

Why do children with ADHD become defiant in the first place? Partly because many tasks are frankly boring but necessary and that boredom is often unpleasant to a child with ADHD, who craves stimulation, fun, and novelty. Or they may become defiant because of all the criticism they received in the past for their lack of persistence; so they learn to balk in circumstances where they fear they'll fail or be criticized yet again. Some adults unwittingly train such children to be oppositional by relying solely on excessive criticism and negative consequences. This is one reason this program emphasizes incentive programs before punishment. Parents also train children with ADHD to become defiant when their response to an initial emotional display teaches the children that resistance, defiance, and negativity are effective means of avoiding work. Also keep in mind that research on social cooperation, sharing, altruism, and concern for others shows that such behaviors develop when a person expects to interact with people again in the future. A child who has a restricted sense of the future, as in ADHD, is less concerned about and motivated to cooperate with others because the child with ADHD lives in "the now" and cooperation is about the social "later" of life: Will that person want to interact with you again in the future?

It is the manner in which you respond to these initial gambits at resistance that determines how excessive and severe they will become. Consequently, by responding to defiance in the manner prescribed here, you can greatly reduce such behaviors in a child with ADHD.

Instructions for Fining Your Child

After you have been using the chip or point system for 1–2 weeks, you can begin to use it occasionally and selectively as a form of discipline. Just tell your child that whenever he is asked to perform a chore or an instruction, he can be fined for not listening to you or following through. From then on, if you give a command and your child does not respond or obey, follow up with "If you do not do as I said on the count of 3, you will lose ____ chips [or points]." Count to 3. If the child still has not begun to comply, deduct from the bank or point book the amount you would have paid for completing the work. If the job is not on the chore list, choose a fine that seems reasonable for the severity of the misbehavior.

You can use fines for any form of misbehavior from this week onward. However, be very careful not to fine excessively or too frequently, or you will wipe out your child's bank account quickly, and the program will no longer work to motivate your child to behave. Consider this: How much would you want to return to work again if your boss took your entire paycheck after the first week because of some minor rule infraction on the job? In general, use the three-to-one rule—for every three times you reward, you can fine the child once. If you find yourself fining your child too frequently and the program has lost its appeal or its ability to motivate your child, stop the program for a month or so. When you start anew, be sure not to fine your child so much.

Instructions for Using Time-Out

Time-out is a frequently used form of punishment for more serious misbehavior. It involves removing the child to a quiet, isolated location to serve a penalty period. Use time-out with only one or two forms of misbehavior during the next week. Choose a type of misbehavior that is not responding very well to the token system you set up in the previous step.

Never give a command that you do not intend to back up with consequences to see that the job gets done. *Always* give your first command to a child in a firm but neutral or pleasant voice. *Do not* yell it at the child, but also do not make it "iffy" by asking it as a favor. You may add "please" to your request or directive, but do not pose it as a favor or question.

After you have given the command, count to 5. You may count out loud, but if you notice that your child gets used to this and waits until the very last count of 5 before obeying you, keep the counting to yourself.

If the child has not made a move to comply within these 5 seconds, make direct eye contact, raise the volume of your voice (but don't yell or scream), adopt a firm posture or stance, and say, "If you don't [do what I ask], then you are going to sit in that chair!" (Point to a chair in the corner.) Once you give this warning, count to 5 again. If the child has not started to comply within 5 seconds, take the child firmly by the wrist or upper arm and say, "You did not do as I asked, so you must go to time-out!"

You should say this in a somewhat louder and even firmer tone of voice, but not with anger. You are raising the volume of your voice to get the child's attention, not out of your own loss of emotional control. Then take the child to the time-out chair. The child is to go to the chair immediately, regardless of any promises she may make. If the child resists, use slight physical guidance if need be. For instance, grasp your child firmly by the upper arm or shoulder and escort the child to the chair. If necessary, take hold of the waist seam at the back of the child's trousers and at the back seam of the shirt collar to guide the child to the chair *without physical harm.* The child is not to go to the bathroom, get a drink, or stand and argue. The child is to be taken immediately to the time-out chair.

Place the child in the chair and say sternly, "You stay there until I tell you to get up!" You may tell the child that you are not coming back to the chair until he has become quiet, but don't say this more than once. Do not argue with the child or let anyone else talk to the child during this time. Instead, go back to your work, but be sure to keep an eye on what the child is doing in the chair. Your child should stay in time-out until three conditions are met:

1. The child must always serve a "minimum sentence" of 1 to 2 minutes for each year of age—1 minute for mild to moderate misbehavior and 2 minutes for serious misbehavior.

2. Once the minimum sentence is over, wait until the child is quiet. This may take several minutes to an hour or longer the first time your child is sent to time-out. You are not to go to the child until she has been quiet for about 30 seconds or so, even if it means the child remains in time-out for up to 1 or 2 hours because she is arguing, throwing a tantrum, screaming, or crying loudly.

3. Once the child has been quiet for a few moments, the child must agree to do what he was told to do. If it was a chore, the child must agree to do it. If it is something the child cannot correct, such as swearing or lying, the child is to promise not to do it again. If the child fails to agree to do as asked (says "No!"), instruct the child to sit in the chair until you give permission to leave it. The child is then to serve another minimum sentence, become quiet, and agree to do what was asked. The child is not to leave the chair until he has agreed to obey the command originally given. When the child has complied, say in a neutral tone of voice, "I like it when you do as I say."

Watch for the next appropriate behavior by your child and praise the child for it. This ensures that the child always receives as much reward as punishment, and it shows that you are not angry at the child but at the inappropriate behavior.

What If the Child Leaves the Chair without Permission?

Many children will test their parents' authority when time-out is first used by trying to escape from the chair before the time is up. Generally, a child is considered to have left the chair if both buttocks leave the flat seat. The child does not have to face the wall. We also consider rocking the chair and tipping it over leaving. The child should be warned about this. If the chair itself routinely becomes a plaything, then just place a small carpet or mat on the floor in the same corner and use that as the time-out location. Or if you live in a two-story home, use the first step of the stairway to the second floor as the time-out location.

The first time the child leaves the chair (mat or stair), put her back and say loudly and sternly, "If you get off that [chair, mat, stair] again, I am going to fine you!" When the child leaves the chair again, take a large number of chips or points—one-fifth of the typical daily earnings—from the child's bank account. Return the child to the chair and say, "Now you stay there until I say you can get up!"

Thereafter, fine the child each time he leaves the chair, even if the child is sent to time-out again for some other misbehavior. If the child leaves the chair without permission, *do not* give the warning again, but go straight to fining. Do not, however, fine your child more than twice during this episode for leaving the chair. Instead, consider using the following penalty for escape: send your child to his or her bedroom for the time-out period. Be sure to remove all toys, video games, TVs, stereos, and other sources of entertainment or play from the room. If it is not possible to clear the room of all attractive play materials, be sure to restrict your child to sitting on the bed.

Some parents and professionals believe that using a child's bed as a place for time-out may result in later sleeping problems, but I am aware of no scientific evidence for this.

Where Should the Chair Be Placed?

The chair should be straight-backed and placed in a corner far enough away from the wall that the child cannot kick it. No play objects should be nearby, and the child should not be able to watch TV. Most parents use a corner of a kitchen, a first-floor laundry room, a foyer, the middle or end of a long hallway, or a corner of a living room (not occupied by others). You should be able to observe the child while continuing your business. Do not use bathrooms, closets, or the child's bedroom (at first). As noted above, sometimes the child can be told to sit on a mat in a corner instead of a chair or on the first step of a stairway going to the second floor. Do not use the steps going into a basement, since many young children have a fear of basements (and the dark).

What Can You Expect This Week?

Typically children become quite surprised and upset when first sent to time-out, in part because you are behaving now in an unexpected way and with firmness. They may become quite angry and vocal or may cry because their feelings have been hurt. For many children, this tantrum only prolongs the first time-out; anywhere from 15–30 minutes is typical but can range up to 1 or 2 hours before they become quiet and agree to do what was asked of them before the first time-out. Gradually your child will begin to obey your first commands, or at least your warnings about time-out, so that the frequency of time-out eventually decreases. However, this may take a week or two. Try to remember during this first week that you are not harming your child but helping to teach her better self-control, respect for parental authority, and the need to follow rules.

What If You Find Yourself Getting Upset?

Most parental anger comes from having to repeat unheeded requests many times over a long time. Few parents I know have found themselves getting upset using this program, because little time elapses between the child's first failure to obey and the next move they are supposed to make. Should you find that you are getting emotionally upset, however, consider the following possible causes:

- Are you repeating your requests too frequently before imposing a consequence for noncompliance? Are you stringing this interaction out so long that you have plenty of time to build anger?
- Are you permitting a problem elsewhere in your life to spill over into your interactions with your child? If so, sit down and try to think of ways to deal directly with that problem. Letting it affect your relationship with your child is grossly unfair to your child and to you.
- Are you becoming persistently depressed or anxious? These emotional states can make your reactions more bitter, hostile, or irritable. Try some of the stress management suggestions in the earlier chapter. Seek help from a qualified psychologist, psychiatrist, or other mental health specialist for evaluation and possible treatment, if necessary.

Hints

1. The child is not to leave the time-out location to use the bathroom, get a drink, or eat a meal (the child can eat afterward). Make no effort to prepare the child a special snack later to compensate for a missed meal, because what makes time-out effective is what your child misses while in the chair.
2. If you want to use the time-out method for bedtime behavior problems, you will need to double the penalty period your child serves, because the child is not missing much of importance to them at bedtime by sitting in the chair.
3. Do not use these punishment procedures out of the home for the next 2 weeks.
4. Be sure to continue the exercises from the previous steps, especially the token system, during the next week.

Step 7: Expand Your Use of Time-Out

Purpose

Just keep using the time-out and fining program. If the particular misbehavior you were targeting for time-out is now declining, target one or two new types of misbehavior this week. Remember, the goal is not to use punishment excessively. Do not extend the use of time-out to any new misbehavior if you're still using time-out fairly frequently (more than two to three times per week) for the last misbehavior.

You can move on to the next step when you have been using time-out for at least 2 or 3 weeks at home and find that the targeted misbehaviors are declining in frequency. You do not need to eliminate or reduce all behavior problems at home to move to the next step. If the child is not responsive, and conflicts are as bad as or worse than when you started, return to your mental health professional for advice or find one who is expert in child behavior management methods like those used here.

Step 8: Learn to Manage Your Child in Public Places

Purpose and Goals

Once you feel that you have your child's behavior under reasonable control at home, you can use these methods in stores, restaurants, churches, others' homes, and other places. Your goal this week is to begin to reduce your child's misbehavior when you're away from home. You can do this fairly easily by using the methods learned up to this point: (1) positive attention and praise for good behavior; (2) praise for complying with directions; (3) effective delivery of commands; (4) tokens or points for good behavior; and (5) fines and time-out for misbehavior.

Instructions

The key to managing children in public places is to establish a plan and make sure your child is aware of the plan *before* you go into the public place. This method has been introduced in Chapter 9. Follow these easy rules:

Rule 1: Set Up the Rules before Entering the Place

Just before you enter a public place, *stop* and review the important rules of conduct with your child. Give your child about three rules that he commonly violates in that particular place, and tell the child to say them back to you. If your child refuses to repeat them, warn your child that he will be placed in time-out in the car. If the child still refuses, return to your car and place the child in time-out.

Rule 2: Set Up an Incentive for the Child's Compliance

While still standing in front of the place, tell your child what she will earn for adhering to the rules. Chips or points can be used as effective rewards for good behavior while out of the home. Or, for a child under age 4, take along a small bag of relatively healthy snack food (peanuts, raisins, pretzels, corn chips, etc.) or some juice to dispense periodically for good behavior throughout the trip. On occasion, you may wish to promise your child a purchase of some sort at the end of the trip, but this should be done only on rare occasions and for exceptionally good behavior so that the child does not come to expect it.

A comment about using food rewards with children: current folk wisdom and pop psychology have it that some children become obese adults because they or their parents used food as rewards for successes or accomplishments. I am aware of no scientific research that supports such conditioning. Nevertheless, use snacks or treats only if other, more social or symbolic rewards (such as praise, tokens, or points) are not effective, and always use healthy snacks when possible, provided that they are ones the child enjoys; this is supposed to be a reward after all.

Rule 3: Set Up Your Punishment for Noncompliance

While still outside the place, tell your child what the punishment will be for not following the rules or for misbehavior. In most cases this will be the loss of points or chips for minor rule violations, and the use of time-out for moderate to major misbehavior or noncompliance. Don't be afraid to use the time-out method in a public place—it's the most effective method away from home. As soon as you enter the public place, look for a convenient time-out location (see sidebar, p. 206) and attend to and praise your child for following the rules.

Give chips or points to your child periodically throughout the trip rather than waiting until the end. In addition, give frequent praise and attention to the child for obeying the rules. If your child starts to misbehave, *immediately* take away chips or points or place the child in time-out. Do not repeat commands or warnings.

The minimum sentence for time-out in a public place should be only half of what it is at home. That is because there is much to be missed while in time-out in public, not to mention some additional embarrassment to the child from public scrutiny. If the child leaves time-out without permission, use your at-home fining method.

Whenever you are out with your child, act quickly (within 10 seconds) so that misbehavior does not escalate into a loud confrontation or a temper tantrum. Also, be sure to give frequent praise and rewards throughout the trip to reinforce good behavior.

Rule 4: Assign an Activity

It is very important when away from home that you provide your child with activities to do, especially if you are making several stops, such as when shopping or running errands. Children often get bored during such outings, and this is particularly true of those with ADHD. Small hand-held computer games, netbooks, tablets, or smart phones that can connect to Netflix or other online libraries of children's

Time-Out Spots in Public Places

In Department Stores: (1) Place the child facing a dull side of an uncrowded display counter or a corner. (2) Take the child to the coats section and have him face the coat rack. (3) Use the gift wrap or credit department area where there is a dull corner. (4) Use a dull corner of a rest room. (5) Use a changing or dressing room if nearby. (6) Use a maternity section (it is not very busy, and there are sympathetic moms there).

In Grocery Stores: (1) Have the child face the side of a frozen foods counter. (2) Take the child to the farthest corner of the store. (3) Find the greeting card display and have the child face the dull side of the counter while you look at cards. (Most grocery stores are difficult for finding an out-of-the-way location, so you may have to use one of the alternatives to time-out listed on the facing page.)

In Places of Worship: (1) Take the child to the "crying room" found in most churches and synagogues. (2) Use the foyer or entryway. (3) Use a rest room off the lobby.

In a Restaurant: Use the rest rooms or one of the alternatives listed in the text.

In Another's Home: Explain that you are using a new child management method and may need to place your child in a chair (or on a stairway step) or in a dull corner if misbehavior develops. If this cannot be done, use one of the alternatives listed in the text (p. 207).

During a Long Car Trip: Review the rules with the child and set up your incentive before the child enters the car. Be sure to take along games or activities for the child to do. Explain that chips can be earned or lost. If you need to punish the child, take away chips or points. If this fails, pull off the road to a safe stopping area and have the child serve the time-out seated on the ground beside the car on a floor mat, with you standing nearby. Never leave the child in or beside the car unattended.

programming are great for this. So are small mechanical drawing toys, like the ageless Etch-A-Sketch. Many restaurants provide crayons and paper, or even pictures to be colored, but don't rely on this. Take along the materials for some diversion that you know your child enjoys. What matters most is that you take something enjoyable and physical to occupy the child's mind and hands while you are busy accomplishing your errands. If you are caught away from home and forgot to take something along for your child to do, see if you can give him something to do that is related to the purpose for the trip. For instance, let your child push the cart in the grocery store or go down toward the end of the aisle and get products off the shelf that you know the child can recognize. Next time you can plan ahead to take something with you to occupy your child's hands, mind, and time.

When Time-Out Is Impractical

There are always a few places where putting your child in a corner for misbehavior is not possible. Here are some alternatives, but use them *only where you cannot find a time-out area:*

1. Take the child outside the building and have him face the wall.
2. Take the child back to your car and have her sit on the back seat. Stay in the front seat or beside the car.
3. Take along a small spiral notepad. Before entering the public place, tell the child that you will write down any episode of misbehavior and he will have to go to time-out as soon as you get home. You will find it helpful to take a picture of him when he is in time-out at home and to keep this with your notepad or in your smart phone. Show this picture to him in front of the public place and explain that misbehavior will put him in time-out when you return home.
4. Take along a felt-tipped pen. Tell the child in front of the public place that if she misbehaves, you will lightly place a hash mark in ink on the back of the child's hand. She will then serve a minimum sentence in time-out at home for each ink mark on her hand.

When Future Behavior Problems Occur

At this point you should find your interactions with your child more positive, particularly in work-related situations, and your child more cooperative with your requests. If you have found no change in your child and the level of conflict is still distressingly high, by all means return to your current mental health professional or someone else who is expert in assisting parents with child behavior management problems.

However, even if you've been successful with these eight steps, remember that all children occasionally develop behavior problems. Fortunately, you now have the skills to deal with these problems. Here are some steps to follow if a new problem develops or an old problem returns.

1. Take out a notebook and begin recording the behavior problem. Try to be specific about what your child is doing wrong. Record the rule that is being broken, exactly what the child is doing wrong, and what you are now doing to manage it.

2. Keep this record for a week or so. Then examine it to see what clues it may give you about how to deal with the problem. Many parents find that at least part of the problem is caused by their return to old, ineffective ways of dealing with the child. Always review your own behavior as well as your child's. Are you:

- Repeating commands too often?
- Using ineffective methods for commands?
- Providing insufficient attention, praise, or reward to the child for following the rule correctly? (Have you stopped your poker chip or points system too early?)
- Not providing discipline immediately for the rule violation?
- Stopping your special playtime with the child?

If you find yourself slipping back to these old habits, correct them. Go back and review the steps from this program to make sure you're using the methods properly.

3. If you need to, set up a special program for managing the problem. Explain to your child exactly what you expect to be done in the problem situation. Set up a poker chip or point system to reward the child for following the rules. Immediately impose mild fines each time the problem behavior occurs.

If the fines don't work, try using a time-out immediately upon the occurrence of the misconduct or defiance. If your notes indicate that the problem seems to be occurring in one particular place or situation, follow the directions for managing your child in public places: (a) anticipate the problem and review the rules just before the problem develops; (b) review the incentives for good behavior; (c) review the punishment for misbehavior; and (d) assign an activity.

A Final Note

The methods described in this chapter should be used immediately and frequently, with little talk or discussion. They should be applied consistently and fairly—and, above all, with the 14 principles from Chapter 9 firmly in mind. Never become so emotionally or personally invested in the program that you cannot maintain a sense of perspective on your child's disability and a sense of humor about your role as parent of a child with ADHD. Most important, don't personalize your child's behavior problems. Practice daily forgiveness of your child's transgressions and your own mistakes.

You stand to reap substantial rewards. Parents who follow this eight-step program find their child's behavior more socially appropriate, cooperative, and friendly. They instill in their child a sense of responsibility and openness to learning from adults through compliance with their advice, rules, and instructions. The child's interactions with siblings also become more positive and cooperative. Some parents even find that their ability to manage other children in the family is greatly improved, as is their marital or couple relationship, now that the behavioral problems of the child with ADHD have been diminished. Certainly most parents undertaking this program report a renewed sense of self-confidence and competence in their roles as parents, teachers, and friends to their children with ADHD. I hope you find that this program does the same for you.

12 Taking Charge at Home

THE ART OF PROBLEM SOLVING

The eight steps in Chapter 11—and the advice in the rest of this book—should prepare you for many different situations, but they cannot cover every possible eventuality. Undoubtedly there will be times when you're not sure how to handle a new problem. When that happens, try some of the following methods.

A System for Solving New Problems

Many of us are already adept at problem solving, but we use this ability somewhat automatically and would not find it easy to call it forth on command. The following seven steps systematize the process so that you can tap this natural resource even when the stress of the situation is clouding your mind. Most of the time they will reveal a plan of action that you might not have thought of otherwise. This process works even better if you go through it with your spouse/partner or a close family friend. Two heads, as they say, are better than one.

Step 1: Define the Problem

Before you can solve a problem, you must define it clearly. For instance, the problem may be that your child does not pick up his toys or do his homework when asked. Either of these descriptions is a better way of stating the problem than "My child won't listen to me" or "Why won't my child do as I ask?" The first approach uses clear and specific terms to define the problem; the second is vague and does not convey what the child is or is not doing or precisely what you expect of the child.

Write down on a sheet of paper exactly what behavior problem you wish to solve.

Step 2: Rephrase It as Positive Behavior

Now rephrase the problem as the behavior you desire from the child instead. "My child does not pick up his toys," for example, could become "My child will learn to pick up his toys when asked to do so." This makes the objective of your behavior management plan very clear.

Let's take a slightly more complicated example. Suppose you originally stated the problem as "My child lies." This is not a bad first attempt, but it could be more specific: "My child lies to me when I confront her about something wrong she has done." This makes it clear that your child does not lie all the time, but only when confronted about some possible misdeed. Then you could rephrase it as "My child will learn to be honest and tell me the truth when I ask her about something she may have done wrong."

This is how educational plans are written for children in special education programs. Rephrasing problems as objectives guides school staff members to help a child by stating more clearly and usefully what they wish to achieve with the child. Doing this has a way of making the means of accomplishing your goal more obvious. When you know what behavior you want to encourage, it's often easier to remember that reinforcing this behavior should be your goal. So the solution could be "I will reward my child when she tells me honestly what she has done" or "I will test my child's honesty periodically throughout the day by asking her what she has been doing. If she gives me an accurate answer, I will reward her for it."

Write down the word *Goal* on your sheet of paper and underline it. Next to this word, write down the positive alternative behavior to the problem behavior you just recorded. You now have two statements on your sheet: the problem, stated specifically; and the goal, the desired alternative to the problem.

Step 3: List Your Options

Here's where you let your creativity flow. Your job now is to brainstorm as many possible options as you can think of to handle the problem behavior and achieve your goal. This sounds easier than it actually is, because many people start to list a possible solution and immediately become critical of their own ideas. When you criticize yourself too quickly, you stop your creative juices from flowing. Leave the criticism until later. For now, your task is to be inventive. Let your mind be free to wonder about anything you like related to your objective, and to wander across the subject. Think about how other parents seem to handle this problem. Think about what you may have seen on TV or in the movies or what you may have read in books about this problem. How would your own parents have handled it? How would your best friends handle it? What do you think a physician or psychologist might tell you?

On your sheet of paper, write down the word *Options* and underline it. Below this, start to write down all possible options or alternatives, no matter how silly they seem. Write down any solution you think others might propose, even if you think you would not handle it their way. Your job right now is to get as many options or solutions on paper as possible.

Step 4: Constructively Evaluate Your Options

Now return to the first option on your list and think about how it will work. What is likely to happen if you try this? Do you foresee any problems? Could those problems be handled easily? Be reasonable and fair in your evaluation. Don't discard an option just because it might take a little effort to implement. It could turn out to be the most effective option on your list.

After you evaluate each option this way, place a number from 1 to 10 next to it, with 1 representing the lowest or most negative evaluation and 10 your most positive evaluation.

Step 5: Select the Best Option

Most of the time, selecting the best option is pretty easy. The numbers next to each item naturally guide your attention to those with the most desirable ratings. Focus on these for a moment. Perhaps you ranked several as equally useful. Reconsider them. Which do you feel is most likely to work for you or to get a positive response from your child? If you cannot decide, just pick one at random to try first. You're simply going to test this idea, as you'd test a hypothesis in a scientific experiment. If it doesn't work, you can return to your list to try the other positive options. If it works, you can continue trying it. The point is that no one is expecting you to pick the "right" answer. No one knows beforehand what is going to be right for a particular child. If you expect to predict accurately all the time, you're asking for much disappointment. Testing the ideas that you believe have merit with an open mind is what we call "scientific parenting"—surely a more realistic, practical, and forgiving approach than striving to be right all the time.

Circle the option you've chosen. If necessary, write it out in more detail so you know exactly what to expect of yourself. Put the solution into practice for a week, and if it seems to be working, continue it for as long as seems necessary. If it does not work very well, look at other possibilities on your list and put another likely solution into effect for a week. Continue this way until you feel you've solved the problem.

Step 6: Compromise on Disagreements

If you've been working at problem solving with another adult, such as your spouse/partner or a close friend, you may disagree on the choice of options. Try not to be too wedded to your own choice in that case. Ask about the other adult's reasoning in more detail and listen carefully to the response. Then briefly explain your own choice. One of you may find yourself convinced.

If you're still deadlocked, give in to the other person—yes, give in! Remember, you are experimenting for a week or so, not changing your family routine for life. You can afford to go along with the other adult's preference for a week. That means being fair too; avoid any temptation to sabotage the other person's choice. If it fails on its own merits, you can go back to your list and try out the one you had chosen.

Step 7: Carry Out Your Plan and Evaluate Its Success

Now that you have a plan, stick to it. Child behavior problems are not likely to be resolved in just a few days. Don't be thrown off the track by failure to see results at the start or by the objections of others—especially those of your child. I have worked with parents who have set up a behavior contract with a child to do homework and then withdrawn it just because the child expressed some initial displeasure. If this happens to you, stay with your plan. Your child's protests may mean that you're right on target—that the child has recognized the need to change behavior to succeed under this new plan, which is exactly what you want. You would not avoid having your child inoculated against disease just because your child dislikes shots; neither should you drop efforts that you know will improve your child's behavior in the long run just because he or she protests the procedure.

After a week or so of consistently following your plan, you can take time to evaluate its success. If it does not seem to be working, go back to your list and select another option. But don't criticize yourself because the first plan did not work. Remember, you are experimenting, and that means there are no guarantees.

Preparing Your Child for Transitions

Knowing that children with ADHD live in the moment and have trouble anticipating and making preparations for the future, you probably are not too surprised when your child has trouble adapting quickly to a new activity. All children get frustrated by adults' control over their use of time, but for children with ADHD making the transitions that even a regular schedule imposes can be a struggle. Typically these children have difficulty switching from a fun, rewarding activity to one they perceive as boring, such as switching from play to homework or to doing chores, or from TV time to dinnertime or bedtime. But they also have trouble switching gears—from active outdoor play, for example, to an inactive long drive in the car. Your child might find switching abruptly to a new set of rules problematic as well: being quiet when a phone call interrupts time spent with a parent, or being courteous and staying in one room when a visitor arrives in the middle of the child's playing freely at home. A child without ADHD may learn to anticipate transitions from, say, TV time to homework time, because that activity transition occurs at about the same time each school day. To a child with ADHD, however, the switch may seem far more intrusive because the child does not learn to anticipate as well.

As suggested in Chapter 11 for managing your child in a public place, the best approach is to help your child prepare in advance for transitions. Here are some recommendations:

1. A few minutes *before* the transition to the new activity must take place, give your child advance notice, such as "Dinner will be ready in just a few minutes. At that time I will ask you to turn off the TV, wash your hands, and come to the table." These statements help to prepare your child for the upcoming transition, and they set the occasion for you to come back in a few minutes and give a firmer command about coming to dinner.

2. Politely ask your child to repeat this warning back to you so you know that the child heard what you said. This is especially important when your child is mentally absorbed in another activity, such as TV or a video game. Simply saying, "Did you hear what I said?" may elicit a "Yes" just so the child isn't scolded for not listening.

3. When the transition time arrives, give the instruction to obey as a direct but neutral, business-like command: "Tommy, as I told you a few minutes ago, it's now time for dinner. Turn off the TV and wash your hands." Ignore any protests and don't argue. Simply restate the command if necessary, then ensure that it is followed, even if that means turning off the TV yourself. Reward your child for following through on the instruction. If your child does not listen, follow the steps given in Chapter 11 for fines, loss of privileges, or time-out.

Using When/Then Strategies

Just as children with ADHD don't anticipate transitions, they are unlikely to anticipate the future consequences of their present actions or to associate these later consequences with what they are now about to do. So spelling out the consequences is very helpful to them. You can also take this a step further: rearrange events so that how your child behaves now does lead to something more rewarding to do a little later.

Arranging artificial links between a child's current behavior and later rewards has been called the *Premack principle,* after Dr. David Premack. According to the Premack principle, any activity or behavior that occurs frequently can be used as a reward for one that occurs less often. (Some people have also called this *Grandma's rule.*) Dr. Charles Cunningham at McMaster University Medical School calls it a *when/then strategy,* and it involves denying the child access to a fun activity until some non-fun but necessary work is done: "*When* you do your homework, *then* you can watch

TV." This is a very inexpensive way of rewarding a child because it transforms activities that are already usually available to the child into privileges to be earned. Because the child is used to having free access to these privileges, however, at first he is likely to protest having to earn them by doing some work. This means sticking to your guns may require some extra diligence from you.

The strategies presented in this chapter all require you to plan ahead to reduce hassles when a problem develops. They can actually be fun to use, can become a natural part of your parenting behavior, and can help your child be happier and more socially cooperative in your family and with others.

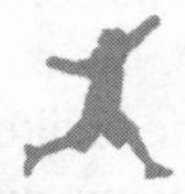

13 How to Help Your Child with Peer Problems

"Andrea called me the other day and said that she didn't want us to bring Bobby to her house for the holidays this year. In fact, he's not welcome at family dinners at all—unless he can learn to 'behave.' I was devastated—this is my own sister!"

"We were really hoping that Girl Scouts would be a positive experience for Samantha, and we tried to explain to the troop leader what she might expect from our daughter. So when she told us Samantha was too disruptive to remain in the troop, all we could think was 'Why couldn't we have worked together on this?' "

"Last week our next-door neighbor arrived at our door with our son in tow and a litany of Tommy's infractions. Each one, of course, was just another way of saying 'Why can't you control this kid?' And I knew then that Tommy would never be invited back. What am I going to do with him after school every day? He's alienated everyone on the block."

"We've tried to keep her from finding out about these things, but kids can be cruel. What do you say to your daughter when she comes to you with tears in her eyes and wants to know why she's the only one in her kindergarten class who wasn't invited to the birthday party—again?"

My colleagues and I frequently hear stories like these at our ADHD clinics. You're probably familiar with this kind of treatment too. If so, you know that peer relationship problems can be the most upsetting of all the problems faced by children with ADHD. As adults you know full well the lifelong value of friendship, yet you also know that you cannot force other children to like and befriend your child with ADHD. Watching your child be rejected over and over by peers can be emotionally devastating. You see the impact that it has on your child's self-esteem and the loneliness it creates. Even though you can work with the child to solve problems at home and have the staff do the same at school, in the social arena you often must stand by helplessly.

I am reminded of a *Dennis the Menace* cartoon in which his mother is kneeling and holding a crying Dennis in her arms as he says that he came home early from school because he needed someone to be on his side. No other picture I have seen captures so well the feeling often expressed by parents of children with ADHD—that they are the only ones, at times, who are on their children's side.

A child with ADHD often has serious problems getting along with other children. The child's overactivity and impulsivity are often considered irritating or aversive by other children, especially if the other children are trying to work or play a game together. Other children will also not like the bluntness or frankness of the child with ADHD, especially if the child makes cruel remarks about them. Certainly other children are threatened by how easily and suddenly the child with ADHD becomes upset, frustrated, or aggressive. When the child is verbally or physically aggressive, defiant, oppositional, or hostile, problems getting along with other children are particularly acute. The end result is a bad reputation for the child among neighborhood peers or classmates.

At the heart of all these social problems is the child's underdeveloped sense of time and the future. Children with ADHD tend to live in the moment—what they can get right now is what's important to them. This means that social skills that generally have no immediate payoff, like sharing, cooperating, taking turns, keeping promises, and expressing an interest in another person, generally do not seem very valuable to them. And because they fail to consider future consequences, they often don't see that their selfishness and self-centeredness in the moment result in their losing friends in the long run. They simply do not understand the concept of building close relationships based on mutual exchanges of favors and interests across time.

Trying to help a child with ADHD who has social problems can be a major challenge for a parent and may not always be fruitful. Parents normally can't be there during their child's interactions with peers, so they can't prompt their child to inhibit impulsive urges or to stop and think about how to behave. For these and other reasons, parents are not likely to have a great deal of influence over their children's social skills or peer relations. Nevertheless, they can have some influence.

"Our son has no friends. What can we do so that other children will like him?"

Experts on the social interaction problems of children with ADHD recommend that parents try (1) working on good social skills with the children, (2) helping the children deal with teasing, (3) arranging for positive peer contacts at home, (4) setting up positive peer contacts in the community, and (5) recruiting help with peer problems from the school.

Working on Good Social Skills

Although it may not carry over into social interactions with other children outside the home, working on social skills within the home or family certainly cannot hurt your child's social relationships. Think of yourself as a "friendship coach" and try doing the following:

1. Establish a home reward program, such as the token or chip program described in Chapter 11, focusing on one or two social behaviors you would like to see increased in your child's daily behavior toward other children. These could include sharing, taking turns, keeping hands to self, speaking quietly, staying seated, not being bossy, or even asking other children what they want to play or how they want to play something. Don't choose too many of these behaviors to work on all at once, or it will be too cumbersome for you and unlikely to succeed.

2. Write the one or two behaviors down on a chart and post them in a place where you and your child can see them, such as on a refrigerator door or the side of a cabinet. Don't make them too obvious a display, especially if you know your child is having company that day because this could embarrass your child and create yet another social problem with other kids. This chart should simply remind both you and your child of what you are trying to work on over the next week or two.

3. Whenever you have a chance to observe your child playing with other children, take the opportunity to stop what you are doing and call your child over to you. Put your arm around the child's shoulder tenderly and then quietly review the two social behaviors you and the child are trying to work on this week. Remind your child that she can earn points or tokens for trying out these new skills and can lose points for unacceptable behavior. This procedure is similar to the strategies discussed in Chapter 12 for preparing for transitions, except that the rules you are reviewing with the child concern how to interact with other children.

4. Now start monitoring your child's behavior during play with others more frequently than you otherwise do. Whenever you notice your child using the new skills (or otherwise behaving well with another child), take a moment to praise your child for this and even award a point or token. In other words, "catch 'em being good." Make sure you wait for a natural break in the action, however. I have found that children are less likely to be embarrassed if you call them away from the play group and reward them out of earshot of the others.

5. On several occasions each week, set aside a few minutes to review with your child the new social skill that you wish to work on that week. During these few minutes you should (a) explain the skill you would like the child to try to use; (b) role-play a situation where you pretend to be a child and model the new skill; (c) have your child try it now, with you pretending to be a child; and (d) then encourage the child to try this new skill the next time he is playing with another child. Act as if you are a social skills "coach" similar to a sports coach in rehearsing the new skill. After this teaching session, be sure to use steps 1 through 4 to observe your child, remind the child to use the skill just before going off to play with others, watch for your child to use the skill, and then reward its occurrence.

6. Try digitally recording or videotaping a sample of your child's play interactions

with siblings or other neighborhood children, but do so discreetly. Many smart phones and netbooks have this option, which can make doing so quite convenient and discreet. It is probably wise initially not to say why you are doing this recording or at least not to call too much attention to it, since you want to capture typical behavior. You can review these recordings with your child to help show the child how he is acting, thereby improving his awareness of his social behavior, and to point out good things he is doing. Of course, you can then use the recording to show the child what may need to be improved in his conduct with other children. Recordings offer a concrete visual display of behavior that can be very useful to children with ADHD since they are often unaware of how they act toward others.

If these recordings are to be an effective teaching tool, however, you must make your review of them positive and constructive, even fun, not preachy or punitive. First point out what you found positive about your child's play with other kids. Make an effort to find several positive things and dwell on these, giving your child lots of positive feedback. Then pick out just one or two inappropriate things your child did. Follow step 5 to teach your child what to do instead. After the review, reward your child with points or a small privilege for taking this time. Once again, follow steps 1 through 4 for monitoring your child to "catch the child being good."

7. Another step you can take to increase your child's positive social skills is to identify another child familiar to you both who seems naturally to use good social skills. Point out what this child is doing that is positive and that your child might want to try when playing with others. But be careful; you can create resentment, especially if your child has had problems with the child you're using as a role model. Also don't use a sibling for this. The last thing most children want is to be compared unfavorably to a brother or sister. You can even use children who are on TV or in a movie as a role model for teaching these lessons.

Whichever of these approaches you try, pay attention to the following areas of social skills that may be a problem for your child: (1) beginning an interaction with another child or group; (2) starting and maintaining a conversation with another child (this includes listening to the other child, asking about the other child's ideas or feelings, taking turns in the conversations, and generally showing interest); (3) resolving conflicts; and (4) sharing things with others.

Dealing with Teasing

Teasing is one of the most common problems encountered by children in their peer group relations. How they deal with it can often determine their future in a peer group. If they deal with it badly, the teasing may increase substantially or even culminate in fights or rejection. Sometimes teasing is just a way that children test another child for the strength of the social bond they have with that child or for the child's emotional control, loyalty to the peer group, or ability to deal with social confrontations. This seems to be particularly so in the peer groups of boys: boys seem to want to see how much they can count on the child being teased in a future crisis situation, where they might need to call on that child for support in dealing with others. They may also want to see just how loyal another boy may be, should their peer group be challenged by another group in some way. Can they count on this boy to be loyal to their group, to remain around and help with the conflict with the other group, to be emotionally controlled and cool under fire, to be able to take taunting and criticism without backing down or blowing up, yet also to be able to negotiate with others if need be? Teasing another to see how the child responds can be a test of the strength of the relationship and if your child reacts badly to it can signal to others that the relationship is weak or tenuous and your child is uncommitted to this group or the relationship. At other times, teasing is certainly a form of social aggression, where the intent is to exact some social cost from another child via humiliation and loss of status and reputation in the peer group. Children of both sexes may use this type of aggression.

How your child deals with teasing is important. Interestingly, when parents advise children how to deal with teasing, they often just tell their child to ignore it. Yet when researchers Drs. Richard Milich, Monica Kern, and Douglas Scrambler at the University of Kentucky interviewed children about how to deal with teasing, they most frequently said that ignoring would not work. In fact, it often increased the teasing, in their opinion. These psychologists found in their research that the best method the children they interviewed had found to deal with other children was a form of responding called *adaptive*, as opposed to ignoring or retaliating with anger and hostility. In adaptive responding, the teased children smiled or even laughed at themselves, acknowledged the message of the tease in a humorous way, turned the teasing into a joke or witty reply, and accepted the teasing but tried to make the situation more humorous.

In other words, teach your child to treat teasing as a kind of social test of her sense of humor and any potential friendship that may exist with the other children, not as a form of aggression. And by all means, help your child avoid showing that the comments hurt her feelings. Instead, help her learn to laugh at herself along with others and even to accept some of her own faults, though these may have been exaggerated in the teasing. For instance, if called "stupid," a child with ADHD might be taught to respond by making a joke of it: "I'm not really stupid; I just got the chance to learn the stuff twice as often as you did." Dr. Milich and his colleagues found that this way of reacting to teasing was likely to be far more effective than just ignoring the teasing or reacting with anger.

Setting Up Positive Peer Contacts at Home

Your child does not have to be the most popular kid in the peer group to have satisfying social contacts or friendships. *Popularity* really refers to social status and is not as important as having friendships. Many children with ADHD are not very popular in that sense, and you will find it difficult to change your child's social status. A better goal for a parent is to encourage friendships. Friendships develop when two people interact frequently, show kindness toward each other, take an interest in what the other person does or likes to do, share a common interest (or experiences), and mutually initiate new efforts to see the other person again (rather than just waiting around for the other person to contact them). By viewing friendships through this more detailed process, you can see where you might be able to advise your child on how to build one or more of them. How can you do this?

1. Encourage your child to invite classmates to your home after school or on weekends. Focus on other children who share an interest with your child, like a sport, hobby, music, and so on. If your child has serious social skill problems, do not leave this playtime unstructured. Plan things for the children to do—going to the movies, playing video games together under your supervision and with some snacks nearby that both children will enjoy, doing crafts or building models together with your assistance, or anything else that you think the other child might enjoy but that has a clear structure and purpose and, above all, your close supervision. These structured peer contacts can be an initial building block toward more positive peer contacts that may foster friendships.

2. When your child has other children over to play, monitor the activities more closely and watch for signs that the interactions may be getting out of control: increasing silliness, horseplay, or roughhousing, or simply louder-than-normal conversations. Of course you should also watch for signs of escalating frustration or hostility. In either case, interrupt the play and have the children take a short break for a snack or a more structured and calmer activity. You could ask the children to tell you things so their attention is focused on you rather than on each other, or you could even shift the location of their play.

3. Make every effort to avoid setting examples of expressing negative emotions or aggressive behavior at home, especially if your child already has problems with both. Watch your own behavior and that of family members to see if you're modeling such behavior unintentionally, whether it's yelling, calling names, arguing loudly, using profanity, or throwing things. You should also more closely monitor your child's TV and movie viewing habits. While exposure to the violence that seems endemic in so many children's programs (including cartoons) usually doesn't increase the aggressiveness of normal children, it can do so for children already prone to aggressive and impulsive behavior, such as your child with ADHD. If you can't limit TV watching, consider occasionally watching TV with your child and pointing out inappropriate aggressiveness that would not be liked by other children.

4. Discourage contact between your child and aggressive playmates or those already socially rejected or isolated for other reasons. The last thing a child with ADHD needs is the reinforcement of her own aggressive tendencies by another child

or even role modeling of aggression from an aggressive peer who may also be experiencing social rejection. Encourage your child to associate with and invite over to your home children who are positive role models for peer relations. Don't be concerned if your child plays with either younger or older children, since many children with ADHD seem to do this. Such children may be more tolerant of your child's social immaturities. Just be sure that these children are positive influences and generally well behaved.

5. If your child has already begun hanging out with a deviant, aggressive, or antisocial peer group, do your best to sever her relationship with this crowd. If that is not possible, give serious attention to moving to a different neighborhood with a better, more prosocial peer group. Research actually shows that moving to a new community and exposing your child to more appropriate peers can do a lot to decrease her risk of delinquency and antisocial activities.

Creating Positive Peer Contacts in the Community

Establishing positive peer contacts in the community will not be as easy to do as the preceding recommendations, but you can still make some efforts that may help your child in this area. Try the following ideas:

1. Enroll your child in organized community activities for his age group: Scouts, clubs, sports, hobby groups, or social groups at your house of worship. Summer camps or day activity programs run by a parks or recreation department can also be useful. The advantage to these is that they offer structured activities under adult supervision, which can limit the likelihood of behaviors escalating out of control for your child. These activities seem to be best if they involve relatively small groups of children, such as a Boy or Girl Scout troop. Children with ADHD often have more trouble in large-group settings, which can backfire and lead to social failure, so make sure the group is not too large and that it is supervised.

2. Try to avoid peer group activities that involve a great deal of coordinated effort with other children or complex rules for success, since these can be overwhelming to your child with ADHD. Also steer clear of activities that involve a lot of passive or sitting time, because your child will find this demand hard to meet. For instance, if your child plays Little League baseball, an infield position will be better than the outfield because the greater action in the infield will help keep the child's attention on the game. Many outfielders with ADHD have become bored and distracted by butterflies or bugs nearby, things happening off the field nearby, or just their own thoughts, only to miss balls that were occasionally hit out to them.

3. Activities that involve more structure (organization) and adult supervision are better than unstructured ones or those with little or no supervision.

4. Experts believe that children with ADHD have more favorable experiences when their peer contacts do not involve a lot of competition, especially in areas where they are not as competent as other children. Competitive events can trigger emotional overarousal, increased disorganized behavior, and frustration. An exception can be made when your child has a clear talent in the area of the activity and can be successful despite its competitive nature.

5. Try arranging for some cooperative learning tasks, even if you have to volunteer to organize them yourself. These involve having a small group of children complete a task as a team working toward a common goal: for example, building a model together, building a camp or tree fort in the backyard, taking guided nature walks (where you are the guide), solving practical problems, running simple science experiments, or engaging in a craft or hobby together. Each child is given a particular assignment within the group that is necessary to achieve the goal. All group members share in the positive consequences of completing the task. Usually children who share in these types of activities display positive feelings toward and an increased liking of each other.

Getting Help from Your Child's School

The peer problems that children have at home and at school can be quite different. School settings involve much larger groups of children. Structured class time is interspersed with free-play or unstructured periods (recess), and schools have a different set of expectations for social behavior. For all of these reasons and others, your child with ADHD may have greater problems with peer relations at school than at home. Consider trying the following recommendations:

1. Attempt to develop better classroom behavior in your child through meetings with the child's teacher or the other methods recommended in Chapter 16. Disruptive and inappropriate classroom behavior is strongly associated with peer rejection of children with ADHD, especially if your child is prone to displays of anger, hostility, or outright aggression. All of your other attempts to help your child socially may be for nothing if they are reversed by disruptive behavior at school.

2. If necessary, consider whether your child should be placed on one of the medications discussed in Chapter 18. The stimulant medications have been found to increase positive peer relationships and status, probably by decreasing the excessive and disruptive behavior of children with ADHD.

3. Do not be overly concerned if your child is receiving some type of special education assistance. Children do not reject others just because they receive some sort of special help at school. Rather, the negative comments or attention of teachers, the greater use of discipline, and more generally the singling out of a child with ADHD at

school for criticism are what can create problems with other children. Other children often take their cue of how to treat another child from the adult authorities around them, so work to reduce any such critical or even humiliating comments of teachers toward your child. Encourage your child's teacher to try some of the behavior change methods in Chapter 16 for developing positive behaviors.

4. Ask your child's teacher to assign special responsibilities to your child in the presence of other children. Experts believe that this permits other children to observe your child in a positive light and enhances your child's feelings of acceptance within the classroom.

5. With your child's teacher, develop a behavior rating card that contains two or three social skills you would both like to see your child using more often at school with classmates. List these two or three behaviors on the left side of the card or sheet of paper. Across the top, create five to seven columns representing the number of times each day the teacher can evaluate the child for performance of these social skills. The columns can reflect the ends of specific subject periods, like reading, math, or science, which provide natural break points for the teacher to provide an evaluation. Or they can represent the different free-play or group activity situations that occur each day and may be problematic for your child, such as arrival at school, recesses, lunch period, in-class play periods, large-group activities, or small-group cooperative tasks. A sample card that you may wish to use for monitoring your child's social behavior at school or in other peer group situations (Scouts, clubs, etc.) appears in Figure 3 in Chapter 16. Feel free to photocopy this one if it is appropriate for your child.

Once you have designed this rating form, make a number of copies so that you can use a new one each day. Have the teacher evaluate your child's behavior in the two or three areas listed on the form at the end of each period of time represented by each column. Your child should expect to be evaluated on interacting with others five to seven times each day. The evaluation can simply involve placing a number from 1 to 5 on the form (1 = excellent, 2 = good, 3 = fair, 4 = below average, 5 = poor). The teacher can also write additional comments on the bottom or back of the form. The teacher can dispense rewards at school geared to how well the child is succeeding in these areas. This form is to go home so that you can reward your child as well. You can do this by assigning a certain number of points, tokens, or chips to each number: For instance, 1 = 15 points, 2 = 10 points, 3 = 5 points, 4 = –10 points, and 5 = –15 points. Add up all the positive points, subtract the negative or penalty points, and let the child use the balance to buy rewards and privileges from a reward list like the kind described in Chapter 11.

6. If your school guidance counselor, psychologist, or social worker provides a social skills training group within the school day several times per week, consider having your child enrolled in this group. Such training groups are likely to be more successful than those run by clinics or other agencies outside of school because they involve your child's natural peer group and take place in normal settings.

Helping a child with ADHD who has peer relationship problems can be a difficult task. Be realistic about your expectations for change in this area and what you can reasonably accomplish. As a parent, you don't see your child for a good part of each school day. Look for any opportunities to arrange for situations in which your child can have a good chance of positive peer contacts. Avoid situations that are likely to lead to social failure. Your efforts should eventually build toward more positive peer contacts and maybe even closer friendships for your child.

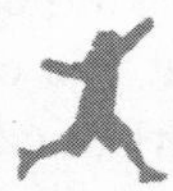

14 Getting through Adolescence

with Arthur L. Robin, PhD

Even strong adults may dissolve into Jell-O when they contemplate the prospect of raising an adolescent with ADHD. The tremendous physical, emotional, and mental changes undergone by teenagers can bring on endless parent–child arguments, demonstrations of disrespect, rebellion against authority, and other behavior that strikes terror in the hearts of adults worldwide. As your child passes puberty, he is faced with a new world of opportunities—alcohol, drugs, driving, employment, and sexual activity among them—and must make smart choices to prevent such opportunities from becoming hazards.

These are just the *normal* challenges of adolescence, and they can be magnified dramatically for teenagers with ADHD. ADHD may hamper your teen's mastery of the developmental tasks facing this age group. Your teen may encounter academic failure, social isolation, depression, and low self-esteem, and may also become embroiled in many unpleasant conflicts with other family members. These often escalating problems can put your family into a state of acute crisis—in which case you may need immediate help from a mental health professional—or at the very least can transform the following areas (and others) into issues of constant conflict:

- Completing schoolwork and homework in a timely and organized manner.
- Performing routine chores around the home.
- Choosing appropriate friends and suitable places to socialize.
- Respecting the rights and privacy of other family members.
- Behaving responsibly while away from home.
- Returning home at established curfew times.
- Using alcohol and tobacco, engaging in sexual activity, and using the family car (for older teens).

Research that Dr. Gwenyth Edwards and I conducted compared the kinds of conflicts and arguments that parents of adolescents with ADHD had with their teens to arguments between parents and typical teens and also examined whether the conflicts differed between mothers and fathers. The study found what you might expect: parents of teens with ADHD reported more conflicts with their teens than parents of normal teens did. Somewhat surprising, however, was the finding that the mothers of the teens with ADHD reported nearly twice as many different kinds of conflicts as did the fathers of those teens. Conflicts between teens with ADHD and their fathers seemed to center most often on the following issues: which clothes the teens wore, playing music too loud, getting into trouble at school, fighting with siblings, and messing up the house. Mothers of teens with ADHD reported having most of the same conflicts, but also got into more arguments about the teens getting to bed on time, getting poor grades at school, the kinds of friends the teens hung around with, and doing homework. Mothers also reported having more severe arguments about these issues than did fathers. All of this illustrates a point made earlier about the stress of raising a child with ADHD: this stress may be borne more by mothers than by fathers in families of children with ADHD. This study certainly bears that out for families of teens with ADHD as well.

The central conflict is, of course, often the one that is at the core of all parent–teenager strife: the adolescent's natural desire to make her own decisions versus the parents' desire to retain decision-making authority. Negotiating this natural transition of a teen to self-determination and handling these conflicts with as little damage to your relationship as possible, while still adequately preparing your teen to eventually move to independence from you in young adulthood, are major challenges in getting through this developmental period.

Golden Rules for Survival

Several "golden rules" can help you improve the quality of life for you and your adolescent:

1. Understand adolescent development and the impact of ADHD on it.
2. Develop a coping attitude and reasonable expectations.
3. Establish clear-cut house and street rules.
4. Monitor and enforce house and street rules, with parents working together as a team.
5. Communicate positively and effectively.
6. Problem-solve disagreements mutually.

7. Use professional help wisely.
8. Maintain your sense of humor and regularly take vacations from your teenager.

Adolescent Development and ADHD: A Crash Course

It may not be obvious from a parent's point of view, but teenagers have a lot of work to do. During these years they are supposed to go from the complete dependence of childhood to equality with their parents as adults. In the course of becoming independent, they are supposed to figure out who they are and what they stand for (that is, identity and values), how to make deep friendships and form lifelong relationships, how to tame their sometimes overwhelming sexual urges, and what they want to do with their lives (education and career goals). Adolescents are supposed to accomplish all of these tasks while being successful in school and getting along with their families.

Imagine a nation establishing its independence, changing from a dictatorship to a democratic republic in which people have greater self-determination. Often there is a bloody revolution. Why should we expect a family to make it through the independence seeking of its children without a disturbance of the peace? A certain amount of conflict is inevitable, especially at ages 12–14, as adolescents push away from their parents yet quickly return when the cruel world mistreats them or they want the resources the parents can provide.

Meanwhile, tremendous physical changes and particularly rapid physical growth and sexual maturation all bring with them increased moodiness, sensitivity to criticism, and fragile self-esteem. Teenagers may have a need to feel omnipotent in order to insulate themselves against the rapid changes they experience and to establish that they can be independent and self-determining people. To admit that they might have any faults may seem catastrophic to them.

Adolescents with ADHD undergo the same metamorphosis in physical maturity and face the same urges and challenges as all other teenagers. Yet they have less executive functioning and so are often less socially or emotionally mature and less capable of self-control than other teens. Consequently, a teen with ADHD may seem even more volatile than a "normal" adolescent, reacting defensively to even the slightest criticism or perhaps anything perceived as criticism. The teen with ADHD may be less ready to assume the responsibilities of independence, but he desires independence as much as any other teenager.

The truth is that as long as this teen remains at home under your care and responsibility, she is likely to require greater assistance and intervention from you than teens without ADHD do, even if you have been working diligently on the child management skills and problem-solving steps discussed in earlier chapters. Remember that the goal of these methods (and the ones discussed in this chapter) is not to "cure" your child, but to lessen conflict and chaos. Ideally, your child will eventually learn those skills and the better forms of social behavior they create, and will come to use them spontaneously as called for in social situations. But you should never expect to stop using these methods entirely.

It's important to understand that while biological maturity will bring some quantitative improvement in inattentiveness, impulsiveness, hyperactivity, and executive functioning (self-control), your adolescent with ADHD will lag behind other adolescents in developing the increasingly complex and sophisticated set of mental abilities that assists them with self-determination and organization, frees them from control by momentary circumstances, and directs their behavior ever farther into the future. The self-restraint, hindsight, forethought, planning, and goal-oriented behavior of teens without ADHD are ever-increasing and coming to play a greater role in their lives, but these abilities will be less mature and slower to emerge in your teen. Deficiencies in these progressively developing skills will be your greatest concerns during adolescence, because, combined with the existing inattentiveness and hyperactivity, they will create a whole new complicated matrix of family conflicts:

- Many teens with ADHD can't seem to stick to agreements made with parents. Is this a manifestation of the disability in attentiveness and self-regulation or true defiance? Often the answer is "both."
- Impulsiveness combined with puberty can make a teen with ADHD more moody, irritable, snappish, "snarky," and unable to tolerate frustration or even to consider the consequences of what they do, which can lead to explosive outbursts, frequent arguments, speedy escalation of conflicts, and even physical confrontations with parents.
- Even motor hyperactivity that persists into adolescence in 30–40% of those with ADHD, when manifested as fidgeting or looking bored during discussions with parents, can easily be misinterpreted as signs of disrespect; this can set in motion an escalating chain of angry and hostile communication.

Coping Attitudes and Reasonable Expectations

These conflicts often converge in the conclusion by parents that a teenager with ADHD has an "attitude problem." The fact is that parents can also have an attitude problem. If you want your teenager to change his attitude, you must first adjust your own thinking.

Expectations versus Demands

It is helpful to expect your teen with ADHD to achieve satisfactory grades and complete homework without a tremendous hassle. It is also helpful to expect him to follow basic rules for living in a family and to treat other members of the family with respect. It is helpful as well to expect him to learn to communicate with you positively and try to resolve conflicts without violence or excessive temper outbursts. Finally, it is helpful to expect that you and your teen's school will need to provide more structure to accomplish these tasks than is necessary for teens without ADHD.

These are *expectations,* not *demands.* Do not expect perfection or total obedience. Do not expect flawless academic performance or compliance with a smile. If you have unrealistic expectations, you will undoubtedly be disappointed, disheartened, and angry much of the time. Your disappointment and anger will prevent you from dealing with your adolescent's problem behaviors in an effective, rational manner. You can easily lose control and impulsively do things you will later regret if you adhere rigidly to unrealistic expectations for perfection and obedience.

Anticipating Ruination

Parents often come to fear that an adolescent who makes too many mistakes will *ruin* her future and that one who has too much freedom will be ruined by failure to handle the freedom responsibly. Will failure to complete homework or clean up his room make your son an aimless, unemployed street person living out of a box? Will being allowed to stay out late or go places without supervision lead your daughter to drug abuse, prostitution, or pregnancy? Many such fears are exaggerated. The problem with exaggerated beliefs is that they can become self-fulfilling prophecies: your adolescent picks up on your lack of trust and reasons that he may as well do the very things you fear the most.

Making Malicious Attributions

If your adolescent fails to take out the trash or make her bed, you may conclude that she is purposely trying to annoy you. Adolescents with ADHD do things for a variety of reasons, some unpredictable, but most of the time the reason is not designed to upset parents. If you interpret many of your adolescent's actions as intentional and malicious, you will stay angry and have a difficult time dealing appropriately with the teen. Are you guilty of unreasonable expectations? Table 4 will help both you and your teenager evaluate your tendency to operate under unreasonable expectations and distorted beliefs.

Changing Your Expectations

If you are having trouble developing reasonable expectations, try the following exercises.

TABLE 4. Common Unreasonable Beliefs

Parents

I. Ruination: "If I give my teen too much freedom, he will ruin his life, make bad judgments, and get into serious trouble."

Examples:
1. Room incompletely cleaned: "He will grow up to be a slovenly, unemployed, aimless, worthless welfare case."
2. Home late: "She could get hurt out late. She could get pregnant, addicted to drugs, and become an alcoholic."
3. Homework incomplete: "He will never graduate from high school, will never get into a good college, will not get a good job, and won't be able to support himself. He will be a drain on us forever."

II. Malicious intent: "My teen misbehaves purposely to hurt me."

Examples:
1. Forgetting to turn the lights off: "She's trying to make me go broke."
2. Talking disrespectfully: "He's talking that way to get even with me."
3. Playing stereo too loud: "She's blasting that stereo just to get on my nerves."

III. Obedience/perfectionism: "My teen should always obey me and behave like a saint."

Examples:
1. Doesn't follow directions: "He can't even take out the trash without me bugging him 10 times. What disrespect/disobedience! If I had done this to my dad, I would have been dead meat."
2. Acting hyper around relatives: "At her age she should be able to sit still and act mature."

IV. Appreciation/love: "My teenager should spontaneously show love and appreciation for the great sacrifices I make."

Examples:
1. "Look what I got after all I've done for you. You don't care about me. You're selfish."
2. "What do you mean you want more allowance? After all the money I give you and all the things I buy, you should be perfectly happy."

Adolescents

I. Unfairness/ruination: "My parents' rules are totally unfair. I'll never have a good time or any friends. My parents are ruining my life with their unfair rules."

Examples:
1. Curfew: "Why should I have to come home earlier than my friends? That's unfair. I'll never have any friends."
2. School: "Mrs. Jones is unfair. She always gives me a hard time. She has it in for me. She's the reason I'm failing math."

II. Autonomy: "My parents have no right to tell me what to do."

Examples:
1. Smoking: "It's my body. I can do whatever I want with it. You have no right to interfere."
2. Chores: "I don't need any reminders. I can get it all done by myself."

III. Appreciation/love: "My parents would let me do whatever I want if they really cared about me."

Examples:
1. "If my parents really loved me, they would let me use the car and go to the concert."
2. "Sarah's mother buys her all those designer clothes. Her parents really love her. Mine hate me and want me to look ugly."

Note. From Robin, A. L. (2006). Training families with ADHD adolescents. In R. A. Barkley, *Attention-Deficit Hyperactivity Disorder: A Handbook for Diagnosis and Treatment* (3rd ed.). Copyright 2006 by The Guilford Press. Reprinted by permission.

Imagine How You Would Feel . . .

Close your eyes and imagine that your teen has come home 2 hours past curfew; have your child do the same thing. Now think of how disrespectful and unappreciative it was for the teen to disregard a rule that already was stretched to the limit to give the teenager as much freedom as you can tolerate. Ask your adolescent to imagine how unfair and embarrassing it was to have to leave a party early and how much parental rules are ruining his social life. Now what do you both feel at that moment? It's likely that very strong anger and frustration will emerge. Ask yourself about the potential outcome of a family discussion when everyone is so emotionally upset. Family members we know usually agree that a "bloodbath" rather than a logical discussion would probably ensue.

This exercise demonstrates that an event (A) gave each of you an extreme thought (B), which made each of you angry (C). Professionals call this the *ABC model of emotions.* It shows that your feelings are really created as much (or more) by yourself and your thoughts as by the event or what someone else did. Consider changing your beliefs about the other person's (your teen's) behavior. You can control how upset the behavior makes you by evaluating and altering your beliefs to be more flexible and reasonable.

The Worst-Case Scenario

What is the worst that could happen if you gave in and compromised with the other person on a point of disagreement? For example, if your teenager is failing to complete his homework, you might think, "If Jim doesn't get his math homework done, he will fail math, fail ninth grade, fail to graduate, get a lousy job, and end up an unhappy adult." Or you could think, "So he gets an F on one of his math homework assignments. It is only one assignment out of many. What's the worst thing that can happen? He could get a lower grade. Didn't I ever fail to get my homework done? I survived, and he will too." The latter is reasonable and flexible, the former unreasonable and illogical.

Remember to be flexible and forgiving with yourself too. Even if you start to think differently, you can slip back into your old rigid or distorted ideas about your teen. You may need to practice a lot at catching distorted beliefs before you will be good at preventing them from influencing the way you react to your teenager.

Consider a father who is very angry because his daughter shows no appreciation for all of the money that has been spent on books, school clothes, supplies, computers, tutoring, and therapy to help her succeed in school and because of the "disrespect and disobedience" she shows by acting restless and bored whenever the topic is brought up (usually in a lecture). This parent might begin to change his own rigidity by pinpointing the extreme belief: adolescents should always express deep appreciation for their parents' sacrifices, and it is a sign of extreme disobedience and disrespect when a teen with ADHD—a teen with a biological deficit in self-control, who has never sat still for more than 10 minutes—fidgets while her dad lectures to her for a half-hour about her lack of caring. Now he might ask himself how much appreciation his daughter's friends are likely to express to their parents or even how much he appreciated his own parents when he was a teen. He could talk to other parents about their children and read a book on normal adolescent development. All of this could lead him to the alternative belief that even though adolescents love and appreciate their parents, they rarely express it.

These strategies are well worth the effort. Ask yourself this question: What is worse, losing a compromise to your teen for a week or losing your relationship with your teen for years? Successfully parenting an adolescent with ADHD is like riding a roller coaster. There may be a thrill a minute, but there are also many bumps and bruises. Try not to overreact to each little bump but to "go with the flow," deciding which issues are high priorities for immediate action and which are trivial and best ignored. Keep in mind your adolescent's relentless quest for self-determination and the impact of ADHD on this process as you try to develop reasonable expectations and accurate interpretations of your teenager's actions.

Establishing House Rules and Street Rules

With young children, parents often resolve conflicts through the use of power, making their positions stick through forceful administration of rewards and punishments. Because of the independence seeking and increased strength of adolescents, simple use of power will not work; your teen will develop the skills to circumvent that kind of parental control. When parents discover that they cannot simply dictate to their teens, they sometimes throw up their hands in desperation and say, "I can't deal with this; do whatever you want and suffer the consequences." Such a laissez-faire approach doesn't work either, because teens with ADHD will do whatever they want, which won't usually include schoolwork and will often include impulsive and even dangerous (if not illegal) activities. When authorities contact the parents about the adolescents' problem behavior, the parents may again crack down in an authoritarian manner. Over time, the parents may alternate between overcontrol and undercontrol, and the teens with ADHD quickly learn to recognize the cycle and to wait out the tight rules and wear down their parents, because freedom is just around the corner.

"My teenager does as he pleases. He comes and goes at all hours of the day and night. He doesn't do anything around the house to help. How can we get him to listen to us?"

Research has found that a more democratic or consensus-building approach, involving the adolescent in the decision making when possible, generally works better than a strict one-sided dictatorial approach. Negotiating solutions that everyone can live with can take more time than issuing ultimatums but is more likely to foster more responsible adolescent conduct, perhaps because the teen sees the reasons for the decisions and has taken part in making them. Most important, the teenager can take this template for solving disagreements outside the home for use in later life.

If your instinctive reaction is that teens with ADHD are too manipulative, defiant, and aggressive to be given any input, understand that there is an important distinction between issues that can be handled democratically and those that are nonnegotiable. Each family has a set of bottom-line rules for living together, which are a function of the parents' values and generalized tenets for civilized living. Before proceeding further, make a list of these rules. Keep it short and simple and divide it into (1) house rules (which apply at home) and (2) street rules (which govern conduct everywhere else). Examples of house rules might include (1) no violence or cursing; (2) no smoking, drugs, or alcohol; (3) you can express dissatisfaction (not anger), but treat people with respect; (4) respect family members' privacy; (5) ask before you take another person's property; and (6) no friends in the house without a parent present. Street rules might include (1) use violence only to defend yourself and only after trying everything else; (2) no smoking, drugs, or alcohol; (3) attend school as scheduled; (4) tell your parents where you are going and call them if your plans change; and (5) come home by a designated curfew time.

Post this list of nonnegotiable rules on the refrigerator. Go over it often with your adolescent. Clarify any ambiguities. Discuss the reasons such rules are necessary, and if need be, ask the adolescent to imagine what life would be like if people didn't follow basic rules like these for living together. Remind your adolescent of the street rules before she goes out with friends.

Monitoring and Enforcing Rules

Enforcement of rules only gets more difficult as children with ADHD get older, so consistency and teamwork remain essential. In any family where parents have inadvertently shown their children that the decisions of one parent can be overruled by appealing to the other parent, a teenager will learn numerous creative ways to divide and conquer. Because parents of a teen with ADHD may need to set more than the customary limits, however, the home is fertile ground for the adolescent's experimentation with such tactics. So communication between parents to erect a united front is paramount (see the sidebar on the facing page). Single parents have a particularly tough job and should enlist the aid of anyone they can count on for *consistent* support, such as a nearby relative or a close friend.

The first step in enforcement is monitoring—keeping track of your teen's compliance with house and street rules, checking up on his general whereabouts, and keeping track of the teen's progress toward completion of any structured task within time

When Parents Unite: A Success Story

Fourteen-year-old Andrew Nordon was having impulsive temper tantrums four or five times a week, often set off by minor provocations at home. When his father refused to take him to the store to purchase a Halloween costume, Andrew squirted a bottle of mustard on his father's $400 suit, ruining it. When his mother refused to give him his favorite dessert, he threw a bottle of pop at her, making a hole in the wall. He terrorized his sister constantly, randomly punching her, pulling her hair, and stealing her money and possessions. Mr. and Mrs. Nordon disagreed vehemently with each other about how to handle their son. Mr. Nordon favored physical punishment ("the belt"), while his wife was afraid that Andrew and his dad would hurt each other. She tried to "reason" with her son and in fact stood between her husband and son to prevent physical confrontations. Aside from reasoning, she did nothing in response to the tantrums.

With the help of a therapist, the Nordons agreed that the "bottom line" would be to call the police and press charges in the event of assaultive behavior and to require financial restitution in the case of destruction of property. They had great difficulty, though, agreeing on how to respond at the time of each impulsive episode. Mr. Nordon insisted on the necessity for corporal punishment, and his wife insisted on doing nothing but having a quiet discussion with her son at a later time. Each parent rigidly accused the other of perpetuating Andrew's tantrums. Andrew downplayed the intensity of his tantrums, claimed he could control them at any time, and objected to his parents' "stupid" rules, perceiving his destructive behavior as "getting even."

The therapist pushed the parents to reach a number of agreements for controlling Andrew's tantrums. The father agreed to refrain from physical violence toward his son if his wife would be more assertive in telling Andrew to control himself or go to his room for 30 minutes until he calmed down. For a month Mrs. Nordon either "forgot" to be assertive or responded to her son in a "mousy manner." Mr. Nordon would at first exercise restraint, but by the third time his wife refused to assert herself, he resorted to physical punishment. Only when her husband actually stood by and coached her every statement was Mrs. Nordon able to begin to respond to her son assertively. An episode when Andrew hit and taunted his sister so intensely that she huddled in the corner sucking her thumb and crying hysterically was the turning point for Mrs. Nordon. She realized how much of a tyrant her son was and began to crack down. Mr. Nordon could not believe she could do it, but he strongly supported his wife. Within 3 more weeks, the tantrums had diminished from four or five to one or two per week. Andrew claimed the change in his behavior was due to his own "willpower"—a fantasy that the therapist did not challenge.

parameters. Monitoring is really just another facet of the structuring that is central to dealing with any individual who has ADHD. Teens with ADHD need closer, more frequent monitoring than other adolescents; you should always know where your teen is. When your teen goes out with peers during free time, you should require an accounting of the teen's destination, including notifying you of any changes in plans. You also need to be awake and waiting at curfew time to keep the teen honest; also stay in the house during homework time if possible.

Just as parents are sometimes prone to undercontrol or overcontrol of their child with ADHD, they run the risk of being disengaged at one extreme or overinvolved at the other. It's wise neither to leave the adolescent at home alone for a weekend nor to show up at a party to check up on your adolescent. Disengagement promotes dangerous behaviors and failure to complete tasks, whereas overinvolvement stifles achievement of self-determination. Striking a balance that respects your adolescent's privacy yet reminds the teen that there is always accountability is, of course, not easy. Here are some suggestions.

Continue Using Positive and Negative Consequences

You can and should adapt many of the techniques described in Chapter 11 for setting up a point system that establishes positive consequences for compliance and negative consequences for noncompliance with house and street rules. The main difference is that the consequences will reflect the age of the child: besides TV privileges and assigning of work around the house, consequences for an adolescent may revolve around use of the family car, use of the Internet, getting an allowance, or having a cell phone, for example.

Project Authority

Parents must project a no-nonsense, controlled, but strong-willed tone to get results. A teen needs to know from a parent's voice tone and mannerisms that the parent means business about the nonnegotiable rules. Be prepared to "go to the wall" in consistently backing each other up and following through on unpleasant consequences with a very angry teen. This is especially important when your teen is accustomed to getting her way. Your new united front will evoke much anger and frustration from the teen, and you'll have to stand firm in the face of such reactions.

Be Prepared to Seek Help

There are times when you may not be able to exert appropriate control over your adolescent and effectively enforce house and street rules. You may need the assistance of a therapist—or, in extreme cases, external authorities such as the juvenile court and the police. Try not to shrink from this recourse if you've tried everything else.

Communicating Effectively

It is very easy for you and your teen to develop bad communication habits. When ADHD compounds the normal conflicts of adolescents, it's no surprise that many parents "lose it" during disagreements with their teenagers, often after school, especially if the parents are also tired from a long day at their own work. Families find that their "discussions" constantly involve put-downs, accusations, defensive remarks, sarcasm, and parental ultimatums. Parents give endless lectures, and teens respond by tuning them out, giving them the silent treatment, or cursing them out. Negative modes of communication can so enrage both parents and teens that the parents act based on hot emotion rather than cool logic and end up with nothing to show for the encounter but regrets.

Take a moment to review Table 5, which lists common negative communication habits and some more constructive alternatives. Try to think about recent events in which these habits came into play. How angry did your teen's negative communication make you? How angry did your teen get, and what happened?

Discuss with your teen how negative communication styles can hurt: how they can offend the other person, even eliciting a counterattack or retaliation. Start by stating some of your own bad communication habits and how you will try to change them the next time you discuss a problem with your teen. Beginning by saying you want to review the teen's bad habits will make your teen immediately defensive.

Next, point out the more positive alternatives, using the examples in Table 5 but also asking your teen to give you examples. Try role-playing these new communication styles. Take care to emphasize that you are not urging your teen to suppress his feelings and hide anger. Instead, you are trying to get the child to express legitimate feelings without offending or hurting someone else's feelings in the process. Don't forget to include nonverbal communication, such as eye contact and good posture.

Make a contract with your adolescent to work on one or two of these communication skills at a time. Then give each other feedback throughout the day about the selected communication habit and try to replay the scene using the more positive behavior. Sometimes digitally recording conversations (such as those at the dinner table) and then reviewing the recordings can be helpful. When your teen tries out new communication skills, you should try to be liberal in praising her efforts.

For example, one mother and her 16-year-old with ADHD decided to focus on impulsive interruptions. They often interrupted each other in midsentence, leading to rapid flashes of anger and immediate arguments. They both agreed to try to let each other finish, no matter how much they wanted to get their own say in. They also agreed to keep their statements short. If one interrupted, the other agreed to say,

TABLE 5. Negative Communication Habits

Check if your family does this:	*More positive way to do it:*
1. _____ Call each other names.	Express anger without hurtful words.
2. _____ Put each other down.	"I am angry that you did ____________."
3. _____ Interrupt each other.	Take turns; keep it short.
4. _____ Criticize all the time.	Point out the good and the bad.
5. _____ Get defensive when attacked.	Listen carefully and check out what you heard—then calmly disagree.
6. _____ Give a lecture/use big words.	Tell it straight and short.
7. _____ Look away, not at speaker.	Make good eye contact.
8. _____ Slouch or slide to floor.	Sit up and look attentive.
9. _____ Talk in sarcastic tone.	Talk in normal tone.
10. _____ Get off the topic.	Finish one topic, then go on.
11. _____ Think the worst.	Keep an open mind. Don't jump to conclusions.
12. _____ Dredge up the past.	Stick to the present.
13. _____ Read each other's mind.	Ask the other's opinion.
14. _____ Command, order.	Ask nicely.
15. _____ Give the silent treatment.	Say it if you feel it.
16. _____ Throw a tantrum; "lose it."	Count to 10; take a hike; do relaxation; leave room.
17. _____ Make light of something serious.	Take it seriously, even if it is minor to you.
18. _____ Deny you did it.	Admit you did it, but say you were accused.
19. _____ Nag about small mistakes.	Admit no one is perfect; overlook small things.

Your negative communication score (total no. of checks) _____

Note. From Robin, A. L. (2006). Training families with ADHD adolescents. In R. A. Barkley, *Attention-Deficit Hyperactivity Disorder: A Handbook for Diagnosis and Treatment* (3rd ed.). Copyright 2006 by The Guilford Press. Reprinted by permission.

"Foul! That's interrupting. Let's start over." It took several weeks to change this pattern, but as they succeeded, they noticed that they had fewer arguments.

Problem-Solving Conflicts with Your Teen

As you begin to practice new ways of communicating with your teenager, you're ready to put your communication skills to use in resolving conflicts and disagreements. The first area to try to improve on is the steps you follow in discussing a problem. Do you skip around to a number of problems in the same conversation without resolving any of them? Are your discussions more for ventilating anger than for arriving at real solutions? Whatever kind of trouble you have with problem solving, consider following the steps for problem solving in Chapter 12. Or start with a couple of sheets of paper and review the problem-solving steps listed in Table 6. Before you begin, be sure both parents and the teenager agree on the following approach:

1. As parents, you will remain calm and business-like throughout the discussion and take an interest in the teen's view.
2. These discussions will feature a mutual give-and-take in which each side is out not to win, but to set up a reasonable plan that both sides can live with.
3. Each party will show a willingness to listen to what the other parties have to say.
4. Start with a topic of disagreement that does not seem to have intense anger or "heat" associated with it.
5. Do not try to resolve all of your disagreements in one meeting. Try working on only one problem area, or at most two, in one session with your teen. Then wait at least a week to discuss any more problems until you have had a chance to put your last plan into action and to evaluate how well it has been working. Only when that area of conflict seems to have been resolved should you proceed further down your list of issues to problem-solve the next one or two.
6. Assign one family member to be the secretary, who will record the information from the discussion. We find it helpful to alternate this responsibility between you and your teen from one discussion to the next.

Step 1: Define the Problem

Each family member defines the problem by making a clear, short statement that pinpoints this member's view of the problem. As each person gives a definition, the others should check out their own understanding of the definition by saying it back to the speaker in the speaker's own words. For instance, in a discussion about curfew you might say to your teenager, "I hear you saying that you would like more time out of the house on weekend nights" or "I get it. It sounds to me like you think the curfew is too strict."

Restating the specific problem that is under discussion sometimes reveals that several different problems are being brought up at once. For instance, during the discussion about curfew, you might raise the fact that your son brings the car back with

TABLE 6. Problem-Solving Outline

I. Define the problem.
   A. Tell the others what they do that bothers you and why. "I get very angry when you come home 2 hours after the 11:00 P.M. curfew we agreed upon."
   B. Start your definition with an "I"; be brief, be clear, and don't accuse or put down the other person.
   C. Did you get your point across? Ask the others to paraphrase your problem definition to check whether they understood you. If they understood you, go on. If not, repeat your definition.

II. Generate a variety of alternative solutions.
   A. Take turns listing solutions.
   B. Follow three rules for listing solutions.
      1. List as many ideas as possible.
      2. Don't evaluate the ideas.
      3. Be creative; anything goes, since you will not have to do everything you list.
   C. One person writes down the ideas on a worksheet (see Figure 2).

III. Evaluate the ideas and decide upon the best one.
   A. Take turns evaluating each idea.
      1. Say what you think would happen if the family followed the idea.
      2. Vote "plus" or "minus" for the idea and record your vote on the worksheet next to the idea.
   B. Select the best idea.
      1. Look for ideas rated "plus" by everyone.
      2. Select one of these ideas.
      3. Combine several of these ideas.
   C. If none are rated "plus" by everyone, negotiate a compromise.
      1. Select an idea rated "plus" by one parent and the teen.
      2. List as many compromises as possible.
      3. Evaluate the compromises as described in steps III-A and III-B.
      4. Reach a mutually acceptable solution.
      5. If you still cannot reach an agreement, wait for the next therapy session.

IV. Plan to implement the selected solution.
   A. Decide who will do what, where, how, and when.
   B. Decide who will monitor the solution implementation.
   C. Decide upon the consequences for compliance or noncompliance with the solution.
      1. Rewards for compliance: privileges, money, activities, praise.
      2. Punishments for noncompliance: loss of privileges, groundings, work detail.

Note. From Robin, A. L. (2006). Training families with ADHD adolescents. In R. A. Barkley, *Attention-Deficit Hyperactivity Disorder: A Handbook for Diagnosis and Treatment* (3rd ed.). Copyright 2006 by The Guilford Press. Reprinted by permission.

an empty gas tank, that he is spending too much money when out with friends, or that you have detected the smell of alcohol or tobacco smoke on his breath when he returns. These are actually separate problems. Write them down on a sheet of paper in a list of problems to be discussed at another time.

Use the second sheet as a worksheet that focuses on the curfew problem only. Set up the worksheet similar to the one shown in Figure 2 and record on it everyone's statement of the problem.

Step 2: Generate Possible Solutions

Now the family members take turns generating a variety of alternative solutions to the problem. Follow these rules for brainstorming: (1) List as many ideas as possible; quantity breeds quality. (2) Don't evaluate the ideas, since criticism stifles creativity. (3) Be creative, even extreme or funny in your ideas, knowing that just because you say it doesn't mean you will have to do it.

Usually parents and adolescents begin by suggesting their original positions as solutions. Gradually new ideas emerge. If the atmosphere is very tense or the family runs out of ideas, try to suggest some outlandish ideas just to lighten the atmosphere with a little humor and spur creativity. Try writing down the most extreme solutions first, so you can see that your own ideas or those of your teen are actually less extreme than you might think. For the curfew problem, you could write down "Stays out all night" and "Does not go out at all on weekend nights." The extremeness of these options helps to suggest that there are degrees of far more acceptable solutions falling in between that can be useful. When you see that there are at least one or two "workable" ideas—ideas that may achieve mutual acceptance—on the list, move on.

Step 3: Evaluate the Alternatives

Now each family member evaluates the ideas and decides on the best one. First think about the consequences of using each solution and then rate it as one you could live with (+ on the worksheet) or do not like (– on the worksheet). Focus only on the person's feelings about the options, avoiding digressions, and continue to restate those feelings to be sure everyone understands.

When the ideas have all been rated, review the worksheet to determine whether a consensus was reached. You may be surprised to find that a consensus can be reached about 80% of the time. Then select one of the ideas rated positively by everyone or combine several such ideas into the solution.

If a consensus was not reached, you are going to have to negotiate a compromise. Look for the idea on which members came closest to agreement. Use this idea as a starting point for coming up with small variations that might be more acceptable to

Name of Family: The Johnsons

Topic: Household chores

Definitions of the problem:

Mom: I get upset when I have to tell Allen 10 times to take out the trash and clean up his room.

Dad: It bothers me to come home and find all the trash still in the house and Allen's records and books all over his room, with my wife screaming at him.

Allen: My parents tell me to take out the trash during my favorite TV show. They make me clean up my room when all my friends are having fun.

Solutions and evaluations:	Mom	Dad	Allen
1. Do chores the first time asked	+	+	–
2. Don't have any chores	–	–	+
3. Grounded for 1 month if not done	–	+	–
4. Hire a maid	+	–	+
5. Earn allowance for chores	+	+	+
6. Room cleaned once by 9:00 P.M.	+	+	+
7. Parents clean the room	–	–	+
8. Close the door to room	+	–	+
9. Better timing when asking Allen	+	+	+
10. One reminder to do chores	+	+	+

Agreement: Nos. 5, 6, 9, 10.

Implementation plan: By 9:00 P.M. each evening Allen agrees to clean up his room, meaning books and papers neatly stacked and clothes in hamper or drawers. Doesn't have to pass "white glove test." Will earn extra $1.00 per day on allowance if complies with no reminders or one reminder. By 8:00 P.M. on Tuesdays, Allen agrees to have trash collected and out by curb. Will earn $2.00 extra if complies.

Punishment for noncompliance: Grounding for the next day after school. Dad to monitor trash; Mom to monitor room.

FIGURE 2. Example of a completed problem-solving worksheet.

From Robin, A. L. (2006). Training families with ADHD adolescents. In R. A. Barkley, *Attention-Deficit Hyperactivity Disorder: A Handbook for Diagnosis and Treatment* (3rd ed.). Copyright 2006 by The Guilford Press. Reprinted by permission.

everyone. Look closely at those parts or details of the option that seem to be creating the disagreement with your teen. Try to work on suggesting substitutes for these parts that might bring you both closer together. Be attuned to the possible role of distorted expectations and be willing to compromise or give in. You can always discuss the problem again next week and try another option.

Step 4: Implement the Solution

Circle or underline the chosen solution, if necessary rewriting it at the bottom of the worksheet. You also must decide who will do what, when, where, and with what supervision to make the solution work. With an adolescent who has ADHD in particular, establishing clear-cut consequences for compliance or noncompliance is very important, as is reminding your teen during the next week to remember to do the things involved in the solution. Whatever consequences you decide on, be sure that they are also written at the bottom of the worksheet so everyone knows what to expect. Then have everyone sign the bottom of the worksheet so it becomes a contract.

Try the solution for at least 1–2 weeks before deciding whether or not it is working. If necessary, you can always come back and renegotiate the contract if it seems unfair or unworkable.

Try this problem-solving approach for several weeks by sitting down once each week to discuss just one or two of the problem areas on your list of disagreements. You may wish to schedule regular family meetings at which you and your adolescent apply problem solving to any disagreements that have accumulated in the past week. (For further suggestions on applying the four-step problem-solving method, see the sidebar below.)

Using Professional Help Wisely

We subscribe to the "dental checkup" model of professional help for adolescent ADHD. By following a preventive regimen, you catch problems before they get too serious, so we advocate establishing a relationship with a professional—a psychologist, physician, or social worker—with whom you meet periodically to review your adolescent's progress. If a problem arises in school or at home, the professional may suggest a more intensive intervention until the problem is resolved; afterward, you may return to the checkup mode of follow-up care. Or if you're applying the "golden rules" in this chapter without success, it may be time to check in with a professional and enroll in some form of therapeutic intervention, such as family therapy. Many of the ideas in this chapter require the assistance of a person outside the family to implement initially if you and your adolescent have a history of serious conflict.

ADHD and Problem-Solving Skills

Experience has taught us that ADHD brings special concerns into problem solving. To apply the four-step method successfully, pay attention to these matters:

1. The adolescent may have trouble paying attention during crucial moments of each discussion. Keep your comments brief and to the point, bring the adolescent into the discussion whenever possible, and talk in an animated and enthusiastic manner with a constructive or positive tone. You can even reward your teen for having the discussion with you the first few times you try it. If your adolescent takes medication, hold the discussions while the medication is active.

2. Some younger teens with ADHD—say, those 12–14 years old—are not always fully able to understand the concepts of problem solving or may not be ready emotionally or developmentally to assume responsibility for coming up with options and negotiating solutions. In such a case, you may have to set up behavioral contracts on your own and then discuss them with your teen. Or you could simplify the steps of problem solving so they can be managed by an immature adolescent. For example, generate a list of alternative solutions and through evaluation boil them down to three options, which you then present to the adolescent for a vote.

3. If either of the parents also has ADHD, volatile discussions may be unavoidable. In that case, consult a professional to get diagnosed and treated yourself and to assist you in carrying out these discussions.

4. An adolescent with ADHD can be so impulsive and distractible that you may feel the need to correct everything the teen does or says. This can create an endless series of issues and negative communication patterns. You need to learn to pick your issues wisely, deciding what to take a stand on and what to ignore. Some families have also dealt with disruptive behavior during the discussions by using a point system to reward positive communication skills.

Taking Vacations and Keeping Your Sense of Humor

The last "golden rule" may well be the most important: maintain your sense of humor and take vacations from your adolescent with ADHD. It can be very difficult to try to see the humor in many parenting situations with your adolescent, but if you try, you will get through your child's adolescence much more easily. And at least several times per year, you and your adolescent need a vacation from each other. Use camps, teen travel, grandparents, friends—whatever it takes—to get away from each other every once in a while. Vacations always help parents recharge their batteries and look at problems with a fresh perspective.

Further Reading

If you wish to read further about the ideas in this chapter, there are several books you can consult. *Parents and Adolescents Living Together,* by Marion Forgatch and Gerald R. Patterson, is written especially for parents. Two books—*Your Defiant Teen* by Russell A. Barkley and Arthur L. Robin with Christine M. Benton; and, written for professionals, *ADHD in Adolescents: Diagnosis and Treatment,* by Arthur L. Robin—may also be helpful. More information about all these books is provided in "Suggested Reading and Videos."

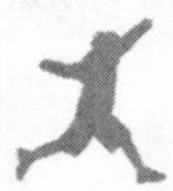

15 Off to School on the Right Foot

MANAGING YOUR CHILD'S EDUCATION

with Linda J. Pfiffner, PhD

If you're among the many parents who first learned of their children's behavior problems through teachers, you already know that children with ADHD have some of their greatest difficulties in adjusting to the demands of school. Numerous studies show that the vast majority of children with ADHD are doing substantially worse in school than typical children in the same grade. A third or more of all children with ADHD will be held back in school in at least one grade during their educational career, up to 35% may never complete high school, and their academic grades and achievement scores are often significantly below those of their classmates. Between 40 and 50% of such children will eventually wind up receiving some degree of formal services through special education programs, such as resource rooms, and up to 10% may spend their entire school day in such programs (known as *self-containing programs*). Complicating this picture is the fact that more than half of all children with ADHD also have serious problems with oppositional behavior. This helps explain why between 15 and 25% of such children will be suspended or even expelled from school because of their conduct problems.

A 2011 study by Dr. Michelle Demaray and Lyndsay Jenkins at Northern Illinois University found that children with ADHD differed from typically achieving children in four major areas in their school functioning: poorer engagement with academic work, poorer social skills, less motivation to learn and do well in school, and worse study skills. Problems in these areas were directly related to the degree of difficulty the children were likely to be having in school.

Teachers frequently respond to the challenging problems exhibited by children with ADHD in these and other areas of school performance by becoming more controlling and directive. Over time, their frustrations with these difficult children may make them more hostile in their interactions as well. While we are not sure how negative child–teacher relationships affect the long-term adjustment of children with

ADHD, experience tells us that they can certainly worsen the already poor academic and social achievement of these children, reduce their motivation to learn and participate in school, and lower the children's self-esteem. All of this may ultimately result in school failure and dropping out.

A positive teacher–student relationship, to the contrary, may improve a child's academic and social adjustment, not only in the short term but also over the long term. Adults who were diagnosed with ADHD as children have reported that a teacher's caring attitude, extra attention, and guidance were "turning points" in helping them overcome their childhood problems.

The fact is that the single most important ingredient in your child's success at school is your child's teacher. It is not the name of the school program your child is in, the school's location, whether the school is private or public, whether or not it is relatively wealthy, or even the size of the class. It is first and foremost your child's teacher—particularly the teacher's experience with ADHD and willingness to provide the extra effort and understanding your child will require for a successful school year. In 2008, Dr. Jody Sherman and colleagues at the University of Alberta, Canada, published a review of the scientific and clinical literature on what factors or characteristics of a teacher were important to the school success of a child with ADHD (*Educational Research,* Vol. 50, No. 4, pp. 347–360). Among the most important factors they identified were teacher patience, knowledge of ADHD, knowledge of useful teaching techniques for managing ADHD in the classroom, ability to collaborate with an interdisciplinary team on the child's treatment, and positive attitude toward children with special needs.

The difference that your child's teacher can make is illustrated in a 15-year-old's poignant account of his school history in the sidebar in this chapter (pp. 248–251). So you should not wait until August to find out who will be your child's teacher for the coming school year. Nor should you allow some computer or school bureaucrat to make a random selection. You should start negotiating with the principal for the best possible teacher for the next academic year as early as March or April.

The main focus of this chapter, therefore, is on how to find the best teacher—and, should the available teachers be unfamiliar with the methods that help children with ADHD succeed in school, on how to help them gain that knowledge to serve your child best. The rest of the chapter addresses secondary matters that are nonetheless commonly of concern to parents: what to look for in a school, classroom structure and curriculum, what type of placement is best for children with ADHD, and whether retention (especially in kindergarten) is likely to serve a child's interests.

What to Look for in a School

A first step in helping a child with ADHD achieve educational success is to choose the right school. In the real world, many of us don't have such a choice. Either economics

Attention Deficit through the Eyes of a Child

by Alan Brown, age 15

I often wondered why I wasn't in group time in kindergarten. The teacher sent me in the corner to play with a toy by myself. Because of being singled out, I didn't have many friends. I was different, but I didn't know why or what it was. Toward the middle half of first grade the teacher called my mom in for a conference. She was telling my mom, "I'm always having to call on Alan. 'Alan, be still, please. Yes, you can sharpen your pencil for the third time. You have to go to the bathroom again?' " That evening my teacher educated my mom. She told my mom about attention deficit disorder (ADD). [*Author's note:* ADD as Alan uses the term here is ADHD (or ADD with hyperactivity, as it was formerly defined by the American Psychiatric Association), not ADD without hyperactivity as described in Chapter 7.] My teacher suggested taking me to the doctor and letting him run some tests. Mom and I went to see the doctor. After some testing the doctor put me on Ritalin. Within about 2 weeks the teacher said I was completing my homework, making good grades, and feeling good about myself. Although we (my mom and I) thought our battle was won, we had no idea what adventures were waiting for us.

Second grade went by. I was doing OK in school. My teacher would usually write on my report card, "Alan worked hard this 6 weeks. Encourage him to read at home." I hated to read; it was so hard to understand what I had read. I loved to play outside, run in the field, and ride on my bicycle. A free spirit.

By the time I got to third grade things were getting off track. I felt like nothing I did was right. I would try to do good work. My teacher would write on my papers, "Needs to concentrate more on answers," "Needs to turn in all work," "Needs to follow directions." I really didn't think my teacher liked me. She was very stern, never seemed to smile, and was always watching me.

Fourth grade was the year everything in my world fell apart! Before school started, my mom took me to see the doctor the way we did every year. The doctor prescribed the same dose as I had taken the year before. He didn't want to raise my dosage unless he really had to.

First 6 weeks passed. I didn't do very well, but the doctor said it might be the new school year or getting settled in and used to a new teacher. My mom told the teacher the doctor was considering raising my Ritalin dosage. The teacher said something had to be done because my grades were low. I wasn't always prepared for class, was slow getting my books out, and always needed to go to my locker because I had forgotten something. My doctor did raise my medication to one pill in the morning and one pill at lunch. Everyone in the room would say, "Dummy has to go take his pill."

My teacher wanted to make me concentrate better, so one day she put my desk in the far corner, separated from the rest of the class. A few days had passed.

I still wasn't finishing my work on time, but I was trying to do the work correctly. The teacher didn't care; it wasn't finished. She then put a refrigerator box around my desk so I couldn't see anyone in class. I could hear as other kids in class would make fun of me. It really hurt; I was ashamed of myself and mad at my teacher. I couldn't tell my mom because I might get in trouble. I hated school, didn't like my teacher, and started not liking myself. Imagine a 9-year-old going through this day after day. It was hard to face the next day. A week had passed, and I poked holes in the cardboard so I could see who was making fun of me. I started peeping through the holes, making the other kids laugh. The teacher would get so annoyed. So I became the class clown. I was expelled for 2 days. When my mom found out what was going on, boy, did she get angry.

She was mad that the teacher would do this and mad that the principal allowed it, and no one could see what this was doing to me.

Mom called my doctor, explained what was going on, asked him to recommend a specialist. We needed some help! I remember my mom cried over the phone. It scared me. I thought I was really in trouble, but instead, she put me in her lap, kissed my cheek, gave me a hug, and said, "You're special to me, and I love you. Together we are going to get through this." It made me feel good because moms can always fix everything.

The next day Mom explained that we were going to meet someone special, someone I could talk to. I was kind of nervous. This person was a licensed clinical social worker. She was nice. I played games while we talked. After a while I felt like she was a friend. It was time to meet with the principal to return to school. Mom and I went to the office. The principal wanted to give my place to a more deserving student, a higher academic achiever. It would make the school look better. At that point Mom asked about my rights as a handicapped student. She didn't like the thought that no one seemed to care what they had done to me, and she said so. At that point the principal made a phone call to one of his friends, also a principal. It had something to do with Mom not going to the school board meeting to discuss this matter.

I was going to a new school, a school close to where my mom worked, thanks to that phone call.

On the way home that day Mom explained to me that what they had done to me wasn't right and they should be ashamed. She said that there were a lot of smart, successful people in this world who were not happy with themselves. She said, "It's more important in life to be happy and know within yourself that no matter what comes your way you can survive. Academics are important, but self-worth is too."

The new school was a more positive atmosphere; my grades came up. The doctor changed my medication to a slow-release pill so I didn't have to leave class to take it anymore.

***Attention Deficit through the Eyes of a Child** (cont.)*

Fifth grade came along. It was great! I had the best teacher; she smiled a lot and was flexible yet had a structured day planned. One day I remember she asked me to go to the closet and get the book *Charlotte's Web*. I went to the closet and found the most wonderful book, *King of the Wind,* a story about a horse. I hid the book *Charlotte's Web* and told the teacher I couldn't find it but that this horse book was there and I really liked horses. All along the teacher knew those books were in that closet. She thought if *King of the Wind* looked that interesting to me, maybe it would be worth doing instead of *Charlotte's Web*. After reading the book, I wrote a report about the story. The teacher was so impressed. She posted the book report in front of the class and made a comment on my report card. I was so proud—proud of myself. I was on track again; life was great. My parents were going to be so proud.

Sixth grade came, and I did fairly well. I had to change classes. It was hard to adjust to better organization skills. I color-coded folders for classes and kept a schedule of where and when classes were.

Seventh grade was a little rocky, but I made it. There were more students. I kind of got lost in the shuffle. By eighth grade it was a struggle every day. More peer pressure to fit in, and I was going through a lot of changes, puberty. I would find myself daydreaming a lot, wanting to be with my grandfather. In the summer I got to spend a lot of time with him. Grandfather owned his own business, and he taught me a lot. Learning was fun that way. It was hands-on learning. Anyway, that year my report card read, "Needs to finish work. Didn't turn in all papers. Needs to show more effort." I dreaded every day. Sometimes I even cried when I was by myself. How could I get these people to understand me? I went to automatic shut-off; everything seemed negative with school.

Summer came. I needed a break; I worked with Grandfather. That summer my family spent a lot of time preparing me for high school.

High school! What a big step! I was growing up. More things were going to be expected of me. I wanted to fit in and not be a jerk or dork.

My parents warned me about wrong crowds and told me high school grades were really important to my future. What pressure! My mom talked to the guidance counselor about my having ADD. The counselor assured her I would do just fine.

I was really nervous the first day, but guess what? All freshmen are. The first 6 weeks went by. Not all of my teachers had taken the time to read my school records. They didn't realize I had ADD. Boy, did things get out of hand.

Later that year, when Mom went in for a conference, one of my teachers said, "I would never have guessed Alan was ADD." Mom looked surprised. The teacher said, "He dresses so nice, has a clean haircut, and shows respect for teachers, not a smart aleck. He doesn't get into trouble." Mom rolled her eyes but didn't say anything until we got into the car. "Alan, that teacher doesn't understand about ADD. It's no respecter of persons. Anyone can get it. It's not a shame to have ADD. At least we know what we are dealing with. Remember, build on your strengths rather than magnify your weaknesses. Ignore that teacher's comment. She needs to be better educated in this field. School isn't just for ABCs anymore!"

I wanted to belong. I acted tough, even started to tell lies. I told stories that made me look big in people's eyes, but everyone knew they were lies. I just made things worse. In high school you are with a lot of people every day. You meet lots of teachers. Some teachers are there just to earn a paycheck, and there are a few who really care about the students they have. I have such a teacher. She took time for me, time to try to understand me better. When I needed someone to stand up for me, this teacher did.

Once, a teacher asked everyone to write a story as if they were in a make-believe world. She asked me about my ideas. I replied, "I deal in the real world." This really puzzled the teacher. I am 15 now. I have to deal in the real world. Dreaming is nice. Being an ADD student takes all my energy to meet the goals I have set for myself.

Through my years in school so far, I've been through a lot. My mom says I have a good heart; I care about those in need. I'm not dumb. You can't always measure smartness by tests. I feel I'm doing better in school. The school psychologist has become an important tool for me. I can talk to him when I get a teacher who doesn't understand, if I disagree with something, or if I'm just having problems. It helps to talk to someone who understands. What I'm trying to say is: No matter what comes my way, I can survive.

I have those who really care, and from that I draw my strength.

rule out private school or the community is not large enough to provide a variety of options. In these cases, you select the options that are available to you, which often can come down again to getting the best possible teacher. Still, more and more parents today—whether their children have ADHD or not—are basing their housing decisions on the local school system, so if your child has ADHD you may want to know what to look for in a school.

1. Speak with principals about their awareness of ADHD as an educational disability, how much in-service training the teachers have had on the disorder, and how receptive the school is to taking in such children.

2. If the school accepts such children, inquire about class sizes. They should be

as small as possible (12–15 is ideal, and 30–40 is absurd). Also, what extra assistance is available to help a teacher? Does the school have school psychologists, psychiatrists, clinical psychologists, and special educators to consult with teachers about children who have problems? Are there master teachers within the school who have extra training in ADHD, learning disorders, or behavior disorders, and who can serve as advisers or mentors to younger, less experienced, or less knowledgeable teachers on classroom management methods for dealing with ADHD?

3. What is the school's attitude toward the use of behavior-modifying drugs by children with ADHD? Some schools believe that medication is neither necessary nor beneficial. These schools are clearly out of touch with the scientific literature and should be avoided. Even if your child is not currently taking any medicine, if at some point she needs it, you will want a school that is knowledgeable and cooperative.

What mechanisms does the school have in place for the administration and monitoring of medication? Most schools have formal policies about such matters. Many schools require, for example, a signed statement from a physician about the type and dosage of medication and the timing of its administration. Public schools also often require the physician to submit a separate approval form to the state department of education before they will permit medicines to be given at school. Fortunately, with the recent development of long-acting ADHD medications, it is becoming less common for children to need to take medication during school hours; a dose of one of these newer medications once in the morning before school can often be enough to get them through the school day with sufficient medication in their bloodstream.

4. Does the school have formal procedures for disciplinary actions and appeals of those decisions? If so, get a copy of the written policies to see what rights your child may have should behavior problems necessitate disciplining him for misconduct. Then determine how comfortable you are with these policies. Be sure they are not just punitive, but also stress the efforts the school is likely to make to help him avoid repeating the offenses.

5. Does the principal encourage open and frequent home–school communication? Will you be welcome to drop by the school periodically to see how your child is doing? Can you request parent–teacher conferences without a lot of red tape? Is the input of parents valued by the school? Some schools will provide daily journals that the children take back and forth between home and school each day. The journal can indicate what was studied in each major subject and what the homework in that subject is each day. The children are often the ones to complete this information after each subject period, and the teacher then adds brief comments. These journals are great for keeping you informed about your child's performance each day. Other schools allow or even encourage teacher–parent contact via e-mail for much the same purposes.

6. If you feel it necessary, is the school staff open to having an outside professional

or expert visit the school with you to discuss your child's ADHD, educational program, and perhaps make further recommendations to improve it? If the school principal or teacher seems defensive about such outside advice, find another school.

7. How many other children entering your child's grade or class also have behavioral, learning, or emotional problems? Most teachers can handle only a few such children in any regular classroom with other typically functioning children. If there are more than two or three per class, ask for a different classroom or find another school.

Choosing a Teacher for Your Child

In making the best possible choice for your child, you need to evaluate teachers on the basis of two factors, as noted in the research review by Dr. Sherman and colleagues above: knowledge and attitude.

How Well Informed Is the Teacher?

Unfortunately, many teachers are uninformed about ADHD or are out of date in their knowledge of the disorder and its management. We have found that some teachers have a poor grasp of the nature, course, outcome, and causes of this disorder. They also may have misperceptions about which treatments are helpful and which are not. When this is the case, little positive change will result from attempting to establish curriculum adjustments and behavior management programs within that classroom. Just as the first step in helping your child was for you to become educated about ADHD, the initial step of school intervention is the education of teachers about the disorder. Armed with the information in this book, you should be able to determine from interviews with the principal and teachers whether a particular teacher is informed on ADHD. If not, you can do a lot to help.

By understanding the methods presented here and in Chapter 16, you become equipped to pass along recommendations to your child's teacher for possible implementation. You can also raise these techniques as suggestions at school conferences about your child's school performance or can even request, when appropriate, that some of them become a formal part of your child's written individualized education program (IEP) if your child is going to be receiving special educational services.

You can also help educate the teacher by providing brief reading materials such as those listed in "Suggested Reading and Videos" at the back of this book or even by sharing this book. In addition, I have made two DVDs (*ADHD—What Do We Know?* and *ADHD in the Classroom*) that summarize the disorder and cover issues of classroom management; many teachers have found them more convenient than reading materials. Finally, we recommend the video *Classroom Interventions for ADHD* by Drs. George J. DuPaul and Gary Stoner. (For full information about all these videos, again see "Suggested Reading and Videos.")

What Is the Teacher's Attitude toward ADHD and Behavior Modification Techniques?

Whether any individual teacher can and will adopt the behavioral programs advocated in this book is greatly influenced by the teacher's educational training and philosophy, as well as by his or her personal experience and beliefs about the educational process. In some cases, intensive training of your child's teacher by a school or clinical psychologist expert in these behavioral programs may be required. Children with ADHD who had teachers who are more domineering in these consultations and less open to the advice and information of the consultant had worse outcomes in school, according to research conducted in 2009 by Dr. William Erchul at North Carolina State University, Dr. George DuPaul at Lehigh University, and collaborators at other universities. Such teachers are substantially less likely to implement any of the consultant recommendations or to make changes in their classrooms for individual children having ADHD. Even with training, "booster" visits by the professional to the school following training may be necessary to maintain the teacher's use of the procedures. Teachers who use a permissive approach to education are often unlikely to use behavior modification, out of misplaced concern that these methods are too mechanical and do not adequately foster a child's natural development and motivation to learn. This is certainly not true. In some cases, these beliefs may be altered through the success of a consultation with a professional trained in behavioral programs. In other cases, such beliefs will not change and may greatly interfere with the effective use of behavioral programs in your child's classrooms. In such a case, a transfer to an alternative teacher with a philosophy more consistent with using behavioral programs may be beneficial.

In cases of poor teacher motivation or a conflicting philosophy, be assertive. Press the school administrators for either greater teacher accountability or a transfer of your child to another classroom or school, rather than waste a year of your child's education. Where this is not possible, you may have to supplement your child's education outside of school through additional tutoring, summer school review programs, and your extra involvement at home in reviewing schoolwork.

Some teachers resist behavioral techniques not because of a conflicting teaching philosophy, but because they believe the problems of children with ADHD are socially based, stemming from conflicts or chaos at home, or that medication is the only solution because ADHD has a biological basis. Other teachers may resent altering their teaching style if they believe this suggests their own behavior is causing a child's problems.

"Her teacher doesn't believe in ADHD. She says that too many children are being labeled and given excuses for their misconduct. How can I deal with her?"

Another important thing to consider is how well adjusted your child's teacher is and whether other parents have filed complaints against this teacher for incompetence, "malpractice," or ineffective teaching. You certainly cannot request that each of your child's teachers undergo a psychological evaluation, but you can seek information from the principal or other school staff members about that teacher's reputation in dealing with children with behavior problems. You can also ask for the names of parents whose children are currently in that teacher's care, so you can call those parents to get a clearer view of that teacher's competence.

What You Can Do to Help

Overall, the importance of a close collaboration among you, your child's teacher, and any professional experts on the treatment team cannot be stressed enough. However, successful collaboration can easily be hindered by attitude—not just the teacher's, but yours as well. Are your efforts being hampered by an attitude formed by a long history of conflicts with school personnel? Or are your expectations unrealistic? Are you waiting for the school to "cure" your child's problems while you remain passive or uninvolved? If your child is having few difficulties at home, have you persuaded yourself that poor teaching or management at school is causing your child's difficulties in the classroom? Be sure to reexamine your attitudes periodically to see if they're hindering the collaborative process.

If antagonism has arisen between you and a teacher, it is quite likely to undermine any intervention. In that case, you may want to ask a professional consulting with you to come to the school to help mediate consultations with the teacher.

Also be aware that in many cases the behavioral programs suggested here will need to be combined with medication to treat the school problems of a child with ADHD. Recent research shows that the combination of behavioral programs and medication produces improvements that are superior to either treatment used alone. Therefore, if your child is having serious problems with school adjustment, you should give thoughtful consideration to using medication (see Chapters 18 and 19).

Finally, when you find one or more good, sensitive teachers for your child, be supportive and praising; assist the teachers in any way you can; be open to the teachers' suggestions of what you can do to help; and convey your approval and admiration not only to the teachers but also to the school principal. This can greatly strengthen your relationship with such teachers, increase their desire to tailor their classroom programs to your child's special needs and abilities, assist you in finding future teachers of similar thinking as your child progresses through that school, and encourage them to come to your defense and your child's when decisions about educational programming must be made by school administrators. Positive attention to your child's teachers builds a stronger relationship with them, just as it does with your child.

Some Advice about Classroom and Curriculum

Various factors related to the structure of the classroom environment, classroom rules, and the nature of work assignments are important to consider if you are to help your child at school. In the past, professionals told parents and teachers to reduce the amount of stimulation in the classroom because it could lead to excessive distractibility in children with ADHD. Research evaluating such measures found, however, that they did not improve classroom behavior or academic performance in such children. Similarly, suggestions that traditional classrooms are too restrictive and that classrooms affording greater freedom and flexibility are best have not been supported by research.

There are several features of the classroom, however, that may need some adjustments when a teacher is working with your child. Keep these things in mind when you are shopping for next year's classroom and teacher for your child. Remember them as well when you meet with that teacher to plan the approach to the school year. Believe it or not, one important point is the seating arrangement in the classroom. Research shows that a traditional desk arrangement in rows facing the front of the classroom, where the teacher typically locates while lecturing, is far better for children with ADHD than modular arrangements, where several or more children share a larger table, especially if they face each other while working. Such arrangements seem to provide too much stimulation and too many opportunities for social interaction with other children, which distract a child with ADHD from attending to the teacher or classwork.

You can also ask that your child be moved closer to the teacher's desk or wherever the teacher spends the most time while instructing the class. This not only discourages classmates from giving your child attention for disruptive behavior, but also makes it easier for the teacher to monitor your child and to dispense rewards and fines quickly and easily. Altering seating arrangements is sometimes as effective as a reward program in increasing appropriate classroom behavior.

Classrooms that are physically enclosed (with four walls and a door) are usually much better for a child with ADHD than so-called open classrooms. Open classrooms are usually noisier and contain more visual distractions. Research shows that noisy environments are associated with less attention to work and higher levels of disruptive behavior in children with ADHD.

A well-organized and predictable classroom routine is also helpful. The posting of a daily schedule and classroom rules can add to this sense of structure. Use of feedback charts at the front of the class that display how children are doing in following rules, behaving, and working may also help your child with ADHD.

In some cases, "nag tapes" are particularly helpful. While this is not really a factor in classroom structure, it is an example of the type of measure the school should be open to using. Before doing work at his desk, the child takes out a small portable digital recorder, puts on an earpiece so the recording does not distract other students, and turns on the player. The child then proceeds to do the work while the recorder plays reminders to him—usually using the father's voice, since we know children with ADHD tend to listen better to their fathers than their mothers—to remain on task, not bug others, and the like. The effectiveness of these tapes will depend greatly on their being combined with consistent methods for enforcing rules and with the use of rewards and punishments for working and proper conduct.

The following additional changes to classroom structure and curriculum are likely to be helpful:

1. As is true for all children, academic tasks should be well matched to the child's abilities. For children with ADHD, increasing the novelty and interest level of the tasks through use of increased stimulation (for example, color, shape, texture) seems to reduce disruptive behavior, enhance attention, and improve overall performance.

2. The teacher should change the style of presenting lectures and task materials to help maintain the interest and motivation of children with ADHD. When low-interest or passive tasks are assigned, they should be interspersed with high-interest or active tasks to optimize attention or concentration. Tasks requiring an active as opposed to a passive response may also allow children with ADHD to better channel their disruptive behaviors into constructive responses. In other words, give a child with ADHD something to do as part of the class lecture, work assignment, or activity, and the child's behavior will be less of a problem.

3. Academic assignments should be brief to fit with a child's attention span. A good rule of thumb is to assign the amount of work that would be appropriate for a child 30% younger. Feedback regarding performance of assignments should be given immediately, and time limits for getting work done should be short. This can be aided by the use of timers, such as clocks or cooking timers.

4. A child's attention during group lessons may be enhanced by delivering the lesson in an enthusiastic yet task-focused style, keeping it brief, and allowing frequent and active child participation. A teacher who pretends to be more like an actor—who is vibrant, enthused, and emotionally charged—will get much more attention than one who drones on about some dry subject.

5. Mixing classroom lectures up with brief moments of physical exercise may also be helpful. This reduces the sense of fatigue and monotony that children with ADHD may experience more often than typical children during extended academic work periods. The teacher can try jumping jacks by the desk, a quick trip outside the

classroom for a brisk 2-minute run or walk, forming a line and walking about the classroom in "conga line" fashion, or other such brief physical activities. These can rejuvenate the attention span not only of a child with ADHD but of other children as well.

6. The teacher should schedule the difficult academic subjects in the morning and leave the more active, nonacademic subjects and lunch to the afternoon periods unless the child is on an ADHD medication. It is well known that the ability of a child with ADHD to concentrate and to inhibit behavior decreases greatly over the school day (see Chapter 4).

7. Whenever possible, classroom lectures should be augmented with direct-instruction materials—short, highly specific drills of important academic skills or, even better, computers with software that does the same thing.

What Placement Is Best for a Child with ADHD?

In many cases, the measures described so far and the programs presented in Chapter 16 will be sufficient, especially for children with mild-to-moderate ADHD symptoms or for children whose inattention and behavioral problems are controlled with medication. However, in other cases, especially those with severe ADHD symptoms and accompanying problems of opposition, aggression, or learning disabilities, alternative educational placements—for example, special education or private school—may be necessary. Ideally, these placements should include classes with a small student–teacher ratio, and the classes should be taught by teachers with expertise in behavior modification.

Special Educational Services

Obtaining special educational services for children with ADHD is often a difficult process. Many such children did not previously qualify for special educational services according to the guidelines specified in Public Law 94-142, the predecessor of the current Individuals with Disabilities Education Act (IDEA). Now they do! If your child with ADHD is failing, he may be eligible for formal special education services under this law under the category known as "Other Health Impaired." Ask your school district to explain the IDEA and your child's rights under it. Keep in mind, however, that your child must be experiencing a significant impairment in school performance because of ADHD to get special education services; a diagnosis alone is insufficient.

Unfortunately, a child with ADHD but without associated problems is likely to be eligible for little special education in most states. When associated problems do exist, such as learning disabilities or emotional disturbances (particularly aggression and defiance), the child will probably be assigned to classes that focus on those problems.

Certainly, children with ADHD who have significant speech and language or motor development problems are likely to receive speech, occupational, and physical therapy, or even adaptive physical education, provided that these developmental problems are sufficient to interfere with academic performance.

Although the situation has improved markedly in the past decade in many school districts, you may need to bring pressure on your school district to abide by the existing laws. Efforts have been underway since 1991 by national parent support associations to force states to follow the recommendations of the federal government to improve services for children with ADHD, but any further improvements may hinge on the need to limit any costs that would escalate for school districts opening their special educational programs to another disabled population.

In the meantime, it is essential that you become familiar with federal, state, and local district guidelines. You can get all of this information from your school district. Other information of help to you can be found in the second edition of *All About ADHD: The Complete Practical Guide for Classroom Teachers* by Dr. Linda Pfiffner, coauthor of this chapter. You can also find sound advice in other books, such as the second edition of *How to Reach and Teach Children with ADD/ADHD* by Dr. Sandra Rief, *Problem-Solver Guide for Students with ADHD* by Dr. Harvey Parker, the *CHADD Educators Manual* by Mary Fowler (second edition by Chris Dendy), *ADD and the Law* by attorneys Peter Latham and Patricia Latham, and *Turning the Tide* by Karen Richards and John Lester. For full information about all of these books, see "Suggested Reading and Videos" at the end of this volume.

In addition, you should become acquainted with the director of special education within your school district. You are only as good as your personal telephone directory or contact list in dealing with the educational problems of your child. A good file of telephone numbers can go a long way toward locating resources within the private sector, such as private schools, formal and informal tutoring programs, and special summer camps. Also contact your local parent support association (for example, your local branch of CHADD or ADDA—see "Support Services for Parents" at the end of the book) for advice on resources in your area for school problems. These organizations can sometimes even send a professionally trained advocate with you to school meetings. In some cases, you may need to get a second opinion about your child's problems because you disagree with the school staff over the nature and extent of those problems and the child's eligibility for services.

It is also important to understand the concept of the "least restrictive environment" as it applies to decisions regarding special educational placement. The IDEA makes it clear that special services are to be provided so that children with disabilities are not unreasonably precluded from interactions with nondisabled peers. School districts are therefore likely to err in the direction of placing children with ADHD in the least restrictive environment necessary to manage their academic and behavioral problems. That is, they may put the children in the program that provides the greatest contact with normally functioning students. Some teachers are not always in agreement with this system. They prefer that even children with mild ADHD be removed to special educational settings, rather than have to adjust their classroom curriculum and behavior management style to accommodate the needs of these children. Parents may be equally biased toward special education, believing that the smaller class sizes, better trained teachers, and greater teacher attention they provide are preferable. School districts are likely to resist these pressures, so as not to violate the rights of children to placement in the least restrictive environment or risk legal action for doing so. Parents may find this frustrating, but must understand the philosophy behind this placement bias and its basis in law.

Should Children Be Retained in Their Grade?

Anywhere from 23 to 40% of children with ADHD will be retained in a grade at least once before reaching high school, mostly in the early elementary years. Therefore, many parents will have to determine whether retention is the solution to their own child's difficulties.

It's understandable that retention would be recommended in so many cases since children with ADHD often display the characteristics of children who are immature for their age. Many teachers might reasonably recommend "another year to grow up." Yet many studies have failed to identify any significant advantages in achievement as a result of delaying school entry, and more recent ones have identified multiple harms that occur to children in association with their having been retained. These adverse effects include loss of interest in school, loss of motivation to learn, increased aggressiveness in boys primarily and increased depression in girls primarily. Retained children are also more likely to be rejected by their peers following retention and are much less likely to complete high school than other children with similar problems who were not retained. School difficulties associated with ADHD are not due just to a brief developmental immaturity, and so repeating the same approach for a second year is not likely to help. It does not, after all, address the specific problems of ADHD. And, in fact, a child who repeats a grade may be bored when reviewing the old material and thus may be doomed to fail. Taken to its extreme, this solution could result in what one mother said was "having him repeating every single grade. At that rate, he would graduate at 30!"

In a study conducted by Dr. Linda Pagani thousands of children in the Montreal public schools were followed for many years of their education. One purpose of this study was to see if grade retention benefited or harmed schoolchildren. The study found that this practice resulted in no measurable benefits to the future of the children who had been retained and that the practice was harmful in many ways. The children who had been retained often lost interest in school and learning, developed further problems with peer relations, and often became more aggressive. My own follow-up study with Dr. Mariellen Fischer found that children with ADHD who had been retained in grade were also more likely to quit school before completing high school. The earlier the grade retention occurred, the more harmful it was found to be. Dr. Pagani's study supports my own recommendation that children not be retained in their grade as a means of dealing with their learning or behavioral problems.

Questions/Options to Consider

While retaining a child in a grade is not advisable once she has started formal schooling, it can be wise to consider keeping a young child in kindergarten an additional year before letting her progress to first grade. What factors should you consider in such a decision?

Academic Status

In general, if a child is mentally capable of completing the work at the next grade level, then a different type of academic environment (for example, greater reinforcement, smaller class) is preferable to retention. If a global delay is identified in academic achievement or intelligence based on psychological testing of the child, retention can be recommended. If not, the child should be promoted, with supportive educational services provided in the delayed areas.

Physical Size and Age

Parents and children have commented on the social problems of retention when the children were bigger than their classmates. So retention might seem wiser when a kindergartener is small in stature and/or has a birthday near the school district's cutoff for first grade.

Emotional Maturity

The impulsivity and low frustration tolerance, among other characteristics, that mark the emotional immaturity of children with ADHD are not likely to be cured by another year in kindergarten or any other grade. Instead, some type of intervention, such as a program of social skills training within the school setting, might be helpful. My colleagues and I have used the social skills training program called *Skillstreaming,* by Drs. Ellen McGinnis and Arnold Goldstein (see "Suggested Reading and Videos"). It has been used successfully by regular classroom preschool and elementary teachers within the typical academic curriculum.

In fact, many of a child's difficulties can be addressed through remedial services provided in the regular classroom as an alternative to retention. Occupational therapy can be used, and recommendations can be given by the occupational therapist for the regular classroom teacher to use in the classroom. Speech and language therapy may also be beneficial, especially when it focuses on communication, in which case such therapy becomes an effective social skills program.

Style and Expectations of the Teacher

As already discussed, teachers vary considerably both in what they expect their students to be able to do and in their attitude toward disorders like ADHD. A number of relatively simple behavioral strategies (discussed in Chapter 16) can be used in the regular classroom by a teacher who is open to this approach, thus eliminating the need for retention. So the choice of a teacher is a critical determinant in the decision about whether to retain a child.

Alternative Classroom Options/Curriculum

In addition to regular kindergarten or regular first grade, there are options that may be available within the school district. These include a language-based kindergarten or first grade, which provides a supportive language-based curriculum and a smaller student–teacher ratio. You could also ask about a K–1 transitional program, which is often used for children who are somewhat slow in development. Because they provide a lot of feedback and do so immediately, computers can be very useful for young children with ADHD. It is a rare child with ADHD who doesn't like computer games. Using such games to enhance learning of academic skills can be a helpful aid to a regular classroom curriculum. A number of computer programs—*Reader Rabbit* and *Math Blaster,* for example—enhance reading and math readiness. So, in general, even when retention is recommended and especially when it is not, considerable attention needs to be directed toward what type of teaching approach was provided last time and what can be done this time to make sure it is more effective.

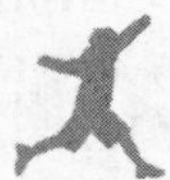

16 Enhancing Education at School and at Home

METHODS FOR SUCCESS FROM KINDERGARTEN THROUGH GRADE 12

with Linda J. Pfiffner, PhD

Now that you've found the best possible setting for your child's education, you can begin to look at specific techniques for maximizing school success on a day-to-day basis. Here is another area where you must become an expert; it may very well be up to you to help plan the intervention and train the teacher(s) in the effective use of classroom modifications and child behavior management programs. It is certainly up to you to see that your child's education is enhanced by what goes on at home. This chapter goes into detail on general principles and specific methods for helping a child with ADHD succeed in school. Even though it focuses on the classroom, this chapter contains many suggestions that could easily be adapted for use at home by parents in getting work done at home and improving the home behavior of a child with ADHD. So as you read it, keep this alternative use of these methods in mind.

Remember to try to involve your child in this process of improving his school success to increase the child's motivation to succeed. Include any child over age 7 in some of your initial planning meetings with a teacher. This gives the child some input into setting goals and determining appropriate and valuable rewards and penalties for behavior. Among the important products of such meetings are behavioral contracts that outline the details of the programs and can be signed by parent, teacher, and child to help maintain the consistent use of the program over time and to clarify each person's role.

General Principles for School Management

Whether or not medication is used, a number of important principles are helpful to keep in mind in developing classroom management programs for your child with

ADHD. These stem from the theory presented in Chapter 2 that ADHD involves an impairment in your child's executive abilities and self-regulation. They are also founded on the principles for managing your child at home given in Chapter 11.

1. Rules and instructions must be clear, brief, and (wherever possible) represented physically in the form of charts, lists, and other visual reminders. Relying on the child's memory and on verbal reminders is often ineffective. Encourage the child to repeat instructions out loud and even to utter them softly to himself while following through on the instruction.

2. Rewards, punishments, and feedback used to manage the child's behavior must be delivered swiftly and immediately, and the entire approach to using consequences must be well organized, systematic, and planned.

3. Frequent feedback or consequences for following the rules are crucial to maintaining the child's compliance.

4. Children with ADHD are less sensitive to social praise and reprimands, so the consequences for good or bad behavior must be more powerful than those needed to manage the behavior of children without ADHD.

5. Rewards and incentives must be put in place before punishment is used, or your child will come to see school as a place where she is more likely to be punished than rewarded. Make sure the teacher waits a week or two after setting up a reward program at school before starting to use punishment. Then make sure the teacher gives away two to three rewards for each punishment. When punishment fails, first determine whether the extent to which rewards are available is insufficient; when it is, punishment will not control your child's behavior.

6. Token reward systems can be kept effective over an entire school year with minimal loss of power, provided that the rewards are changed frequently. Children who have ADHD become bored with particular rewards faster than other children, and teachers who fail to recognize that fact often give up on a token program too soon, believing it has stopped working when it is just boredom with the specific privileges children can purchase with their tokens that is the problem.

7. Anticipation is the key with children who have ADHD, especially during times of transition. To ensure that your child is aware of an impending shift, ask the teacher to follow the strategies presented in Chapter 12: (a) review the rules *before* going into the new activity; (b) have the child repeat these rules, including rewards for good behavior and punishment for misbehavior; and (c) follow through on this plan once the activity begins. *Think aloud, think ahead* is the important message for educators here.

You can also share some of the principles from Chapter 9 with your child's teachers: (1) strive for consistency, (2) do not personalize the child's problems, (3) maintain a disability perspective on the child, and (4) practice forgiveness. With these rules in mind, a creative teacher can easily devise an effective management program for your child with ADHD.

8. But sometimes children with ADHD may need extra help outside of school to stay on pace with typical children in getting school homework done or keeping up their academic skills and knowledge. Some parents step in and play the role of tutor to the child, which in some cases can work very well. We have found, however, that many parents make poor tutors or find that issues between the parent and child that arose in other situations carry over to adversely affect the time set aside for this tutoring. For these reasons, and others, we often encourage parents to hire a formal tutor to work with their child several times a week. In addition to such a tutor, or instead of one, parents should check out the self-taught courses on the Internet at Khan Academy *(www.khanacademy.org)*. These are courses designed for children and teens to complete on their own and cover many of the academic subjects that children and teens are likely to be taking at school. They use a better and self-paced format that seems beneficial for the child with ADHD. Parents (or a tutor) can also work together with the child or teen on these courses initially. The courses are free.

Behavior Management Methods for the Classroom

Positive and negative consequences are the most effective tools for behavior management in the classroom, just as they are at home. Positive consequences usually include praise, tokens and tangible rewards, and special privileges. Punishments commonly are ignoring, verbal reprimands, fines or penalties in a token system, and time-out. The greatest improvement in classroom behavior and academic performance is likely to come only from a combination of strategies.

Using Positive Consequences

Teacher Attention

Praise and other forms of positive teacher attention such as a smile, nod, or pat on the back are some of the most basic management tools teachers have at their disposal. Positive attention is valued by most children, including your child, though attention alone is rarely enough to manage all of the problems children with ADHD may have at school.

"The teacher asked me, 'Why should I give your child lots of rewards for behaving well when I don't do this for the children who behave normally? They'll resent it.' How can I respond?"

Giving praise and acknowledgment may seem simple, but the organized and systematic use of such attention requires great skill. The teacher must be specific about what is praiseworthy and must convey genuine warmth. Praise must be delivered quickly and must vary in wording to have the best strategic effect. Effective use of praise also requires increased monitoring or supervision, so the teacher can "catch the child being good" more often and give the positive consequences earned. But this is easier said than done. The demands on a teacher's time and attention in the average classroom are considerable. Supervising your child more closely inevitably competes with monitoring all the other children and teaching the curriculum. Some teachers may even feel that your child does not deserve this extra attention and supervision—that the other children in the class do not get this kind of attention for behaving well, so it is not fair to give it to your child for misbehaving. If your teacher makes such remarks, share your knowledge as discussed in Chapter 15, so the teacher understands that ADHD is a disability—not simply naughtiness or laziness. Society often makes exceptions for people with disabilities, and in this case children with ADHD are no exception. Also, note that other children may not require so much feedback to continue to perform well, while the child with ADHD may fall behind and do poorly in school without it. The fact that we don't need a ramp to get over a curb in the roadway or up the stairs into a building doesn't mean that people with physical disabilities shouldn't have them available, nor does it mean we will resent such people with disabilities for having them available. So this line of argument by a teacher really doesn't make any sense.

Using Cues to Provide Consequences

Several devices can be used to help a teacher remember to provide frequent feedback to a child with ADHD: (1) Smiley face stickers can be placed about the classroom at points where the teacher may frequently glance, as reminders to check out what the student with ADHD is doing and praise the child if it is at all positive. (2) The teacher can also set the timer on her smart phone or even set a simple spring-wound cooking timer to go off periodically as another reminder to stop and monitor the ADHD student. (3) A soft tone can be put onto a digital recorder at random intervals (more frequently for the first week or two and then spaced out farther) over a 90-minute or 120-minute period to remind the teacher to check on the student and provide praise as appropriate. For students 8 years old and up, the teacher can even use this type of cueing program to teach self-monitoring. The student gets a small white file card divided down the middle to form two columns with a plus sign (+) or smiley face over the left column and a minus sign (–) or frowny face over the right column. Whenever the child hears the tone, he can record a point (hash mark) in the plus column for obeying instructions or one in the minus column for being off-task. The teacher's job is to check quickly on the child's behavior when the tone sounds and make sure the student is recording accurately. Self-monitoring is enhanced when an easel at the front of the classroom lists five or so rules for each class period, so the teacher can flip to the appropriate page throughout the day. (4) The teacher can also start a class period with about 10 bingo chips in, say, a left pocket, moving a chip to the right pocket whenever positive attention has been given to your child. The goal is to move all 10 chips to the right pocket by the end of that class period.

Tangible Reward and Token Programs

Despite the usefulness of praising good behavior and ignoring misbehavior, these procedures are often not enough by themselves. A variety of more powerful rewards, often in the form of special privileges such as helping the teacher, earning extra recess, playing special games, having computer time, and doing art projects, can be given. It's important that a long list of choices be available to prevent boredom. Also, because frequent rewards are important to helping a child with ADHD, some of these rewards should be possible to earn a few times a day. More valuable rewards, like a pizza party or special class outing, should be earned over longer periods of time, such as weekly.

Using token, point, or chip programs to earn rewards can also be very effective (see Chapter 11). The teachers may find it helpful to interview the child with ADHD about the kinds of activities or other rewards the child would like to earn, as well as selecting some based on observation of the child. If few powerful enough rewards are available at school, you may have to set up a home-based reward program, as discussed later in this chapter. Or you could donate a favorite type of toy or piece of play equipment from home for the teacher to use with a classroom reward system.

One very powerful reward kids seem to like these days is to be allowed to play video games. We have been successful in approaching local civic clubs for donations of such games or some funds to offset the expense of buying handheld inexpensive ones by giving presentations on the seriousness of classroom behavioral problems and the critical need for such rewards in the management of disruptive children. Teachers can also check the local Goodwill store for any used older generation gaming systems and games that may still be quite desirable to have in the classroom as a source of rewards, or parents can find them at such stores and donate them to the classroom.

Token programs can also be used for a group of children, with all class members earning rewards based on the behavior of one or more of the classmates or of the entire group. Group programs can be particularly effective when peers are rewarding a child with ADHD for disruptive behavior by laughing or joining in the inappropriate conduct. In some group programs, the performance of a student with ADHD serves as the standard for determining how much reward is given to the entire class. In other cases, tokens or points are given to each child in the classroom, including the child with ADHD, based on how the student with ADHD has done. This has the advantage of motivating the other children in the class to help the student with ADHD behave well, follow the rules, and get work done. A different form of this program involves breaking the class up into small teams, which earn or lose points depending on their behavior. The team with the greatest number of positive points or fewest negative points earns privileges for that entire team. The group approach has the advantage of not singling out the child with ADHD, but this benefit must be weighed against the potential for the child with ADHD to be vilified for causing the whole class to be penalized when the student with ADHD does poorly.

Token programs can also be used to increase your child's academic productivity and work accuracy. In one program we set up, the token system involved children earning checks on an index card for each correct answer, with the checks redeemable for a large variety of backup rewards at school (such as candy, free time, school and art supplies, picnics in the park, etc.) later in the day. This program sharply increased math and reading scores, and it reduced disruptive behavior to a level similar to that seen when the children had previously been on medication.

In another, very novel program, tokens were given for successful completion of four tasks: two that involved learning to read and using new vocabulary words in sentences and two that involved teaching these tasks to another student, called *peer tutoring*. When a token had been earned for completion of each of these four tasks, it was exchanged for 15 minutes of play on a pinball machine or electronic game in the classroom. Additional game time was earned whenever a child passed a subject's unit test, such as a chapter in the reading assignment. This token program dramatically increased both the completion of schoolwork and the accuracy of the work. It also improved the students' performance on the school district's weekly reading exams. This program was carried out by just a single teacher.

The types of goals selected for token programs are critical to their success. Giving rewards for outstanding performance works for other children, but many children with ADHD need affirmation for lesser achievements. At the start, therefore, rewards should be given for smaller accomplishments—such as for completing a part of the work when the child has a long history of failing to complete work or for being quiet for part of the day when the child is often disruptive throughout the day.

Tokens also need to be adjusted for the age of the children involved. Tangible tokens, such as poker chips, are very important in managing 4- to 7-year-olds, while points, numbers, or hash marks on a card can be used through high school. With preschool or kindergarten children, however, using plastic chips may actually serve as a distraction, so we have often used a small fabric pocket pinned to the back of a child's clothing. When tokens are dispensed, the teacher reaches out to the child, slips the token into the child's "knapsack," and gives a light affectionate squeeze to the child's shoulder. Several times each day, the pocket is removed and emptied, and the child can exchange the tokens for various classroom privileges.

Using Negative Consequences

Ignoring

Ignoring is often used as one of the first treatments for mild misbehavior, especially when children's misbehavior seems to be encouraged by teacher attention.

Unfortunately, it is not easy to distinguish the cases when a child with ADHD is trying to get attention by misbehaving from those in which the child is not. Most misbehavior stems from your child's biological deficits in inhibiting behavior and sustaining attention. Ignoring does not mean simply failure to monitor a child's behavior; it means *contingent withdrawal* of teacher attention when the misbehavior occurs. It works best in combination with praise—for example, praising the children who stay in their seats while withdrawing attention from a child with ADHD who is wandering around the classroom. But even when a powerful reward program is used as well, ignoring may not be sufficient punishment to teach a child with ADHD to stop misbehaving. In these cases, additional negative consequences appear necessary. Ignoring is also not indicated in cases of aggression or destruction—acts of misconduct that deserve swift, certain punishment to discourage their repetition in the future.

Reprimands

The reprimand is probably the most frequently used negative consequence in the classroom, but its effectiveness can vary considerably. Brief, specific reprimands given swiftly, without much emotion (business-like), and consistently backed up with other punishment if not heeded can be effective for your child with ADHD. Reprimands that are vague, delayed, long-winded, emotional, and not backed up with other consequences are not helpful. Reprimands mixed with positive feedback also fail, as do inconsistently delivered reprimands. For example, children who are sometimes reprimanded for calling out but other times responded to as if they had raised their hands are apt to continue, if not increase, their calling out. Reprimands also appear to be more effective when delivered with eye contact in close proximity (nearby) to a child. In addition, children respond better to teachers who deliver consistently strong reprimands at the outset of the school year than to teachers who gradually increase the severity of their discipline over time. In summary, reprimands, like praise, are not always sufficient to change your child's behavior. More powerful backup consequences may be necessary.

Behavior Penalties or Fines

Penalties, or what professionals call *response cost,* involve the loss or removal of a reward based on the display of some misbehavior. Lost rewards can include a wide range of privileges and activities or even tokens in a token system (fines). Fining can easily be adapted to a variety of behavior problems and situations; it is more effective than the use of reprimands alone and seems to increase the effectiveness of reward programs.

In one research study, the teacher deducted one point every time she saw a child not working. Each lost point meant a loss of 1 minute of free time. A digital counter was placed at each child's desk to keep track of the child's point totals. One child's counter consisted of numbered cards that could be changed to a lesser number each time a point was lost. The teacher had an identical counter on her desk where she kept track of point losses. The child was instructed to match the number value on his counter with that of the teacher's frequently during the class. A second child had a battery-operated electronic "counter" with a number display, called the *Attention Trainer* (you can see it at *www.addwarehouse.com* or just enter the name in your Internet search engine, like Google, to learn more about it). The teacher simply took away points for off-task behavior on the display by using a remote transmitter like that used in an electronic garage-door opener.

Both of these methods increased the time the children paid attention to their work and their academic performance. The results were almost as good as when the children had been on stimulant medication. The swiftness with which the consequences were delivered in either procedure certainly helped to make the program work. In addition, these procedures were very easy to use, practical, and efficient for the teacher.

As with other punishments, however, the use of fines or penalties has raised some concerns about possible negative effects. Ways to reduce these are discussed later in the chapter. We have found that giving lots of rewards in class and avoiding unreasonably strict standards can reduce the number of penalties that need to be used.

Time-Out

Time-out was discussed for use at home in Chapter 11. The term really means the time during which positive reinforcement or rewards are not available. It is frequently recommended for use at school with children who have ADHD and are particularly aggressive or disruptive. Time-out can be applied in several ways. One of these, often called *social isolation,* involves placing the child in a chair in an empty room for a few minutes. It has come under much criticism lately. Now professionals generally recommend just removing the child from the area of rewarding activities rather than from the entire classroom. This may involve having the child sit in a three-sided cubicle or sit facing a dull area (for example, a blank wall) in the classroom. In other cases, children may be required to put their work away (which eliminates the opportunity to earn rewards for academic performance) and to put their heads down (which reduces the opportunity for rewarding interaction with others) for brief periods of time.

Another time-out procedure uses a good-behavior clock. Rewards (penny trinkets, candy, etc.) are earned by a child and by the class based on that child's behaving appropriately for a specified period of time. A clock runs whenever the child is paying attention, working, or behaving appropriately. The clock is stopped for a short period of time when the child is disruptive or off-task. Studies have found dramatic decreases in hyperactive and disruptive behavior as a result of this method.

Most time-out programs set specific rules that must be fulfilled before the child can be released from time-out. Typically, these rules involve the child being quiet and cooperative for a specified period during time-out. In some cases, extremely disruptive or hyperactive children may fail to comply with the typical procedure. They may refuse to go to time-out or escape from the time-out area before finishing their penalty period. To reduce problems in these cases, children may earn time off their penalty period for good behavior or for complying with the procedure (that is, the length of the original time-out is reduced). Alternatively, when a child refuses to follow the time-out rules, the length of the original time-out may be increased for each rule infraction. In another approach, the child may be removed from the class to serve the time-out elsewhere (for example, in another class or in the principal's office). Failure to comply with time-out may also be responded to with a penalty or fine in the class token system. For instance, activities, privileges, or tokens may be lost for uncooperative behavior in time-out. One strategy that may be particularly effective for reducing uncooperativeness with time-out involves having children stay after school to serve their time-out when they are not cooperative in following time-out rules during school hours. The use of this procedure, however, depends on having staff members available to supervise after school.

Some teachers may keep children in from recess to serve time-out or to complete their schoolwork when it has not been completed during normal class time. We do not recommend this procedure because children with ADHD need their periodic physical exercise as much as or more than typical children and because research shows that physical exercise can help to reduce subsequent ADHD symptoms for a while.

There are cases when a child's problem behavior typically increases during time-out. This requires the teacher to intervene or restrain the child to prevent harm to the child, to others, or to property. Alternative procedures to time-out may be needed. Most schools have some guidelines for the types of punishment they permit. Parents may want to ask for copies of these so they can be familiar with what limits the school district may place (or not place!) on these methods.

School Suspension

Suspension from school (usually from 1 to 3 days) is sometimes used as punishment for severe behavior problems, but it should be used with much caution. Many children may find staying at home or in full-day day care more enjoyable than being in school. Suspension is also undesirable when the parents both work and cannot supervise the child when they are at home during suspension, when they may not have the management skills needed to enforce the suspension, or when they are overly punitive or abusive to a child due to the suspension. Given that many parents now work during school hours, it is better for a school to develop an in-school suspension program where students who are suspended for a day or two for misbehavior can go to an alternative location in the school that is under stricter supervision and with work that must be done in order to be returned to the regular classroom.

How to Limit the Effects of Punishment

Despite the overall effectiveness of punishment, some unpleasant side effects may occur if it is used improperly. These unwanted effects include the escalation of the problem behavior, the child's dislike of the teacher, or (in rare cases) the avoidance of school altogether. Drs. Lee Rosen and Susan O'Leary from Stony Brook University, offer several guidelines to reduce possible adverse side effects:

1. Punishment should be used sparingly. Excessive criticism or other forms of punishment may also make the classroom unpleasant or aversive. Frequent harsh punishment may even increase a child's defiance. This is especially likely in cases where a teacher mistakenly serves as an aggressive model—that is, the teacher's use of punishment teaches the child to be aggressive like the teacher.

2. When negative consequences are used, children should be taught and rewarded for alternative appropriate behaviors that are not compatible with the inappropriate ones. This practice will help by teaching the children appropriate skills, as well as by decreasing the potential for the occurrence of other problem behaviors.

3. Punishment involving the removal of a reward or privilege is to be preferred to punishment involving the use of an aversive event, such as isolation or physical punishment. In fact, the use of physical punishment is often limited in schools for ethical and legal reasons.

Getting Results to Last and Carry Over to Other School Situations

Despite the substantial success of behavioral methods in school, there is little evidence that the gains made by children under these programs last once the programs are stopped. Also, the improvements that may occur in one setting where the programs are used (say, reading class) often do not carry over to settings where the programs are not being used (say, math class or recess). This can be very disappointing to both parents and teachers.

One current solution is to use management programs wherever the child's behavior is a problem, but this approach has practical limits. Most programs won't be easy to carry out at recess, for example. Instead, withdrawing the management methods gradually—by reducing the frequency of feedback (fading from daily to weekly rewards) and substituting more natural rewards such as praise and regular activities for token rewards—may increase their endurance. One study found that the abrupt removal of punishment, even when a powerful token program was in use, led to a dramatic deterioration in class behavior, but when punishment was removed gradually, high levels of paying attention and hard work were maintained.

One particularly effective way to fade out a management program involves changing the places in school where the programs are in effect on any given day. The child is never quite sure when or where the programs will be used and learns that the best bet in these circumstances is to keep behaving well.

Even though research continues on these issues, the difficulties have not been resolved. Specially arranged treatment programs for children with ADHD simply may be required across most school settings. For now we know these must be kept in place for long periods of time over the course of a child's education to be helpful. This observation may seem discouraging, but given our view that ADHD is a fairly chronic developmentally disabling condition, it is no surprise.

Having Classmates Help with Behavior Management

The disruptive behavior of children with ADHD often prompts their peers to respond in ways that promote or maintain the problem behavior. On the one hand, classmates may reward such a child's clowning and silliness with smiles and giggles. On the other hand, they may also retaliate against the child's teasing or intrusiveness. Either way, the child gets a bad reputation among peers. As discussed previously, using group-based reward programs may be effective in counteracting peer attention for misbehavior by a child with ADHD. However, some studies show that classmates can also intervene directly to produce good behavior in a fellow student with ADHD.

One of the most powerful ways classmates can help is by being encouraged to ignore the disruptive and inappropriate behavior of the child with ADHD. Peers can also increase this child's appropriate behavior by giving the child praise and positive attention for it. We see this in action during sporting events, when team members cheer and congratulate each other for successful plays, and it can be extended to praising one another for being a good sport, getting a high grade on an exam (or accepting a low grade without a tantrum), contributing to a class discussion, or helping another student. Token programs, in which classmates monitor the behavior of the child with ADHD and give or take away tokens for good or bad behavior, can also be successful as long as they are supervised by a teacher.

Of course, these classmates should usually be rewarded for their own efforts. Otherwise, what's in it for them? In some cases praise is sufficient, but the teacher can also use tangible rewards or a token program. Rewarding these children not only reinforces their efforts, but also ensures that the program is carried out well.

The use of classmates as "behavior sheriffs" has practical advantages. It provides an alternative to the teacher being compelled to observe everyone all the time, and it may require less time than traditional teacher-mediated programs. It may also serve to improve the behavior of the "sheriffs" and to encourage the transfer of the improved behavior into other situations where the same peers are present. However, programs carried out by classmates are successful only to the extent that these classmates have the ability and interest to learn the methods and to carry them out accurately. The teacher should train and supervise classmates carefully and should not let them get involved in the punishment aspects of any program.

Home-Based Reward Programs

In a home-based reward program, the teacher sends home an evaluation of how the child with ADHD behaved in school that day and the parents use it to give or take away rewards available at home. This method has been effective in modifying a wide range of problems that children with ADHD have at school. Because of its ease of application and the fact that it involves both the teacher(s) and parents, it is often one of the first interventions you should try.

Behavior Report Card

The teacher's report can consist of either an informal note or a more formal report card. We recommend the use of a behavior report card. The card should show the "target" behaviors that are to be the focus of the program listed on the left side. Across the top should be numbered columns that correspond to each class period at school. The teacher gives a number rating reflecting how well the child did for each of these behaviors for each class period. Examples of daily school behavior report cards are shown in Figures 3, 4, and 5. Figure 3 illustrates a card designed to assist in managing classroom behavioral problems. Figure 4 shows a card designed to help with a child who has behavioral problems during free time, such as recess or lunchtime. And Figure 5 is a blank card that can be tailored to whatever behavioral problems parents and teachers wish to focus on in this type of treatment program. Parents can feel free to photocopy these figures for use with their own children, with permission of the publisher. These teacher reports are typically sent home daily. In some cases, notes are sent home only when a child has met certain goals for behavior or academic work that day. In other cases, a note can be sent home on both "good" and "bad" days. As the child's behavior improves, the daily reports can be reduced to twice weekly, then weekly, and then twice monthly, finally being phased out altogether.

A variety of home-based programs may be developed and tailored for your child. Some of the behaviors targeted for the program may include both social conduct (sharing, playing well with peers, following rules) and academic performance (completed math or reading assignments). Targeting low academic performance (poor production of work) may be especially effective. These home-based school report cards have resulted in improvements in both academics and social conduct. Examples of behaviors to target include completion of all (or a specified portion) of the work, staying in an assigned seat, following teacher directions, and playing cooperatively with others. Negative behaviors (for example, aggression, destruction, calling out) may also be included as target behaviors to be reduced by the program. In addition to targeting class performance, homework may be included. Children with ADHD often have difficulty remembering to bring home their homework assignments. They may also complete their homework but forget to return the completed work to school the next day. Each of these areas may be targeted in a note-to-home program.

We suggest that you target only four or five behaviors to work on. Start out by focusing on just a few behaviors you wish to change to help maximize your child's success in the program. When these behaviors are going well, you can add a few more. The daily ratings of each behavior may be global and subjective (for example, "poor," "fair," "good"). However, it helps to make them more specific and objective (for example, frequency of each behavior or the number of points earned or lost for each behavior). We recommend including at least one or two positive behaviors that the child is currently doing well with, so that the child will be able to earn some points during the beginning of the program.

Typically children are monitored throughout the school day. However, to be successful with frequent problem behaviors, you may want to have your child rated for only a portion of the school day at first. As the child's behavior improves, the ratings may be increased gradually to include more periods/subjects. In cases where children attend several different classes taught by different teachers, the program may involve some or all of the teachers, depending on the need for intervention in each class. When more than one teacher is included in the program, a single report card may include space for all teachers to sign. Different report cards may be used for each class and organized in a notebook for children to carry between classes. Again, the cards shown in Figures 3–5 can be helpful, because they have columns that can be used to rate the child by the same teacher at the end of each subject or by different teachers if more than one is involved.

The success of the program depends on a clear, consistent method for translating teacher reports into consequences at home. Some programs involve rewards alone; others use both positive and negative consequences. Some studies suggest that a combination of positive and negative consequences may be most effective. One advantage of home-based programs is that a wide variety of consequences can be used—praise and positive attention as well as tangible rewards, both daily and weekly.

Overall, home-based reward programs may be even more effective when combined with classroom-based programs, which give the parents frequent feedback, remind parents when to reward a child's behavior, and forewarn parents when behavior is becoming a problem at school. Furthermore, the type and quality of rewards available in the home are usually far more extensive than those available in the classroom—a factor that may be critical for children with ADHD, who need more powerful rewards. Aside from these benefits, note-to-home programs generally require much less time and effort from your child's teacher than do classroom-based programs. As a result, teachers who have been unable to start a classroom management program may be far more likely to cooperate with a note-to-home program. Despite the impressive success of note-to-home programs, the effectiveness of such a program depends on accurate evaluation of the child's behavior by the teacher. It also hinges on the fair and consistent use of consequences at home. In some cases children may attempt to

Daily School Behavior Report Card

Child's name ______________________ **Date** __________

Teachers:

Please rate this child's behavior today in the areas listed below. Use a separate column for each subject or class period. Use the following ratings: 1 = excellent, 2 = good, 3 = fair, 4 = poor, and 5 = very poor. Then initial the box at the bottom of your column. Add any comments about the child's behavior today on the back of this card.

	Class periods/subjects						
Behaviors to be rated:	1	2	3	4	5	6	7
Class participation							
Performance of class work							
Follows classroom rules							
Gets along well with other children							
Quality of homework, if any given							
Teacher's initials							

Place comments on back of card.

FIGURE 3. A daily school report card for managing ADHD behavior problems during class time at school, used with a home-based token reward system.

undercut the system by failing to bring home a report. They may forge a teacher's signature or fail to get certain teacher signatures. To discourage these practices, missing notes or signatures should be treated the same way as a "bad" report (for example, a child fails to earn points or is fined by losing privileges or points). The child may even be grounded for the day (no privileges) for not bringing the note home.

Some Examples of Note-to-Home Programs

The cards shown in Figures 3–5 contain five areas of potential problems for children with ADHD. Columns are provided for up to seven different teachers to rate a child in these areas or for one teacher to rate the child many times across the school day. We have found that the more frequent the rating, the more effective is the feedback to the child and the more informative is the program to you. The teacher initials the bottom of the column after rating the child's performance during that class period, to ensure against forgery. When getting the correct homework assignment home is a problem for a child, the teacher can require the child to copy the homework for that class period on the back of the card before completing the ratings for that period. In this way the teacher merely checks the back of the card for accuracy of copying the assignment and then completes the ratings on the front of the card. For particularly

Daily Recess and Free-Time Behavior Report Card

Child's name ______________________ **Date** __________

Teachers:

Please rate this child's behavior today during recess or other free-time periods in the areas listed below. Use a separate column for each recess/free-time period. Use the following ratings: 1 = excellent, 2 = good, 3 = fair, 4 = poor, and 5 = very poor. Then initial at the bottom of the column. Add any comments on the back.

	Daily recess and free-time periods				
Behaviors to be rated:	1	2	3	4	5
Keeps hands to self; does not push, shove					
Does not tease others; no taunting/put-downs					
Follows recess/free-time rules					
Gets along well with other children					
Does not fight or hit; no kicking or punching					
Teacher's initials					

Place comments on back of card.

FIGURE 4. A daily school report card for managing ADHD behavior problems during free time at school, to be used with a home-based token reward system.

Daily School Behavior Report Card

Child's name ______________________ **Date**

Teachers:

Please rate this child's behavior today in the areas listed below. Use a separate column for each subject or class period. Use the following ratings: 1 = excellent, 2 = good, 3 = fair, 4 = poor, and 5 = very poor. Then initial the box at the bottom of your column. Add any comments about the child's behavior today on the back of this card.

	Class periods/subjects						
Behaviors to be rated:	1	2	3	4	5	6	7
Teacher's initials							

Place comments on back of card.

FIGURE 5. A blank daily school report card for managing ADHD behavior problems at school, to be used with a home-based token reward system. The problem areas can be filled in beforehand by parents or teacher(s), so as to focus the card system on whatever specific behavior problems are of concern for a particular child.

negative ratings, we also encourage teachers to provide a brief explanation. Teachers rate children using a 5-point system (1 = excellent, 2 = good, 3 = fair, 4 = poor, and 5 = very poor).

The child takes a new card to school each day. These can be kept at school and a new card given out each morning, or you can provide the card as your child leaves for school, whichever is most likely to be done consistently. Upon returning home, you should immediately inspect the card, discuss the positive ratings first with your child, and then proceed to a neutral, business-like (not angry!) discussion with your child about any negative marks and the reason for them. Your child should then be asked to formulate a plan for how to avoid getting the negative mark tomorrow. You are to remind your child of this plan the next morning before your child departs for school. You should then award your child points for each rating on the card and deduct points for each negative mark. For instance, a young elementary-age child may receive five chips for a 1, three chips for a 2, and one chip for a 3, while being fined three chips for a 4 and five chips for a 5 on the card. For older children, the scale might be 25, 15, 5, –15, and –25 points, respectively, for marks 1 to 5 on the card. The chips or points are then added up, the fines are subtracted, and the child may then spend what is left on privileges from the home reward menu.

As these cards illustrate, virtually any child behavior can be the target for treatment.

Training Children with ADHD to Think Aloud, Think Ahead

Many treatment programs for children with ADHD have used methods that teach the children to talk to themselves out loud, give themselves instructions on what they should be doing, and reward themselves verbally for how they did. These methods are often called *cognitive behavior modification, self-instruction,* or *self-control programs*.

One such program involves teaching children a set of self-directed instructions they should follow when they are doing their work. Self-instructions include (1) having the children say out loud to themselves what the task or problem is they have been assigned to do; (2) saying what plan of attack or strategy they will use to approach the problem; (3) keeping their attention on the task; (4) describing their plan as they follow it through to completion; and (5) telling themselves how they think they have done. This may also include giving themselves a reward, such as a point or token, for getting the problem correct. In the case of an incorrect answer, the children are taught to say something encouraging to themselves, such as "Next time I'll do better if I slow down."

At first an adult trainer typically shows a child how to do the self-instruction while performing the work. The child then performs the same task while the trainer provides the instructions. Next, the child performs the task, repeating the self-instructions aloud. This talking aloud is then faded to silent speech (or whispering). Rewards are typically provided to the child for following the procedure as well as for selecting the correct solutions. Children can use these methods for virtually any type of schoolwork or even on their homework.

Despite the apparent promise of these methods for children with ADHD, who are obviously impaired in self-control, many research studies have failed to show strongly positive results. In general, the results of these programs are modest or do not seem to last once the program is stopped. The results also do not carry over into other classes, places, or situations where the methods are not being taught or where the children are not rewarded for their use.

For these reasons, we strongly recommend that this approach never be the only program used, that it not be the principal approach in the child's classroom, and that it be used in the classroom by the teacher—not taught by someone else outside the classroom, where it is not likely to carry over back into the classroom.

Managing the Academic Problems of Adolescents with ADHD

All of the recommendations made so far apply as much to adolescents with ADHD as to younger children. However, the changes that take place in high school—the greater number of teachers involved with each student, the shorter class periods, the increased emphasis on individual student responsibility, and the frequent changes in class schedules from day to day—are likely to result in a dramatic drop in educational performance as many children with ADHD enter high school. This is compounded by the fact that there is little or no accountability of teachers for a particular student at this level of education. Only when a teen's misbehavior becomes sufficiently serious to attract attention, or academic deficiencies are grossly apparent, will someone take notice. Usually the response of the school is punitive rather than constructive.

"You say that my daughter needs more structure and supervision in high school, but the principal says this is just coddling her, that if we keep doing this she will never learn self-discipline or self-management. She says it is time for Sarah to sink or swim, to experience the natural consequences of her mistakes and disorganization. Is that true?"

It is very easy for average adolescents with ADHD to fall through the cracks at this stage unless they have been involved with the special educational system before entering high school. Those who have will have been "flagged" as in need of continuing special attention. But the others are likely to be viewed merely as lazy and irresponsible. It is at this age level that educational performance becomes the most common reason adolescents with ADHD are referred for professional help.

"Our son won't go for extra help from his teachers. He says he doesn't need it, that he can bring up his grades on his own. He refuses the medication you recommended too. What can we do?"

Dealing with large schools at this age level can be frustrating for parents and for a teenager with ADHD alike. Even the most interested teacher may have difficulties mustering sufficient motivation among colleagues to be of help and keep the adolescent out of trouble at school. Here are a few ideas that may help:

1. If your teenager is failing or doing poorly and has never had special education, immediately request a special education evaluation if one has not been done before or within the past 3 years. Federal law (the Individuals with Disabilities Education Act) requires a reevaluation every 3 years that a child is in special education. Special educational services will not be forthcoming until this evaluation is completed, and this can take up to 90 days or longer in some districts. The sooner it is initiated, the better.

2. Adolescents with ADHD usually require counseling about the nature of their disability. Although many have already been told that they are "hyperactive" or have ADHD, a lot of them have not come to accept that they actually have a disability. Counseling can help these teenagers learn to accept their limitations and find ways to prevent their disability from creating significant problems. Such counseling is difficult, requiring sensitivity to the adolescents' desire to be independent and to form their own opinions of themselves and their world. It often takes more than a single session to succeed, but patience and persistence can pay off. Find a counselor or other professional who knows about ADHD and ask this professional to spend a few sessions counseling your teen about the disorder. Your teen is more likely to listen to the professional than to you.

3. Counsel the adolescent on the advantages of returning to medication if it has been used successfully in the past. Medication can improve school performance and help the teen obtain those special privileges at home that may be granted as a result of such improved performance (use of the car, later curfew, higher allowance, etc.). Adolescents who are concerned about others learning that they are on medication should be reassured that only they, their parents, and the physician will be aware of this. Be prepared for resistance to the idea of medication and consider setting up a behavior contract by which the teen earns certain rewards (money, extra free time, etc.) for taking the medication daily.

4. Schedule a team meeting at the beginning of each academic year, and more often as needed, at the teenager's school. This meeting should be attended by the teachers, school psychologist, guidance counselor, principal, parents, *and the adolescent with ADHD.* Take with you a handout describing ADHD to give to each participant. If you think it is helpful, ask a professional to go along with you to give advice. Briefly review the nature of the adolescent's disorder and the need for close teamwork among the school, parents, and teen if the teen's academic performance is to be improved. Get the teachers to describe the current strengths and problems of the teen in their classes, and to make suggestions as to how they think they can help with the problem. Some of these might include being available after school a few days each week for extra assistance; reducing the length of written homework assignments; allowing the teen to provide oral means of demonstrating that knowledge has been acquired, rather than relying on just written, timed test grades; and developing a subtle reminder system to alert the teen when she is not paying attention in class without drawing the whole class's attention to the fact.

At this conference, the teen then makes a public commitment to doing specific things to improve school performance. The team should agree to meet again in 1 month to evaluate the success of the plans and troubleshoot any problem areas. Future meetings may need to be scheduled depending on the success of the program to date. Meetings should be scheduled at least twice a year to monitor progress and keep the school attentive to the needs of this teen. The adolescent always attends these meetings.

5. Introduce a daily home–school report card as described earlier. These are often more critical for teens than for any other age group to provide daily feedback. Also, a home point system must be set up that includes a variety of desired privileges that the teen can purchase with the points earned at school. Points can also be set aside in a savings book to work toward longer term rewards. Remember, however, that it is the daily, short-term privileges and not these longer term rewards that give the program its motivational power. So don't overweight the reward menu with long-term rewards.

Once the adolescent is able to go for 3 weeks or so with no 4's or 5's (negative ratings) on the card, the card is cut back to once or twice a week. After a month of satisfactory ratings, the card can either be faded out or reduced to a monthly rating. The adolescent is then told that if word is received that grades are slipping, the card system will be reinstated.

6. Get the school to provide a second set of books to you, even it means putting up a small deposit, so that homework can be done even if the teen leaves a book at school. These books can also be helpful to any tutor you've hired.

7. Get one of the teen's teachers, the homeroom teacher, a guidance counselor, or even a learning disabilities teacher to serve as the "coach," "mentor," or "case manager." This person's role is to meet briefly with the teen three times a day for just a few minutes to help keep him organized. The teen can stop at this person's office at the start of school. At this time, the manager checks to see that the teen has all the homework and books needed for the morning's classes. If a behavior report card is being used with this teen, it can be given to the teen at this time. At lunch, the teen checks in again with the manager, who checks that the teen has copied all necessary assignments from the morning classes, to help the teen select the books needed for the afternoon classes, and then to see that the student has the assignments that are to be turned in that day for these afternoon classes. If the behavior report card is being used, it can be reviewed by the "coach" at this time and discussed with the teen. At the end of school, the teen checks in again with the manager to see that he has all assignments and books needed for homework. Again, the behavior report card can be reviewed by the coach and discussed with the teen before sending it home for further review by parents and conversion into the home point system. Each visit takes no more than 3–5 minutes, but, interspersed as they are throughout the school day, these visits can be of great assistance to organizing the teen's schoolwork.

8. If you feel you can't help with homework, then consider a private tutor as discussed above or have your teenager attend any extra help periods that the school requires the teachers to hold at the end of the school day. The student can go to one extra help period per week for each course. And don't forget about the Internet self-taught courses at Khan Academy *(www.khanacademy.org)* discussed above that can be as beneficial for teens as for children with ADHD.

9. Set up a special time each week to do something alone with your teen that is mutually pleasurable. This provides opportunities for parent–teen interactions that are not work-oriented, school-related, or fraught with the tensions that work-oriented activities can often involve for teens with ADHD. These outings can contribute to keeping your relationship with your teen positive. They can also counterbalance the conflicts that school performance demands frequently bring to families. You'll find more on making sure you don't stress schoolwork at the expense of your relationship with your child in the next chapter.

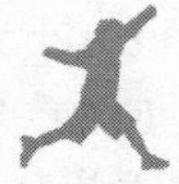

17 Keeping School Performance in Perspective

You may recall the story of Steve's mother (in the Introduction), who had come to our clinic because she was having trouble with her 8-year-old son. When I asked her (as I usually do) what had brought her to us, she threw me for a loop when she said simply, "Help me. I'm losing my child." It was a plea, and an interview, that I have never forgotten, for it summed up in a few words the excruciating pain felt by so many parents of children with ADHD.

In the rest of my interview with her, I learned that the problem with her son had begun innocently enough, with a teacher conference about her son's poor classwork, lack of attentiveness, and erratically completed homework early in first grade. It was further nurtured by her natural desire to help her son do better in school. Her mission at that level had been accomplished very well indeed. But she was not celebrating this achievement. To her, the schoolwork that had seemed so important and was now being done well seemed a hollow victory. Something more primal was being lost in the process here that made academic success rather paltry by comparison.

As a result of that first teacher conference, Steve's mother began to set aside virtually all of her other activities and responsibilities after school and in the early evening to spend with Steve on schoolwork. Initially Steve enjoyed the time with his mother, and initially she thought that helping her son complete his unfinished classwork and do his homework would take only about an hour a day. But of course his carelessness and inattention complicated matters, and soon it was not uncommon for them to be spending several fitful hours on this work every day.

Despite some teaching experience she had to support her efforts, Steve's mother quickly became frustrated, angry, and bitter in the face of her son's failure to respond to her "help." From being upbeat, cajoling, prodding, and joking, she moved to threatening to withdraw privileges. He might work then—sometimes with tears faintly visible in his eyes, at other times angry and resentful at having to do so much schoolwork. Later in the year he also began to challenge her about the nature of assignments, even though the goal was clear.

In time, sporadically at first, Steve began to avoid his mother after school, sometimes lying to her about what work he had to do. When the work was finished, he would retreat from her quickly to his room or the family room. Gradually the arguments and conflicts began to permeate other daily activities that involved the two of them, like mealtimes and bedtime.

Over the year, Steve's grades improved, and he finished first grade with an above-average grade, to the delight of his mother. The sarcasm and withdrawal that had grown over the school year abated during the summer, though Steve went to great lengths to avoid the weekly tutoring sessions his mother imposed. When second grade began, bringing a return to the rigors of the first-grade after-school schedule, Steve began to dig in his heels in earnest. Now it was his father, who had only nominal responsibility for schoolwork, he sought out for company at home. When Steve's mother tried to hug or kiss him good night, he merely stiffened at her embrace, turned his cheek, and replied in a monotone, "'Night, Mom," with little feeling. She was devastated. She would retreat to her bedroom to cry quietly or complain bitterly to her husband that while he still had a son, she did not seem to have one anymore.

Once again Steve finished the school year with excellent grades. She set about tutoring him again that summer, but it was the worst summer of their life together.

Why was she losing Steve? she asked herself. Couldn't he see how hard she was working on his behalf? Didn't he realize how important school was to his future? Where was his sense of priorities?

This crisis ultimately led her to call me for an appointment at the beginning of third grade. She did not think she could go through another academic year following the same course. She was growing increasingly depressed. She envied her husband's closeness with Steve and resented his limited involvement with schoolwork, though she knew she had volunteered for this role. She tried to assuage her sadness with the consolation that Steve was succeeding at school. It didn't work. She now realized that something very precious was being taken from her, probably in part by her own doing. She was no longer sure she wanted to pay the price she was being asked to pay for creating her son's academic success.

My interview with Steve only affirmed what his mother had already sensed: he was consciously avoiding her, in a sense really letting go of her. All his mother thought of, he said in essence, was school and how well he was doing and so forth. When asked if he was pleased by his report cards, he shrugged his shoulders. "So what?" he seemed to be saying, as if they were his mother's grades, not his. The bitterness and anger were almost palpable, but I also detected a substantial degree of forlornness like his mother's. He too appeared to realize at some (not fully conscious) level that something precious was being taken from him.

Steve's mother and I both knew, and his father agreed once we brought him into our meetings, that the job before us was difficult. What textbook tells you how to repair a damaged parent–child bond? What trite little management technique or notebook organizer could reorganize this situation? What medicine corrects that underlying social and emotional substrate so absolutely crucial to a parent's and a child's life with each other?

From here these parents and I proceeded not as doctor and patients, but as a team searching for possible solutions to a problem for which none of us were well prepared. What we learned to do is explained later in this chapter. Along the way, however, we all learned several major lessons in family life.

Lessons in Family Life

Lesson 1

A parent's relationship with a child is a sacred bond and trust and ultimately must be appreciated by both parents and teachers as having a higher priority to and serving as a fundamental underpinning of any academic priority. Consciously acknowledge its existence. Give it full respect. And don't trample it with unnecessary or excessive stress, such as the pressures of unfinished schoolwork that is sent home to complete with a parent.

Lesson 2

The failure to cultivate and sustain this relationship can have devastating emotional consequences for both parties.

Lesson 3

School staff members often may be too quick to let parents take over academically related responsibilities, to the detriment of family life and the parent–child relationship. When homework is assigned to an elementary-age child, in all honesty it is assigned to that child's family, and particularly to a parent working with that child—not to the child alone. Thus assigning homework should be viewed as a delicate balance to be negotiated between the need to further the child's education and the need of that child to have a well-rounded and fulfilling relationship with parents apart from schoolwork.

Research has repeatedly demonstrated that homework does not boost children's academic achievement or success compared to children not given such homework. It is only in the high school years where a relationship between amount of homework and academic achievement can be detected as significant, and even then the relationship is a small one. Experts recommend that homework in high school be limited to 1½–2½ hours per night in total. There is no measurable benefit of homework above this range on school success. Yet with each passing year many schools, especially private ones, give more and more homework to younger and younger children as if it were not only essential to their academic success (it isn't), but also a badge of prestige and exclusivity for the school. All the while this results in a progressive erosion of family life as schoolwork comes to dominate all weekday and Sunday evenings during the school year, displacing time families previously spent together building important family bonds and conveying family values, culture, and heritage as well as in joint leisure, hobbies, games, informal sports, and so on.

Furthermore, most of us as parents are lousy tutors and are mediocre in simply supervising homework. Late in the day we, like our children, are tired, sometimes irritable, and impatient—we simply want to get the homework done at all costs. Few of us even think of the impact of unfinished classwork and excessive homework on family life. Fewer still choose to raise this issue with a teacher as a reason for limiting such assignments.

Lesson 4

Even without confrontations over schoolwork, you may not be nurturing a relationship with your child or preventing harm being done to it. Your child may be filling this time with TV, video games, or time away from home just hanging out, and you may be permitting this to happen. Your relationship with your child does not sustain itself by its own momentum; it must be actively encouraged and fueled by your ongoing investment of love, intimacy, contact, attention, role modeling, respect, and acceptance of your child.

Lesson 5

The natural, gradual individuation of our children from us need not be accompanied by a loss of our emotional bond to them. We can, however, lose this bond or relationship prematurely by overemphasizing one priority of parenting to the near-exclusion of all others. Schoolwork, while it is critical among the developmental tasks a child must master, is not singularly so.

Lesson 6

As the example of Steve and his family shows, if damage to a parent–child relationship has begun to occur because of an excessive emphasis on schoolwork, it is not irreparable, at least not if resuscitated within the first few years of the discovery of this destructive process. Probably such damage can be partially reversed even years later. But relationship repair will not happen of its own accord.

Priorities for Parents

Our first step in trying to repair the bond between Steve and his mother was to identify what parents' priorities should be in raising a healthy, well-rounded, well-adjusted child, so we could see which areas were being sacrificed to the priority of academic achievement. This is the list we came up with:

1. The active promotion of the physical survival and well-being of the family unit and its members, through the provision of adequate food and shelter to sustain life and the provision of safety to its members.

2. The instilling of a sense of family, and of membership within it as a needed, loved, valued, respected, and responsible participant in its successful functioning. As Craig Knippenberg said so well in a column for the *ADDvance* newsletter years ago, there are two things we as parents give our children; one is roots, and the other wings.

3. Providing the foundation for a child's moral development. This means making a commitment to the preparation of children to be socialized to enter society and benefit from the wisdom of its members. Morals are the "rules of the road" for how to live among, respect the rights of, and interact with other members of society that contribute to its smooth and peaceful functioning, limiting conflict as much as possible and resolving it peacefully and fairly when it arises.

4. The instruction in and development of interpersonal skills that lead to adaptive and successful social transactions, acceptance, and enduring friendships. Learning to wait, take turns, share, listen to, praise, forgive, problem-solve, and cooperate with their peers and others are just a few of the skills that parents must take time to teach their children, apart from the daily demands of school homework. This area can be a major problem for families of many children with ADHD, given the social interaction problems such children are likely to have. Evidence for the importance of this domain of children's development can be found just by looking at the pain many parents experience vicariously through their children with ADHD when they have no friends and have never received an invitation to a birthday or slumber party.

5. The instruction of our children in a sense of community and our obligations to it as a member of a larger society. Whether we depend on formal organizations like scouting, houses of worship, or schools to assist us, we as parents carry the major responsibility for introducing our children to and eventually sponsoring our children's entry into this larger community.

6. The proper development of our children's physical and mental health and well-being—not just diet, exercise, hygiene, and the like, but also the acquisition of self-help and adaptive skills to permit the children to become self-sufficient. Moreover, this means seeing that there is adequate time for and attention to the pursuit of

happiness and self-satisfaction for the children through leisure, recreation, hobbies, and informal sports. Sometimes we forget that children need a break too.

7. Instilling a sense of belonging to a larger humanity, of fulfilling our obligations to it, and of being an inhabitant of a finite planet with progressively diminishing resources. How we introduce our children to the multitude of ethnic, religious, and cultural groups in our world affects how well they will be integrated into a larger society.

Do you still think doing unfinished classwork is the highest priority of a parent in raising a child? Then think about the pictures in your family photo album or your collection of home videos of your children. Are any of them of you and your child doing schoolwork together? Probably not. Why not? Think about it.

Once Steve and his family—remarkably, without much effort—articulated these priorities, the importance of academic work began to shrink in relative significance. Ultimately Steve's parents agreed that excellent grades, while laudable, were not to be mandatory; average ones would do just fine.

But that left the problem of the extensive unfinished schoolwork and homework. In a meeting with the teacher, we came to an agreement that Steve's inability to finish classwork was itself a symptom of a larger problem *in that classroom,* not a problem in the home. If the problem was to be truly solved, the solution would have to occur *in that classroom.* This led us to the types of modifications of classwork typically made for children with ADHD and discussed in Chapters 15 and 16. Similar compromises were made on homework.

The next step was to divest Steve's mother of much of the burden of schoolwork by having his father take equal turns at this task, and to shift her relationship with her son away from the solely academic. We also discussed using an academic tutor with Steve if necessary so that neither parent needed to play the role of schoolmaster. We began scheduling recreational outings at which discussing schoolwork was forbidden and encouraged her to give nondirective attention to Steve with positive feedback (but never feigned or excessive praise). Things did not change quickly. Steve seemed naturally suspicious of the changes we were attempting to make. Even so, as the changes became the routine, the edginess, sarcasm, and oppositional stance he took toward his mother began to subside. He even began asking to go places with her again and seemed faintly pleased by her presence at his scouting and sports events. Within a few months his mother reported that she sensed a reestablishment of her old relationship, but that its closeness was not yet where it had once been. Still, she was hopeful, as was I. Steve's grades dropped somewhat, to C's with occasional B's, but his mother felt this was acceptable while they worked on their home relationship. When last I met this family, Steve and his mother were getting along well, and she felt their relationship was pretty much back to normal. The affection they naturally had felt for each other returned, and they were striving to keep academic work in perspective, relative to the other areas of family life and parent–child relations of equal importance. They seemed to have accepted Steve's ADHD as a disability and to have adjusted their expectations of academic success accordingly, realizing that average students with ADHD can nevertheless be well rounded, morally upright, and just plain terrific apart from their class standing.

And so, as you pursue the academic achievement that your child can aspire to, do not lose sight of the other, equally compelling priorities of raising children. Do not sacrifice your parent–child relationships and emotional bonds on the altar of academic performance. If the academic wolf does come calling at your door, which it most certainly will, greet it and accord it just due, but by all means do not relinquish your children to it.

Part IV

Medications for ADHD

18 The Approved Effective Medicines

STIMULANTS AND NONSTIMULANTS

Medication is probably the most widely publicized, most hotly debated treatment for ADHD. This chapter discusses the drugs that have received approval from the U.S. Food and Drug Administration (FDA) for the management of ADHD: the stimulants and the nonstimulants atomoxetine (Strattera) and guanfacine XR (Intuniv). As a whole, hundreds of studies indicate that these medications can be of great help to those with ADHD.

The Stimulants

The stimulants, the drugs most commonly used, have been shown to be effective in improving behavior, academic work, and social adjustment in anywhere from 50 to 95% of children with ADHD. How well your child responds may depend, however, on the presence of other problems. The truth is that medication does not help everyone. For that reason—and because medication is no exception to the rule that misinformation about ADHD abounds—you should gather as much background knowledge as you can before agreeing to a trial of medication for your child. This chapter gives the most up-to-date information available on the stimulant medications. These chemicals are methylphenidate and amphetamine. The brand names of the methylphenidate medications available in the United States are Ritalin, Concerta, Medadate CD, Focalin, and the skin patch Daytrana. The brand names for drugs using amphetamines are Dexedrine, Adderall, Adderall XR, and Vyvanse. The nonstimulants Strattera (atomoxetine) and Intuniv (guanfacine XR) will be discussed later in this chapter. The antidepressants and clonidine are reviewed briefly in Chapter 19.

As a supplement to this chapter, one source you can turn to is the *Physicians' Desk Reference* (PDR), available at most public libraries and on the Internet (*www.pdr.net* for physicians and *www.pdrhealth.com* for consumers). This reference book includes information on all commercially available drugs—what the drugs are most useful for treating (indications), when they should not be used (contraindications), and the unwanted reactions (side effects) of the medications. Although the PDR is updated annually, it does not usually keep pace with the latest findings from drug research, especially with respect to the main effects and side effects of the drugs. It also will not tell you how likely it is that your child will experience side effects; it merely lists all side effects that have been reported. This can mislead you to think that all these negative effects are common, which is not the case. The best way to use the PDR is as an introductory reference. Don't believe that everything it tells you *may* be a problem *will* be a problem with your child.

A better source of information is your family doctor or pediatrician—as long as the doctor has kept up to date by reading the medical journals reporting on such research. Ask your doctor, "How familiar are you with this class of medicines, and how often do you prescribe them for children with ADHD?" (Also ask the questions in the sidebar on the facing page before agreeing to a trial of medication for your child. In particular, request a copy of any fact sheets or patient information forms the doctor or manufacturer may dispense to parents.)

Another excellent source that may also help you learn what you want to know about medications book is *Straight Talk about Psychiatric Medications for Kids* by Dr. Timothy E. Wilens. For full information about both these books, see "Suggested Reading and Videos" at the end of this volume.

What *Not* to Believe

"Isn't Ritalin a dangerous drug? I've heard a lot of bad stories about this drug. Isn't it addictive? Won't it make my son more likely to take drugs later?"

Before you read on about how the stimulants work and what they may be able to do for your child, let's clear up a few misconceptions about these drugs.

MYTH 1: Stimulant drugs are dangerous and should not be taken by any child. During the 1980s and again in the mid- to late 1990s, an inaccurate and regrettably successful media propaganda campaign against the use of stimulants, particularly Ritalin (methylphenidate), with children was waged by a fringe religious group, causing a dramatic rise in media coverage of this medication. The 1990s campaign was fueled by the release of misleading, alarmist, and biased information about stimulant medication abuse in the United States by the Drug Enforcement Administration as part of an effort to prevent Ritalin from being reclassified as a nonaddictive drug—a change that would have made prescribing this medication more convenient for physicians. As a consequence, the use of these medications for children with ADHD continues to be controversial in the public's mind, although there is absolutely no controversy among the scientific community as to the safety and effectiveness of these medications.

What to Ask Your Physician about Medication

If your doctor recommends a trial on any medication for treatment of your child's ADHD, ask at least the following questions, many of which are answered in this chapter:

1. "What are the effects and side effects, both short term and long term, of this particular medication?"
2. "What doses will be used, and by what schedule should they be given?"
3. "How often should you see my child for reevaluation while he [she] is taking this medication?"
4. "When should the medicine be stopped briefly to see if it is still required for treatment of ADHD?"
5. "Are there foods, beverages, or other substances my child should not consume while taking this medication because they will interfere with its effects in the body?"
6. "Will you be in contact with the school periodically to determine how my child is responding to the medication in that environment, or am I expected to do that?"
7. "If the child accidentally takes an overdose of the medication, what procedures should I follow?"
8. "Do you have a fact sheet about the medication that I can have to read?"

Unfounded fear of these drugs is unfortunately perpetuated by a few physicians who require that parents sign a consent form indicating that they have been informed about the medicines and their side effects and have agreed to have their child placed on one of them for treatment of the child's ADHD. *If your doctor asks you to sign such a form, don't assume it means the drugs are dangerous*. These forms were introduced only in response to the highly publicized threats of malpractice suits by the religious sect mentioned above, and some doctors still feel the need to protect themselves in this way. Fortunately, this practice has declined substantially in the last decade, and so you may never be asked to sign such a form these days. Up-to-date information on possible side effects is given later in this chapter. If you are asked to sign a consent form, read it carefully since it will contain information about the medicine, but do not let it make you afraid of the stimulant medicines or of signing the form.

MYTH 2: Stimulants just cover up the "real problem" and do not deal directly with the root causes of the child's ADHD. Many parents come to us with the concern that stimulants do not treat the "real problems," but it is simply untrue. Critics of these medications mistakenly assume that a child's ADHD symptoms stem from purely social causes, such as poor discipline or lack of love at home. As previous chapters have indicated, there is no scientific evidence that purely social causes are at the root of a child's ADHD. We now know that ADHD is largely a genetic disorder associated with deficiencies in the functioning of certain regions in the brain related to inhibition, attention, and self-control. The stimulants deal directly with the part of the brain that is underactive and gives rise to the outward symptoms of ADHD, as explained later in this chapter. In this sense, the stimulants are no different from using insulin for a child with diabetes. Unfortunately, like insulin, stimulants have only a temporary effect, which leads some people to believe they're masking the problem rather than helping it. Like a diabetic who needs insulin, your child may have to take stimulant medicine daily for a long time, but these drugs are a way of tackling the problem directly. *Stimulants are the only treatment to date that normalizes the inattentive, impulsive, and restless behavior in at least 50–65% of children with ADHD.* However, even though the stimulants do *improve* the behavior of 70–90% of all children with ADHD, the stimulants do not *normalize* the behavioral problems of all of these children who respond positively to medication. For approximately 30–45% of children with ADHD, their behavior will be significantly improved but not normalized by this medication.

MYTH 3: Stimulants make children "high," as illegal drugs do, and are addictive. You may have heard that adults who take stimulants often have a sense of elevated mood, euphoria, or excessive well-being. This is true only if people crush the drug and inhale it nasally as a powder, inject it into a blood vessel, or take exceptionally high doses. Euphoria in children taking the prescribed forms of these medications by mouth is exceedingly rare. Some children do describe feeling "funny," "different," tense, irritable, or, on rare occasions, dizzy. Others actually become a little bland in their mood, and a few even report feelings of sadness. These mood changes occur a few hours after the medicine is taken and occur more often among children treated with higher doses. In most children, these changes are very minor.

Parents are often also quite concerned about the risk of addiction to stimulants and about an increased risk of abusing other drugs when the children become teenagers. There are no reported cases of addiction or serious drug dependence to date with these medications, and the many studies that have examined whether children on these drugs are more likely than those not taking them to abuse other substances as teenagers show that they are not. Indeed, several separate studies conducted by me at the Medical College of Wisconsin, by Dr. Timothy E. Wilens and colleagues at Massachusetts General Hospital (Harvard Medical School), and by Drs. Howard Chilcoat and Naomi Breslau, then at Henry Ford Hospital in Detroit, found that taking stimulants during childhood did not predispose children with ADHD to an increased risk of substance use or abuse as teenagers. In fact, Dr. Wilens's study found that adolescents with ADHD who had remained on their medication during the teen years had a significantly lower likelihood of substance use or abuse than did children with ADHD who were not taking medications during adolescence. Thus the scientific literature to date should reassure parents that they are not predisposing their children to the potential for later substance use or abuse by giving stimulants to their children for the management of ADHD. Parents should know that the most important factors in determining a child's risk for adolescent substance use or abuse are (1) early onset of conduct disorder or antisocial behavior in the child, (2) poor monitoring by parents of the child's or teen's whereabouts in the community, (3) the affiliation of the child or teen with other teens who are using or abusing illegal substances, and (4) the degree to which the parents may also be using alcohol, tobacco products, or illegal substances.

MYTH 4: Stimulant medications stunt children's growth, and their use is strictly limited by age. Some studies in the early 1970s seemed to suggest that children taking these medicines might be stunted in their height and weight gain. More recent and better studies have shown that this is not as much of a problem as was once thought. Your child's eventual adult height or skeletal size is not likely to be affected by taking the medicine, although recent studies suggest that in the first year or two of taking the medicine the child may fail to grow by 1 centimeter on average. The effects on your child's weight are also likely to be minimal, resulting in a failure to gain 1 or 2 pounds during the initial year of treatment. No effects on height or weight are typically evident by the third or later years of treatment. Keep in mind that children respond very differently to these medicines, some experiencing no weight change or failure to gain height and others losing more than just a few pounds. Your child's growth should be followed by your physician to make sure that any weight loss or failure to gain height is not serious.

The initial belief in the 1970s that stimulants might stunt the growth of children with ADHD led to the common practice by physicians of recommending that children take these medications only for school days and stop taking them on weekends, on school holidays, and during summer vacations. Because we now know that the risk of growth problems arising from these medications is much less than was originally believed, it is not necessary that all children taking stimulants have such drug holidays. Many can continue to take medication throughout the weekends and summers. They will derive benefits from doing so in their relations with peers; their participation in organized clubs, sports, and summer programs; and their general behavior at home. Parents whose children experience significant behavioral problems during these and other weekend and summer activities, and whose children are not having growth problems from the medication, should discuss with the children's physicians the possible value of continuing the children's stimulant medication during these periods.

MYTH 5: Stimulants can be used only by young children. Contrary to what you may have heard, stimulant medicines can be used throughout the life of a person with ADHD, not just during childhood. There was widespread concern in earlier decades that the stimulant medications could not be used once puberty started because they would no longer be effective. This was a fallacy, and we are now seeing a dramatic increase in the prescribing of these medications for teenagers having ADHD. We are also witnessing an increase in the use of these drugs with adults who have ADHD.

MYTH 6: Stimulants do not result in lasting benefits to a child's academic achievement. The argument that stimulants have no lasting positive effects on academic achievement is a misleading one, concocted as part of broader efforts to dissuade parents from considering the use of stimulants for their children with ADHD. If one takes a simplistic view of the term "academic achievement" and expects stimulants to directly and immediately increase the amount of academic knowledge and skill in a school subject matter that a child acquires, then of course the stimulants will disappoint in the short run. The pills do not contain any knowledge that is automatically placed in a child's brain when consumed. A child with ADHD who does not know her multiplication tables today, while not taking any medication, will not automatically know them tomorrow after taking a dose of stimulant medication. To expect this kind of change would be silly and demonstrates the flaws in this criticism of stimulants.

What the stimulants do is help the child with ADHD show what she knows during performance of school assignments by improving the child's attention span, concentration, resistance to distraction, and thoughtful, reflective behavior. They also make the child more available to learn what is being taught in school by reducing the child's off-task, disruptive, and otherwise inattentive behavior. Given these gains, several years of medication does result in the child having more academic knowledge than she would have had without medication.

If we view the term *academic achievement* more broadly, as how well the child is behaving at school, getting along with peers, following classroom rules and teacher directions, completing assignments, and completing them accurately and so getting better grades, the evidence is overwhelming that the stimulant medications produce significant improvements in these areas of school functioning. Even if the stimulants do not increase a child's academic knowledge, the fact that they result in improvements in many other areas of school functioning is sufficient justification for parents to consider the possible use of these medications with their children. Such changes not only can boost self-confidence and self-esteem in the classroom setting, but can make the child more likable to the peer group and therefore give him more opportunities to make or keep classmates as friends. They can also reduce the amount of censure, punishment, and rejection the child experiences at school from both peers and teachers, and may well preclude the child from needing to be retained in grade or placed in formal special education classes due to substandard academic achievement. For all of these reasons, the improvements in school adjustment and success that result from the stimulants are frequently the most common reasons for prescribing these medications for children with ADHD.

MYTH 7: Stimulants like Ritalin cause cancer. Despite what you may have read or heard, there is absolutely no evidence in any scientific journal that Ritalin or any stimulant medication causes cancer in humans. No such reports have ever been filed with the manufacturer or with the FDA, which monitors the safety of medications used with children and adults. This charge against Ritalin is based on a single study by Drs. Dunnick and Hailey using a strain of laboratory rodents that are bred specifically to be prone to liver tumors. When these rodents were given doses of medication that were in excess of three times or more the recommended doses for humans, they were more likely to develop the tumors than if they had not been given Ritalin. The results were not replicated by those authors when other species of rodents were used. A paper published in 2005 by Dr. El-Zein and associates also suggested that children taking Ritalin may have a higher occurrence of genetic (chromosome) abnormalities in their blood cells and speculated that this might put them at greater risk for cancer. But the study used fewer than 15 children and did not provide much information on how the children had originally been chosen for this study. Also, these children did not have cancer, but the authors thought they might be at greater risk for it later in life. Such a small single study cannot be used to draw any conclusions about cancer risks associated with taking stimulant medication. A subsequent larger and better-conducted study by Dr. Tucker and colleagues in 2009 found no such evidence of abnormalities in the blood of children treated with these medications, showing that the first study was incorrect in its findings. Indeed, the stimulants have been used for 30–70 years (depending on which type), and there have been no reports of increased cancer among users of this medication, nor have any of the many follow-up studies of children with ADHD observed up to adulthood found any such link. There is no scientific evidence anywhere in the literature on humans that stimulants cause cancer in children or adults.

MYTH 8: A child who takes stimulants will never be able to serve in the military. My colleague Dr. William Hathaway, now at Regents University of Virginia, interviewed the surgeon general for each branch of the military and learned that a childhood history of stimulant use alone would not prevent a young man or woman from enlisting in the military. Typically, those with ADHD are permitted to enlist as long as they meet all other eligibility criteria. What might lead to disqualification from military service is use of medication for any psychiatric disorder during the last few years prior to enlistment because it would indicate an ongoing mental disorder serious enough to require medical treatment.

MYTH 9: Stimulants cause sudden death in children and adults. From time to time, parents may hear reports in the popular media that a child or adult may have died suddenly while taking one of the stimulants used to treat ADHD. Yet every time such deaths are further investigated by experts on the matter as well as by the FDA, no link can be made between the sudden death and the medication. Parents need to keep in mind in trying to understand these sorts of news reports that up to seven people in every 100,000 will die suddenly each year, often related to problems with their heart. Thus, if 500,000 people are taking a particular stimulant drug, like Adderall

XR, up to 35 of them might die each year from sudden death—deaths that have nothing to do with taking this medication.

Late in 2011, the two largest studies of this issue ever conducted were published in scientific journals and included hundreds of thousands of patients treated with these medications over long spans of time. The one involving children published in the *New England Journal of Medicine* by Dr. William Cooper and colleagues used more than 1.2 million children and young adults with ADHD taking stimulants. Both studies concluded that there was no evidence of any significant association of taking stimulant medications with any serious cardiovascular events, such as sudden death, heart attack, or stroke. While it is important to identify any risk of sudden death (or other serious side effects) that a drug may cause, it is just as important not to leap to false conclusions about a medication's doing so when these events occur at the same rate in the general population without use of the medication. Falsely blaming drugs for particular adverse events that they actually do not cause can lead to banning drugs that have proven helpful in treating thousands of cases of ADHD, thereby unnecessarily depriving people of a useful treatment.

How the Stimulants Work

The stimulants are so named because of their ability to increase the level of activity or arousal of the brain. Then why don't they make people more hyperactive? Because it seems that the areas of the brain they activate are responsible for inhibiting behavior, maintaining effort or attention to tasks and goals, and more generally creating self-regulation. That seems to be why they are so helpful to those with ADHD.

The two most commonly recommended stimulants for ADHD are the drugs *d*-amphetamine (as in Dexedrine) and methylphenidate (as in Ritalin, Metadate CD, Concerta, and Daytrana). Several more recently invented stimulants are either just the *d*- isomer or methylphenidate (Focalin) or are simply a combination of the *d*- and *l*-isomers of amphetamine (Adderall, Adderall XR, and Vyvanse). More information on these medicines can be found on the Internet at *www.nlm.nih.gov.* Because caffeine (found in coffee, tea, soft drinks, and other foods) is a stimulant, some parents ask whether this drug or the beverages containing it will help their children with ADHD. Although there were some early reports in the popular press in the 1970s that caffeine might be useful, the scientific studies done on this subject have not borne this out. This is probably because caffeine works on a very different neurotransmitter in the brain from the ones most likely involved in ADHD. Therefore, it is recommended that you consider only the stimulant drugs just listed.

Over the past decade or more, exciting and important technological developments have created new delivery systems that allow children to get longer lasting relief from ADHD symptoms while taking these stimulant medications than was available with the regular immediate-release forms of amphetamine or methylphenidate. These new long-acting and once-daily medications are called Concerta, Metadate CD, Focalin XR, Ritalin LA, and Daytrana, all of which contain versions of methylphenidate, and Adderall XR and Vyvanse, which are extended-release forms of Adderall. These are not really new drugs. They are new delivery systems that help to maintain a continuous level of medication in the body for 8 to 12 hours and so need to be taken only once a day in most cases. Concerta, for instance, is in the form of a small water-based pump that contains a thick liquid form of methylphenidate that is slowly squeezed out of the capsule over a period of 10–12 hours after being swallowed. This eliminates the need for a child to take the old form of immediate-release methylphenidate, such as Ritalin, two to three times each day because that old form lasted only 3–5 hours. Metadate CD is a capsule containing little beads of methylphenidate, each bead being coated with a different time-release outer shell. Some of the beads dissolve immediately after being swallowed while others dissolve in 1 hour, 2 hours, 3 hours, and so on, so that the medication stays in the body for a longer period of time. For children who don't like to swallow pills, Metadate CD capsules can be opened and sprinkled on food without changing the manner in which it works in the body. Some other sustained-release forms of these medications (such as Adderall XR) work by a similar method. Vyvanse is an amphetamine like Adderall except that it is combined with another chemical (lysine) so that the amphetamine does not become active until that other chemical is split off. This takes place in the human gut and surrounding blood vessels, where a naturally occurring enzyme separates the amphetamine from the lysine, allowing the former drug to work as usual. It has the advantage of being less likely to be abused by drug users who ordinarily would try to inhale or inject such a drug. It also appears to last a few hours longer than Adderall XR, and so for adults or older teens it may provide somewhat longer management of their ADHD symptoms across the waking day. The advantages of these new delivery systems are obvious, and in the short time they have been on the market they have become the most commonly used forms of the stimulants for treating ADHD.

The stimulants work primarily by increasing the action of certain chemicals that occur naturally in the brain. The way the brain handles information is based on how these chemicals that are produced in the brain cells (neurons) are released from them to communicate with (influence) other nerve cells nearby. Although we don't know all of the chemicals that are influenced by the stimulants, we do know that two of them are dopamine and norepinephrine, both of which occur naturally throughout the brain but are concentrated very heavily in the prefrontal region and related brain areas, which we believe may be one of the primary sites causing the problem in ADHD (see Chapter 3). By increasing the amounts of these chemicals that are released from nerve cells into the intercellular space or by keeping the released chemical there longer, the stimulants increase the action of these brain cells, which seem to be those most responsible for inhibiting our behavior and helping us use self-control.

Therefore, it's not surprising that hundreds of studies conducted on how these drugs change the behavior and learning of children with ADHD show that between 70 and 90% of children treated with one of the stimulants improve in their behavior.

Still, that leaves as many as 10–30% who show no positive response to any one drug, or whose behavior in rare cases might even be made worse. So you can't assume that your child will necessarily benefit from medication, and we all must recognize that medication is no panacea for all the problems that come with ADHD. There are some cases in which medication alone is enough or is the only practical way to address the concerns you and the child's teacher(s) have about your child's ADHD. For most cases, though, the greatest benefit of stimulant therapy seems to come from a combination of these drugs with other psychological and educational treatments.

What Do the Drugs Do for Behavior and Emotions?

Unquestionably, the stimulants produce positive effects on sustained attention and persistence of effort to work. The medicines also reduce restlessness and gross motor activity in children. In many cases a child's attention to assigned classwork is so greatly improved that her behavior appears normal. Most children taking the medicine are far less impulsive and have fewer problems with aggression, noisiness, noncompliance, and disruptiveness. Overall the drugs improve an individual's executive functioning and with it his capacity for self-regulation. You can see why these medicines are so often recommended for children with ADHD.

How Do the Drugs Change Learning and Academic Performance?

Numerous studies have been conducted on the effects of stimulants on children's intellect, memory, attention, and learning besides their behavior. The studies show that the stimulant medicines are very likely to improve a child's attention, impulse control, fine motor coordination, reaction time, working memory, and planning and problem-solving abilities. When children with ADHD have to do learning tasks, the medicine seems to help them perform more efficiently and in a more organized manner but especially results in their being more productive (getting more work done). As discussed above under Myth 6, no medicine can actually improve intelligence or knowledge, but the stimulants increase your child's ability to show what he has already learned. In general, the drugs produce their greatest influence in situations that require children to show self-control, restrict their behavior, and concentrate on assigned tasks—situations like school.

Stimulant medications are not likely to initially improve your child's scores on school achievement tests, which measure the grade level or difficulty of the material children have learned. The medicines do, however, result in substantial increases in the amount of work a child is able to produce and in some cases increases in the accuracy of the work as well. Over a few years of staying on the medication, some research now indicates that a child's academic achievement (knowledge) may well start to improve.

Do the Medicines Change Social Behavior?

Treatment with stimulant medication has definitely been found to reduce the intensity and improve the quality of social interactions between children with ADHD and their parents, teachers, and peers. Stimulants increase the children's ability to comply with parents' commands and to maintain that compliance over time. The medicines also reduce behavior that competes with getting work done, such as inattention, distraction, restlessness, and forgetfulness. In turn, parents and teachers respond by reducing their level of control and their degree of supervision over the children.

They may also increase their praise and positive reactions to the children. There has been some concern among a few professionals that these medicines may reduce a child's interest in socializing with others. Recent studies have not shown this to be a problem, but it may be possible in rare cases if the child is taking a very high dose.

The degree of improvement differs among children, and each child should be expected to have a unique response. We've seen no overall difference between boys and girls. We do expect to see greater improvement with moderate or higher doses, but your child's physician will have to try your child on several different doses before discovering which one is best, and may also have to try more than one drug or delivery system.

How Long Do the Effects of the Drugs Last?

It depends on the type of medicine and the preparation or delivery system being used to get the drug into the body and bloodstream. Stimulants are almost always given orally when used for ADHD. However, Daytrana (transdermal methylphenidate) is a skin patch that can be worn on the shoulder or buttocks for the waking day and then removed several hours before bedtime. It contains the drug methylphenidate and other chemicals that allow the drug to be absorbed through the skin. Regardless of how they are delivered into the body, these drugs are swiftly absorbed into the bloodstream and cross into the brain quickly and easily. They are also eliminated from the body within 24 hours. This means you can rest assured that if your child has an undesirable reaction, it will usually last only a few hours to a day. But it also means your child must take this medication at least once daily every day.

The older immediate-release forms of these medicines, such as Ritalin or Dexedrine, reach their peak in improving behavior within 1–3 hours and may control behavior for 3–6 hours, but each child reacts somewhat differently, and each drug acts differently. Some changes in behavior are noticeable within 30–60 minutes after taking the medicine, again depending on which drug is being taken.

Besides these immediate-release fast-acting tablet forms of methylphenidate and amphetamine (Ritalin and Dexedrine), both come in sustained-release preparations. These latter preparations reach their peak influence somewhat later than the fast-acting forms (usually in 3–5 hours) and may produce effects that last somewhat longer (typically 8–12 hours). Also keep in mind that amphetamines, like Dexedrine and the newer compound Adderall, are nearly twice as potent as methylphenidate preparations, like Ritalin. As a result, they may produce greater changes in behavior and their effects may last an hour or two longer than methylphenidate preparations are likely to do. Because they are stronger or more potent, they are typically given in somewhat lower doses (usually half as much as Ritalin or generic methylphenidate), so as to avoid overdosing or excessive side effects.

Parents often ask whether children develop a tolerance to stimulants so that the current dose becomes ineffective over time. Though some physicians have reported that a few children in their practice seemed to develop some tolerance (loss of effect) over a long period of use, research studies have not been able to document such an effect. Usually if the dose is losing its effectiveness it means that the child may have grown since being on the medication. That increased body mass would require that the dose be increased to get the same effects on behavior. Other parents ask whether their child will need to have regular blood tests to monitor the amount of the drug in their bloodstream. This is not a requirement for taking the stimulant medications. The amount of drug in the bloodstream does not seem to be related to how well it works to control behavior, so there is no need for such tests.

Wasn't There Once Another Stimulant Available Called Cylert?

Yes. Pemoline (brand name Cylert) was available for more than 20 years but is no longer on the market. It worked a little differently than the other stimulants. It was associated with a small but significant increase in risk of liver toxicity and even failure and death, all of which required physicians to monitor liver functioning several times per month in a child taking this medication. This risk along with the inconvenience of liver testing requiring blood samples led to a dramatic decline in the use of Cylert for managing the disorder. Ultimately, the manufacturer (Abbott Labs) discontinued manufacture of the drug. Pemoline was available for a while in generic form, but even that has been pulled from the market because of safety concerns. It is not available in the United States except for "compassionate use" purposes that require a physician to file for government approval of use of the drug in each specific case.

The Side Effects

There are a number of side effects that children can experience when taking these medicines, but the vast majority are minor, though some can be annoying. Again, keep in mind that if any of these are bothersome enough to warrant stopping the medication, they will likely go away once the medicine "washes out" of a child's body—within 24 hours. Most of these side effects are clearly related to the dose of medicine the child is taking: higher doses produce more side effects. It has been estimated, however, that from 1 to 3% of children with ADHD cannot tolerate *any* dose of *any* stimulant medication.

It's impossible to predict whether your child will have any of the side effects discussed here. If any family members had an adverse reaction to the drug, there may be a genetic basis to expect that the child might have a similar reaction. So please tell your doctor if this is the case in your family when any of the ADHD medications are being recommended for use with your child.

How likely are the specific side effects? We do have some revealing research findings: over half of children with ADHD I evaluated with my colleagues at the University of Massachusetts Medical School ADHD clinic showed decreased appetite, insomnia, anxiousness, irritability, or proneness to crying. *However, many of these side effects (especially those associated with mood) were present when the children took a fake pill (called a placebo). This means that these side effects may represent problems that are associated with ADHD rather than with the medicine.* In most cases the actual side effects were quite mild. Stomachaches and headaches were reported in about a third of the children, but these were also mild.

Decreased Appetite

All of the stimulants seem to reduce a child's appetite to some degree—temporarily and mainly in the late morning or early afternoon, which explains why over half of all children on these drugs may eat little of their lunch while on the medicine. For many children their appetite comes back (sometimes with a vengeance!) by evening. That is why you should make sure that a child who is on this medicine has a chance to eat adequate types and amounts of food each day to grow well.

Increased Heart Rate and Blood Pressure

Your physician may find that your child's heart rate and blood pressure increase a little while taking these medicines. These changes are minor and do not place most children with ADHD at any risk. However, if your child is one of the rare children who have high blood pressure already, you should make sure your doctor takes this into consideration before deciding to prescribe one of the stimulants.

Increased Brain Electrical Activity

Many studies have found that brain electrical activity increases while a child is on these medicines. These changes are associated with the increased attentiveness and self-regulation experienced by the child. You wouldn't know about this directly unless your child were to have an EEG done for some reason, but you will notice this indirectly because your child's behavior will be improving in conjunction with these changes in brain activity, as discussed earlier.

Insomnia

From one-third to nearly one-half of all children placed on medication may notice that it is harder to fall asleep at bedtime (insomnia) after taking these medicines during the day. Most children fall asleep within an hour or so later than their typical bedtime before starting medication. If the insomnia persists longer than this or you are concerned about this problem for your child, tell your physician so that the problem can be addressed. Sometimes this is done by reducing the dose or taking the medicine earlier in the morning. In other cases, a different medication may have to be tried that does not cause this side effect, such as the nonstimulants discussed below. Some research has found, however, that 20–35% of children taking stimulants during the daytime actually fall asleep better than they did prior to taking medication. As I said above, each child is unique, and so the profile of side effects they may (or may not) experience is often unique as well.

Nervous Tics and Mannerisms

One side effect that you should be somewhat concerned about is the possibility of nervous tics—abrupt twitches of small muscle groups around the face or, less likely, in other parts of the body. Nervous blinking, squinting, or making faces are just some of the tics that can be seen. Other tics are vocal—abrupt noises such as repeated sniffing, throat clearing, or sharp, loud utterances. In its extreme form, the combination of multiple body tics with these vocal noises is called *Tourette syndrome.* You should know that 10–15% of typical children will show some sort of tic or nervous mannerism during childhood, so simple or occasional tics are nothing to worry about if they develop and may have nothing to do with the stimulant medication your child is taking. Some research has shown that such tics in children with ADHD may be made worse by the medicine in a minority of cases (about 35% or fewer). If this happens, in my experience the tics return to their normal level within a week or so after the medicine is stopped. In about 20–25% of other cases, however, the tics the child may have had prior to starting the medication may actually get better on medication. In about half of the cases, the tics remain unchanged from their premedication level. Evidence suggests that the amphetamine preparations, such as Dexedrine, are more likely to result in a worsening of tics than are those containing methylphenidate.

A few children have developed the full Tourette syndrome, though it is not clear in research studies that the medicine actually causes the disorder. It may have worsened it or hastened its appearance in a child who was prone to get the disorder in the first place. But this is quite rare. In most cases, as I discussed above, children with a history of tics or Tourette syndrome can take the stimulants safely with no worsening of their tics. Should that occur, however, the medication can be stopped, whereupon the tics often return to their previous levels, and a nonstimulant medication can be considered for ADHD management.

A physician should ask whether a child with ADHD has a personal or family history of tics or Tourette syndrome before trying a stimulant drug with that child. If so, it is recommended that the children start out on a lower-than-usual dose of medicine to see how such children may react to these drugs. When these medications are used and tics develop, the treatment should be stopped immediately. The tics will usually subside within 7–10 days. Treatment can then be resumed at a lower dose if the child's behavioral adjustment has deteriorated dramatically. If the tics return even at the lower dose, trying an alternative medication (such as the nonstimulants discussed below) may be successful. Failing this, parents should be warned not to have their children treated with stimulants in the future without alerting the treating physician to this history of tic reactions to the stimulant medicines.

We have noticed that up to 15% of children placed on stimulants may develop other simple nervous mannerisms, such as nail biting, skin picking, lip biting, or hair twirling, even if they did not have them previously. Again, withdrawing the medicine usually corrects the problem in a week or so. Your doctor may then consider using one of the nonstimulants discussed below to manage your child's ADHD symptoms.

Temporary Psychosis

This is a very rare side effect at the typical doses used for managing ADHD. All of the stimulant medications have the potential to produce temporary symptoms of psychosis (thought disorganization, rapid speech, skin hallucinations, extreme anxiety, supersensitivity to noises, etc.) at very high doses. In rare cases this can happen at low doses. Such reactions occur in fewer than 1% of the cases, being slightly more common in very young children and less so in older ones. If this occurs, the problem often lasts only until the dose wears off. Even so, the reaction can be frightening to some parents. If so, take your child to a hospital emergency room and tell the attending physician what has occurred. The physician can, if desired, administer another medication to your child that counteracts the effect of the stimulant and can make this reaction diminish more quickly.

Long-Term Effects

Critics of stimulant use for treating ADHD have contended that the stimulants pose a high risk because we have no long-term rigorously controlled studies on the potential long-term negative effects that might be caused by persistent use of the medications. The critics are right that we have no such studies, and here is why: the studies needed to address this issue are unethical in the United States. We simply cannot put some children randomly on stimulants for their ADHD for years, while putting just as many children with ADHD on a placebo for years, and then follow their course. This would be patently unethical because the stimulants have so much research demonstrating their usefulness in the management of ADHD and their short-term safety that professionals cannot withhold drug treatment from children and keep them on a placebo for more than just a few weeks. Moreover, the exorbitant costs associated with doing such research, not to mention the extraordinary time delays in completing them, would ensure that no medications would be approved for use until at least one generation of children had been followed for life after receiving these medications.

So, to evaluate the stimulants' long-term safety, we must turn to other, somewhat less direct sources of information. First, parents must understand that the stimulants have been on the market for 50–70 years. In that time, millions of children and now adults with ADHD have been treated with these medications, many for several years or longer. In none of these cases have any reports of significant long-term side effects been reported to either the pharmaceutical companies or the FDA that could be conclusively associated with taking the stimulant medication.

Second, we have to look at the short-term studies. Do their results imply that long-term side effects would be likely? The answer is no. More than 500 scientific studies have appeared in journals testifying to the relative safety of these medications and their clear effectiveness in helping 70–90% of children with ADHD who have been placed on them. Certainly, some side effects do occur, as noted in this chapter. But these are relatively benign, last only a few hours to a few days at most for many children, are not harmful or life-threatening, and are easily managed by adjusting the dose of medication downward or discontinuing the drug. None of the findings give even a hint that long-term problems are likely to occur following sustained use of the medications for several years or more. As I note under Myth 4 above, even significant problems with growth have now been shown to be a relatively transient occurrence and the failure to grow as much as expected is usually relatively minor for most children. In exceptional cases where growth retardation does occur to a degree that is of concern to parents or physicians, it can be easily managed with drug holidays—ceasing the use of the medication on weekends during the school year and for the summer vacation. Such holidays are the exception, not the norm any longer, because most children do not experience serious growth problems and because ADHD can pose significant risks of harm for children in various ways when they are off their medication (accidental injuries, family conflicts, peer rejection, driving risks, etc.).

Finally, we have to look at what is known about the neurochemical actions of these medications in the brains of children and animals. So far, findings from both types of studies have not shown any clear indications that long-term or enduring side effects would be expected from extended oral medication use. In view of these three sources of information, we can only conclude that at the moment there seems to be no significant likelihood that long-term problems will emerge in children treated with stimulant medications. Can this be guaranteed? Of course not. There are no guarantees in life, including that our children will be safe from all harm when we use over-the-counter medicines or send them out the door to go to school or take them for trips in our cars, yet we do so without pause. The risks of harm from doing so are far higher than those found to be associated with the stimulants. What is important is that our understanding of the risks associated with the use of medications be well informed. As of this writing, the stimulant medications are safer and more effective than for nearly every other class of medication used in psychiatry, and that is all that can be said at the moment.

Should Your Child Receive Stimulants?

You and your doctor will have to consider many factors in making this decision. You'll also have to remain alert to your child's reactions, so that you can quickly recognize when a trial of medication has failed and should be ended. The stimulant medications are the most commonly used psychiatric drugs employed with children, especially in cases where inattentive, hyperactive, or impulsive behavior is sufficiently severe to create problems with school or social adjustment. It has been estimated that between 1 and 2 million children annually, or between 1 and 2% of the school-age population, may be using stimulants for behavior management. Traditionally most of these children were between 5 and 12 years of age, but as we've mentioned, many of them are now older. So you can enter this decision-making process confident that we know more about this form of treatment for ADHD than any other.

Unfortunately, there is no foolproof way to predict who will do well on stimulant medication. So far, the most helpful criterion we have is the degree of inattention and impulsiveness in the child. The more severe these symptoms are, the better a child is likely to respond to the medicine. We have also learned that the more anxious a child is, the less likely she will be to have a positive reaction to the medicine. But even that predictor is controversial, as some studies have now shown that children with ADHD and anxiety disorders do just as well on medication as those who don't have an anxiety disorder. The evidence at the moment is mixed. For that reason I recommend that physicians treating children who have both disorders do so more carefully, starting with lower doses and adjusting those doses upward more gradually than usual while having parents monitor both the ADHD symptoms and those of anxiety more carefully, perhaps with a rating scale of those symptoms completed periodically. Some studies have also found that the quality of the relationship between a parent and the child may predict the child's drug response: the better the parent–child relationship, the greater the response to medication. It may be that parents who are more appreciative and rewarding of the behavior changes brought by the stimulants produce further gains in their children from the medicine. Of course, it could also be that better parent–child relations are just a marker for the child having milder ADHD, which may explain why those children may have done better on the medication.

Your doctor will also take into account the following factors:

1. The percentage of children with the primarily inattentive form of ADHD (sometimes called ADD or sluggish cognitive tempo, SCT; see Chapter 7) who respond well to the medication may be somewhat lower—20–55%—than that of children with the more typical forms of ADHD. And the magnitude of the response they have to the medicine may not be as impressive. On the plus side, the necessary dose when benefits are found may be lower than that used with more typical forms of ADHD.

2. Stimulants may help children with ADHD who are also developmentally delayed (previously called "mental retardation") only if the general delay is not too severe. In one study, children with mental ages greater than 4 years or IQs above 45 often had positive responses, whereas those with lower mental ages or IQs generally responded poorly.

3. Children with ADHD who have seizures may have more side effects (behavior problems) while on the stimulants than are seen in children with ADHD who do not have seizures.

4. Some children with brain injuries from trauma or open head wounds or those who develop ADHD symptoms after being treated with radiation and or chemotherapy for head and neck cancers or leukemia may develop symptoms of ADHD to a degree that warrants a possible trial on stimulant drugs. These children may also respond well, but both some research and my experience suggest that the probability of a good response is lower in this group of children with these types of causes of their ADHD.

As you have undoubtedly discerned by now, *a diagnosis of ADHD should not constitute an automatic knee-jerk recommendation for drug treatment.* If your doctor seems to be taking this approach, we suggest you find a new doctor. The following rules might help you in making a decision about trying medication, but remember—this applies to both parents and physicians—to remain flexible to the unique needs and circumstances of each case.

1. *Has the child had adequate physical and psychological evaluations?* Medications should never be prescribed if the child has not been directly examined in a thorough manner.

2. *How old is the child?* Drug treatment is somewhat less effective or leads to somewhat more frequent side effects among children 2–4 years of age than those 5 years and older. This does not mean such medications cannot be tried in this preschool age group, only that it be done more conservatively, with an eye out for these potentially greater problems, and only after behavior management training of the parents has been tried.

3. *Have other therapies been used?* If this is your family's initial contact with a professional and your child's ADHD is mild and not complicated by another disorder, the prescription of medication might be postponed until other interventions (for example, parent training in child management skills) have been attempted. Alternatively, when the child's behavior presents a moderate-to-severe problem or your family cannot participate in child management training, medication may be the most viable initial treatment.

4. *How severe is the child's current misbehavior?* In some cases, the child's behavior is so unmanageable or distressing that medication may prove the fastest and most effective manner of dealing with the crisis until other forms of treatment can begin. Once progress is made with other therapies, some effort can be made to reduce or terminate the medication, but it's not always possible.

5. *Can you afford the medication and associated costs* (for example, follow-up visits)?

6. *Can you adequately supervise the use of the medications and guard against their abuse?*

7. *What is your attitude toward medication?* If you are simply "antidrug," don't let your doctor pressure you into agreeing to this treatment, because you probably won't be able to comply wholeheartedly with the regimen. But you should also seriously scrutinize your own opinion to ensure that it is based on balanced, unbiased sources of information about the pros and cons of taking stimulant medications. Talk with your doctor or other experts on ADHD, read more about the medications at reliable websites like *www.help4adhd.org, www.nlm.nih.gov, www.aap.org,* or *www.aacap.org,* and review other resources and videos listed at the end of this book to be sure your opinions are well informed before making any blanket decisions.

8. *Is there a delinquent or drug-abusing family member in the household?* In this case, stimulant medication should not be prescribed, since there is a high risk for its illegal use or sale.

9. *Does the child have any history of psychosis or thought disorder?* If so, the stimulants are not indicated, because they may worsen such difficulties.

10. *Is the child highly anxious, fearful, or more likely to complain of bodily symptoms?* Such children might be less likely to respond positively to stimulant medications, though this is arguable at this time. As I recommended above, in these cases if stimulant medications are to be used, then physicians should simply start lower (doses), go more slowly (titration), and monitor the child more closely for potential side effects. Alternatively, consider using one of the nonstimulants discussed below that do not have this potential to worsen anxiety or pose other side effects and may even treat the anxiety symptoms.

11. *Does the physician have the time to monitor medication properly?* In addition

to an initial evaluation of the drug's effectiveness with a child for establishing the optimal dosage, the physician needs to see the child periodically to monitor the child's response and side effects. We recommend that a child taking stimulants be seen by the physician every 3–6 months for this monitoring.

12. *How does the child feel about medication and its alternatives?* With older children and adolescents it is important that the use of medication be discussed and the reasons for its use fully explained. In cases where children are "antidrug" or oppositional, they may resist efforts to use it, such as refusing to swallow the pill. If that is the case, have the child or teen discuss his concerns with the physician so he can be reassured that many of his concerns are either unfounded or possibly exaggerated.

How Stimulants Are Prescribed

The procedures described here are those typically followed by my physician colleagues in the ADHD clinics I have supervised and also used by many physicians elsewhere. Even so, your own physician may follow a somewhat different procedure based on the unique needs of your child, as well as the doctor's own training and preferences.

The first choice of medication is typically one of the new extended-release forms of methylphenidate (Concerta, Focalin XR, Ritalin LA, Medadate CD, Daytrana, etc.) or the amphetamines (Adderall XR, Vyvanse). A child's failure to respond to one stimulant may not rule out a positive response to another stimulant, however, so we recommend a trial of the second type of medicine (methylphenidate, amphetamine) if a poor response to the first type was evident. If this trial fails, we suggest switching to atomoxetine (Strattera). If this too fails, then a trial of guanfacine XR (Intuniv) is in order. Keep in mind that children under age 6 who show a poor response to stimulants may well respond positively to them a year or two later.

With generic methylphenidate (or Ritalin), the usual practice is to start a child at a low dose such as 5 milligrams (mg) (2.5 mg for children under age 5) in the morning and at noon, though some physicians recommend starting with just one dose in the morning. The dose is then increased by 5 mg (or 2.5 mg) every week until a good response is found or a dose of 1 mg/kg (1 mg for every 2.2 pounds [1 kilogram] of the child's weight) is reached. Children who wake up early in the morning or who eliminate the drug more rapidly from their bodies may require doses three times per day. The dose used rarely exceeds 20 mg per dose, two to three times daily, because of the risk of more severe side effects at higher doses. Some professionals use daily doses as high as 60–70 mg. Nevertheless, because every child responds differently, some children may need higher doses. If yours does, don't be alarmed. So long as no serious side effects are occurring, your child is in no danger. Giving the doses with or after meals may lessen the appetite problems or stomachaches sometimes associated with these drugs. Where such side effects are not a problem, the medications can be given 30 minutes before mealtimes.

With generic *d*-amphetamine (or Dexedrine) or Adderall doses are typically given that are about half the size of those of Ritalin because of its greater potency. Like generic methylphenidate, these amphetamines often have to be given several times a day because their beneficial effects typically last only 3–6 hours.

As discussed earlier, the extended-release forms of methylphenidate and the amphetamines, such as Concerta, Adderall XR, or Vyvanse (and others noted above), may be more effective than the shorter acting immediate-release forms of these medications. They also negate the need for a noontime dose and thus enhance confidentiality for the child, since schoolmates will not have to know that the child is taking a drug.

Although no research has studied whether they differ from the brand-name drugs in effectiveness, some physicians have told us that the generic forms do not work as well for some children.

These drugs can be given according to various schedules, depending on the type of delivery system (short-acting or sustained release), the severity of a child's ADHD, and the associated difficulties. Many children find that the side effects they initially experience decrease over the first few weeks as they become adjusted to a drug's presence in their body. For this reason (if the medicine is stopped over the weekend, side effects may reappear on Mondays), and because weight loss is not a problem for many children, it is no longer recommended that a child stop the medicine on weekends during the school year. Practitioners these days are also less likely to stop the medicine during the summer months, unless a child's ADHD has been mainly affecting school performance. Many children benefit from staying on their medicine throughout the summer, especially if they're going to be busy with sports, camps, Scouts, summer school, tutoring, or other structured activities.

If your child is taking the immediate-release forms of these medications, it is frequently necessary to use the medicines twice a day or even three times a day if the effects disappear quickly. This problem is often noticed by a child's teachers, who may observe that the morning dose has essentially worn off by midmorning. In such cases a breakfast dose can be given at 7:00–8:00 A.M., a second dose at 10:30–11:00 A.M., and a final dose at 2:00–3:00 P.M. Only when a child's behavior problems are *exceptionally severe* is a dose closer to the dinner hour recommended, because a late dose increases the odds of decreased appetite at dinnertime and insomnia at bedtime. Closer attention to behavior management programs is a better alternative. However, adolescents may need this third dose late in the afternoon to help them concentrate during their homework. Your physician can try your teen on this third dose to see whether or not it can be tolerated well. Because of the inconvenience associated with using these immediate-release medications in this manner, most children taking stimulants are now on the once-daily extended-release forms of these medications. I recommend these be tried first before moving to the immediate-release types of medications to avoid the need to take medicines during school hours or on such a frequent schedule.

In general, the dose should always be the lowest possible and should be given only as many times per day as necessary to achieve adequate management of the child's behavior.

Parents should never assume they have the physician's permission to adjust the dosage of medication without consultation with the physician.

In the near future, parents may find that some new stimulant drugs will be available for use in the treatment of children with ADHD. As research increases our understanding of the genetics of ADHD and how those specific genes work in controlling brain neurochemistry, new medications may be invented that may be more precise in controlling ADHD symptoms with fewer side effects, and so may prove more helpful for those with the disorder.

When Should the Medicines Be Stopped?

There are no firm guidelines for stopping stimulant treatment. The medicine can be used until it no longer seems necessary. Up to 20% of children may be able to stop taking medication after a year or so, for several reasons. Some children have only mild cases of ADHD and may mature to a point where the medication is not needed. Other children with ADHD may improve to the extent that they also do not need medication, even though some symptoms of their ADHD remain. Still other children may continue to have significant symptoms of ADHD, but they have a better teacher for the new academic year, and their symptoms do not hamper them as much as they did with previous teachers. However, some children with ADHD may need to return to medication later that year or in subsequent years, depending on the demands for sustained attention and behavioral inhibition made on them at school or elsewhere. Most children with ADHD, however, will need to remain on their medication for years.

Treatment can be stopped annually for a few days to a week—usually done a month or so after the beginning of the new academic year, to give the child time to get used to the new school year and the teacher to get to know the child before the medicine is stopped. When a doctor waits to see if a child who has been off medication for the summer has trouble in school without it, the child is put in the position of developing a bad reputation with the teacher and classmates—an image he must then overcome after going back on the stimulants. It's better to get the school year off to a good start with the medication and then stop the medication briefly during October. If there is a decline in school performance, the child can be kept on medication during that school year.

Strattera (Atomoxetine)

Strattera (atomoxetine) is a nonstimulant medication developed for the treatment of ADHD. It is known as a specific norepinephrine reuptake inhibitor because it slows down the reuptake or reabsorption of the neurotransmitter norepinephrine back into nerve cells in the brain, once that chemical has been released during activation of that nerve cell. A number of studies have now been published that demonstrate the effectiveness of atomoxetine in the treatment of ADHD (see *www.Strattera.com*). There is also extensive research available on the safety of the medication when used with children, teens, and adults who have ADHD.

The FDA approved the use of atomoxetine for children and adults with ADHD in 2003. Since then more than 5 million patients have taken this medication. Evidence indicates that the drug not only improves the symptoms of ADHD, but also reduces oppositional and defiant behavior and anxiety. Parents of children on atomoxetine have reported fewer emotional difficulties and behavioral problems as well as greater self-esteem in their children and less emotional worry and fewer limitations on their personal time in themselves. However, research comparing this drug to the stimulants typically finds that the degree of improvement in ADHD symptoms is somewhat less, though the percentage of children who respond positively to it is about the same as the stimulants, around 75%.

What Are the Side Effects of Atomoxetine?

Unlike the stimulants, atomoxetine does not result in insomnia or difficulties falling asleep in the evening. It also does not appear to exacerbate motor or vocal tics in children who have tic disorders. The side effects include mild loss of appetite and sleepiness or sedation, particularly during the first few weeks of use of the medication. The drug also results in mild increases in diastolic blood pressure and heart rate but with no significant changes on electrocardiogram patterns (ECG intervals). Fewer than 10% of patients treated with this medication required stopping the medicine because of significant side effects. Research has now followed treated cases for more than 3 years and supports the long-term efficacy, safety, and tolerability of atomoxetine for the treatment of childhood and adult ADHD.

How Is Atomoxetine Prescribed?

Currently, the most recent guidelines for using the medication recommend that atomoxetine be initiated at 0.3 mg/kg/day for 10 days, then increased to 0.6 mg/kg for another 10 days, and then finally increased to a target dose of 1.2 mg/kg/day with a recommended maximum dosage of 1.4 mg/kg/day or 100 mg/day. (Note: To figure out your child's weight in kilograms, or kg, divide his or her weight in pounds by 2.1.) Further improvement may occur in some cases at doses up to 1.8 mg/kg/day, but this dose has not received approval from the FDA. Atomoxetine is effective when given once a day. But it can be divided into two doses for use twice a day (morning and bedtime) if annoying side effects occurred with the single-dose schedule. The drug should not be used in combination with fluoxetine, paroxetine, or monoamine oxidase inhibitors.

Didn't I Hear Something about Liver Problems with Atomoxetine?

From 2003 to 2010, just two cases of severe liver injury were reported to the manufacturer and the FDA out of more than 5 million patients who have taken atomoxetine since its FDA approval. These patients recovered with normal liver function after discontinuing the medication. It is not clear in one of these cases that the liver problem was related to the medication, while in the second case it may have been. The medication should be discontinued in any patients with jaundice (yellowing of the skin or whites of the eyes) or laboratory evidence of liver injury. Experts and the manufacturer recommend that patients on atomoxetine be cautioned to contact their doctor immediately if they develop pruritus, jaundice, dark urine, upper-right-sided abdominal tenderness, or unexplained "flu-like" symptoms. However, any risk of liver problems appears to be exceptionally rare.

Intuniv (Guanfacine XR)

Intuniv (guanfacine XR) is the latest drug to be developed for the management of ADHD in children and adolescents (ages 6–17 years), having received approval from the FDA in 2009 for that purpose. Guanfacine was originally used to treat high blood pressure by reducing heart rate and relaxing the walls of blood vessels, allowing the flow of blood more easily. And so it is classified as an *antihypertensive* drug. It was marketed under the brand name Tenex. Unlike other antihypertensive drugs (see clonidine in Chapter 19), this drug has weaker effects in reducing blood pressure and other effects on heart functioning and so is generally considered to be safer for use with children than the more potent alternative clonidine. The extended-release (XR) form of guanfacine is called Intuniv and has been formulated to have a sustained release across the waking hours. This is done by making the drug into pellets and covering the pellets in coatings that dissolve at different intervals. To avoid destruction of the time-release coatings, parents should be sure their child does not crush or chew the tablet but swallows it whole.

This long-acting drug is considered to produce its effects in the brain by influencing small mechanisms on nerve cells called alpha-2 receptors. These receptors appear to adjust the strength or purity of an electrical signal that flows through the nerve fiber when it is activated by opening or closing these little valve-like mechanisms on the nerve. Intuniv seems to work in ADHD by reducing the degree of "noise" (openness of the valve-like receptors) and thus enhancing the electrical signal in the nerve cells, especially in the prefrontal lobes of the brain, where such receptors occur more than elsewhere. As you learned in earlier chapters, these parts of the brain are involved in sustained attention, impulse control, and the other executive functions that provide us with self-regulation. Studies have now been published that clearly show this drug to be effective in reducing ADHD symptoms in children. There is also good evidence available on the safety of the medication when used with children who have ADHD. For more information on Intuniv, visit *www.Intuniv.com, www.nlm.nih.gov,* or *en.wikipedia.org/wiki/Guanfacine.*

As with atomoxetine, evidence indicates that the drug not only improves the symptoms of ADHD but also reduces oppositional, defiant, and aggressive behavior, anxiety, and even nervous tics and the other symptoms of Tourette syndrome.

What Are the Side Effects of Guanfacine XR?

Guanfacine XR is quite different in its side effects from the stimulants discussed above. For instance, it is unlikely to result in insomnia or difficulties falling asleep in the evening and may even promote earlier sleep onset because of its association with increased drowsiness or sleepiness if taken at bedtime. It also does not appear to exacerbate motor or vocal tics in children who have tic disorders and may even reduce them, which is why guanfacine (Tenex) has been used to treat tic disorders or Tourette syndrome. The most common side effects of this medication are feeling lightheaded or dizzy because of the often mild reductions in heart rate and blood pressure, and so the drug should not be used in children who may already have difficulties with low blood pressure or heart functioning. Children taking the drug should be encouraged to drink plenty of water as these symptoms can be exacerbated by dehydration or exposure to foods and beverages that have some diuretic effects, such as caffeine and alcohol. The drug is also usually associated with increased sleepiness or sedation, particularly during the first few weeks of use of the medication. The most serious side effects are rare but include fainting, blurred vision, skin rash, and significant reductions in heart rate and blood pressure. Should these occur, call your prescribing doctor immediately. Other side effects include dry mouth, fatigue, weakness, headache, irritability, stomachache, loss of appetite, gas pains, nausea, vomiting, constipation or diarrhea, nasal congestion, and, for adults, decreased sexual ability. Fewer than 10% of patients treated with this medication require stopping the medicine because of significant side effects. Parents are warned as well not to cease use of the drug with their child abruptly as there is the rare potential to cause serious problems with your child's blood pressure and heart functioning by doing so.

Research has now followed treated cases for several years and supports the longer term efficacy, safety, and tolerability of this drug for the treatment of childhood ADHD.

How Is Guanfacine XR Prescribed?

Guanfacine XR (Intuniv) is available in 1-, 2-, 3-, and 4-mg tablets. The most recent guidelines for using the medication recommend that it be started at 1 mg per day and then gradually increased every week or so, with typical doses eventually being 3 mg or 4 mg. Intuniv is effective for managing ADHD symptoms when given once a day and should be given at the same time each day. Do not skip doses or adjust the medication without first consulting with your prescribing physician. The manufacturer warns against consuming the drug with any high-fat meal. The drug should also not be consumed with grapefruit or grapefruit juice due to potential adverse interactions between them. The drug is also contraindicated if your child is taking certain other medications, such as sedatives, antipsychotics, anticonvulsants, or antidepressants, or even herbal supplements, such as St. John's wort. Be sure to tell your physician about any other medications or nutritional or herbal supplements your child may be taking.

In summary, the past decade has seen the development and FDA approval of two new medications for the management of ADHD in children (atomoxetine, guanfacine XR) and adults (atomoxetine). The availability of these medications certainly broadens the ability of clinicians to treat the diversity of patients who have ADHD and provides alternative treatments for those cases that may be having significant side effects from the use of stimulants (for example, insomnia) or who may have coexisting disorders that could potentially be worsened by stimulants (anxiety, tic disorders, insomnia, low appetite).

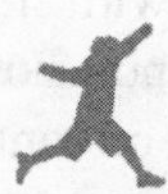

19 Other Medicines

ANTIDEPRESSANTS AND ANTIHYPERTENSIVES

Although they are not as effective as the stimulants, several drugs called *antidepressants* and another antihypertensive drug called *clonidine* can be of some benefit to those with ADHD. But keep in mind these drugs have not received FDA approval for use in the management of ADHD, and so the FDA-approved drugs discussed in Chapter 18 should always be tried before considering the use of these medications with your child. With the development and government approval of atomoxetine (Strattera) and the safer antihypertensive drug, guanfacine XR (Intuniv; see Chapter 18), for the management of ADHD, there has been a marked decline in the use of antidepressants as well as clonidine for managing ADHD. That is because atomoxetine and guanfacine XR have been studied more extensively and have been found to be safer medications with fewer significant side effects on heart functioning than seems to be the case for the tricyclic antidepressants or clonidine. Therefore, atomoxetine or guanfacine XR should be tried before using a tricyclic antidepressant or clonidine for the management of ADHD symptoms. If your doctor recommends any of these medications, or any other for that matter, be sure to ask the questions listed in the sidebar in Chapter 18.

Tricyclic Antidepressants

The brand names (with generic names in parentheses) of the antidepressant medicines that were used most frequently with ADHD before 2003 are Norpramin or Pertofrane (desipramine), Tofranil (imipramine), Elavil (amitriptyline), and Wellbutrin (bupropion hydrochloride). The first three of these belong to the class of drugs known as *tricyclic antidepressants*. There are other tricyclic antidepressants as well, such as Pamelor or Aventyl (nortriptyline) and Anafranil (clomipramine), but clinical scientists have not studied their effects on ADHD very well, so they are not discussed here. Because Wellbutrin is very different from the tricyclic antidepressant drugs, I discuss it in a separate section.

Norpramin, Tofranil, and Elavil were all developed primarily to treat depression. However, they have also been used to treat some children with ADHD as well as children with anxiety or panic reactions, some with bed-wetting problems, and others with sleep problems such as night terrors. They are useful when a child with ADHD has not shown a good response to the stimulants or nonstimulants discussed in Chapter 18 or cannot tolerate taking those medications. Like all other drugs that modify behavior, these drugs change behavior by altering the brain's chemistry in certain locations. We believe that in ADHD they increase the amount of the chemicals norepinephrine and dopamine available for work within the brain, especially the prefrontal area, as do the stimulants. The tricyclic drug most frequently studied for treating ADHD is Norpramin, but it is likely that the other tricyclic antidepressant drugs would produce similar benefits.

Sometimes the changes in behavior related to ADHD can be seen within a few days of starting these medicines, while in other cases it may take several weeks. If the medicines are being recommended to treat depression in a child with ADHD, ask your doctor about more modern antidepressants known as SSRIs (selective serotonin reuptake inhibitors) for this purpose. They are likely to be safer medications, causing fewer problems with heart functioning than may occur with the tricyclic medications. If you and your doctor do finally decide to use a tricyclic drug, several weeks will be needed to judge how well a dose of medicine is working. The dose will be increased or decreased, depending on the results of the first trial, and then a few more weeks will have to pass before the benefits of the new dose are noticed. This means your child may require a considerably longer trial to find out whether a tricyclic will work for her than that needed for the stimulants discussed in Chapter 18.

Studies have found that children with ADHD who are given this type of drug are likely to show mild to moderate improvements in their ability to pay attention and control their impulses. They may also be somewhat less restless or hyperactive. Often the most obvious result is an improvement in mood. The children may seem less irritable or quick to anger, somewhat happier or in better spirits, and less anxious or worried. These drugs are not as effective at changing the symptoms of ADHD as the FDA-approved drugs discussed in Chapter 18, which is yet another reason the approved medications should always be tried first.

Like the stimulants, the tricyclic antidepressants are taken by mouth once or twice a day (mornings and evenings). Unlike the stimulants, they do not wash out of the body very quickly and must build up in the bloodstream over longer periods of time. This means that once a useful level of the drug is reached its effects last throughout the day, but it also means that it can take several weeks to gradually withdraw the child from the medication if necessary. Missing a dose or stopping the medicine abruptly may not be dangerous, but it could cause a headache, stomachache, nausea, or aching muscles. The child could also show some emotional or behavioral reactions, such as crying, sadness, nervousness, and problems with sleeping.

What Are the Side Effects?

Slower Heart Rate

One of the problems with tricyclic antidepressants is that they can slow down the transmission of the electrical signal in the heart, causing problems in the heartbeat or heart rhythm. For this reason, every child who is to be tried on such an antidepressant, such as Norpramin, Tofranil, or Elavil, should first be given an electrocardiogram (EKG or ECG)—an easy test that measures how well the heart is beating. If the test gives any abnormal findings, the child should not be placed on any of these medicines. Also, any family history of sudden cardiac (heart) arrest should be a warning to avoid these medicines in most cases.

In fact, because these medicines can have serious effects on the heart, *they must be kept out of reach of children or anyone else who might accidentally take too much of the medicine; an overdose could be fatal.*

Seizures

Another problem with these medicines is that they may increase the risk of seizures or convulsions, particularly if the child has a history of seizures, has had a serious head injury, or has had some other serious neurological problem. In such cases, it is probably best not to use these medicines.

Minor Physical Effects

The most common side effects of Norpramin, Tofranil, or Elavil seem to be a feeling of dry mouth, which can be handled by giving a child some sugar-free gum to chew, and constipation, which can be dealt with by using stool softeners or adjusting the diet so it contains more fiber or bulk. Some children may also experience blurred vision or even nearsightedness. Occasionally children have had difficulty getting their flow of urine started when they try to urinate. None of these is a serious problem, and they can all be handled by lowering the dose of the medicine.

Rare Side Effects

Some of the side effects of tricyclic antidepressants are rare but can be very serious. Besides the slowed heart rate and increased risk of seizures already mentioned, some children may have a psychotic reaction in which they have disturbed thinking, highly excessive speech, seriously increased activity level, and even hallucinations. Also at high doses, some children experience mental confusion. Where any of these side effects occur, the child's physician should be informed immediately and the medication discontinued under the physician's guidance. Increases in blood pressure can occur, although they are mild, and can be of concern if the child already has a history of high blood pressure.

Also rare but not as serious are the occasional cases of rash that have been reported. These are probably the result of an allergic reaction to the food coloring (tartrazine) used in making the pills, and not to the medicine itself. Changing to a different form of the medicine that does not contain the food coloring can solve this problem. Very rarely, children taking these medicines may show some nervous tics. If this occurs to a significant or frequent degree, the medicines can be stopped, and the tic reactions will usually go away. The drugs can also increase the sensitivity of the skin to sunlight, requiring that a child wear strong sunscreen more often or better protective clothing than normal when active outdoors.

Drug Interactions

Because these medicines can interact with a number of other medicines in undesirable ways, it is best to ask your physician which medicines should be avoided while a child is taking Norpramin, Tofranil, and Elavil.

How Are These Drugs Used with Children?

The best doses of Norpramin, Tofranil, and Elavil are 1–5 mg for each kilogram (about 2.2 pounds) of body weight per day. For instance, if your child weighs 80 pounds (38 kg), the lowest probable dose for this child would be 38 mg and the highest 190 mg. Some children may respond well between 1 and 3 mg/kg (between 38 and 117 mg in the example), whereas others will need more medicine to receive any benefit from the drugs. Sometimes, when a child is taking these medicines for the treatment of depression, blood tests may be necessary to see if enough medicine is getting into the bloodstream to benefit the child. This is usually done when the dose seems adequate but the child either is not responding or is showing signs of having too much medication. Even then, however, it is not clear from research that knowing the blood level of the medicine is of much help in determining the best dose.

Unlike with the stimulants, children can build up a tolerance to the tricyclic antidepressants, so typically they cannot take these medicines for more than a year or two. Sometimes these antidepressants begin to lose their effectiveness after only 4–6 months. In these cases, the medicine may have to be stopped for a few months before it can be tried again.

Wellbutrin (Bupropion Hydrochloride)

Wellbutrin is a relatively new type of antidepressant medication that has been found in several studies to be of some benefit in the management of ADHD symptoms in both children and adults. It is not chemically related to the tricyclics or other types of antidepressants and so does not share the same risks or side effects that were noted above, especially those related to heart functioning. Like other antidepressants, however, the medication does require several days to several weeks to build up in the bloodstream before its effectiveness can be judged. The drug is available in both its regular form and a long-acting preparation. It is typically prescribed so as to be taken several times during each day. There is a very slight risk that the drug may induce seizures, particularly at high doses and more likely in children with a prior history of seizures. Other side effects of the medication include edema (swelling), skin rashes, irritability, loss of appetite, and difficulty falling asleep. Typical doses range from 3 to 6 mg/kg per day, or about 140–280 mg for a 100-pound child.

Didn't I Hear Something about Antidepressants Possibly Causing Suicide?

Yes, you more than likely have heard in the media questions being raised about whether antidepressant medicines like the tricyclic antidepressants, the SSRIs (selective serotonin reuptake inhibitors like Prozac), and Wellbutrin might increase suicidal thinking or even suicide attempts in children and teens taking these medications. Parents should understand that the evidence here is not as clear as the sensational stories in the media sometimes portray it to be. Typically, these sorts of problems have been reported occasionally in children who are being treated for depression with the medicines. Those children and teens already would have a higher than normal likelihood of having suicidal thoughts or of making suicide attempts given their depression. In an examination of the records of patients with depression or mood disorders who had been treated across seven different studies of these medications, Dr. Bridge and colleagues found the risk for suicidal thinking was 0.7% higher than in children taking placebo in these studies. No completed suicides occurred in these trials. Nevertheless, on October 15, 2004, the FDA issued a public health advisory to warn physicians prescribing these medicines about a potential for increased suicidal thoughts or actual attempts in children being treated for depression with these medicines. If your child is taking one of these medications or any other medication not discussed in this book, see Dr. Timothy E. Wilens's *Straight Talk about Psychiatric Medications for Kids*, which offers more information on the FDA warning and the surrounding controversy and advises parents on appropriate precautions to take to protect children and teenagers being treated with these medications.

Clonidine

Another type of medicine shown to have some benefit for children with ADHD is clonidine, a drug frequently used to treat high blood pressure in adults. (Clonidine is marketed under the trade name Catapres by one drug company, but it is usually sold and referred to by its generic name.) Clonidine is similar to guanfacine XR (Intuniv), the antihypertensive drug discussed in the preceding chapter that has received FDA approval for use in treating children with ADHD. The fact that both drugs can produce changes in behavior and mood make them of some benefit to children with ADHD who have problems with or get no beneficial effects from the stimulants or with atomoxetine. These two antihypertensive drugs differ in that guanfacine produces much less adverse effects on heart functioning and blood pressure than does clonidine and so carries less risk for side effects (fainting, dizziness, nausea) that may be related to them. Guanfacine XR is also sustained longer in the bloodstream and so requires fewer doses during the day, as the XR in its name implies (XR = extended release). For these reasons, if an antihypertensive drug is to be considered for use with a child with ADHD, then guanfacine XR would be the preferred choice over clonidine. Other disorders for which clonidine has been used include migraine headaches, schizophrenia, bipolar disorders, obsessive–compulsive disorder, panic disorder, and serious eating disorders like anorexia nervosa. It has also been used in treating the tics, vocal noises, and other involuntary movements seen in Tourette syndrome.

When used for children with ADHD, clonidine may reduce the motor hyperactivity and impulsiveness seen with the disorder. It may also increase a child's cooperativeness with tasks and directions and increase the child's tolerance for frustration. Dr. Robert Hunt of Vanderbilt University, a nationally recognized expert on the use of this drug with children with ADHD, reports that clonidine may not be as effective as the stimulants in improving such a child's sustained attention or reducing distractibility. However, it may be as effective as the stimulants in reducing aggressive and impulsive behavior or the tendency to become overaroused very quickly. Dr. Hunt believes that this medication may be best suited for those children with ADHD who are very oppositional or defiant or who have conduct disorder.

When taken by mouth, clonidine may produce changes in behavior that can be noted within 30–60 minutes and may last for 3–6 hours. It also comes in an adhesive patch that can be worn on the skin. When this skin patch is used, changes in behavior may not be noticed for several days. However, it usually takes several months before one can tell just how much benefit the drug is producing in the management of a child's behavioral or emotional problems.

What Are the Side Effects?

The most common problem children have with clonidine is sedation or a feeling of tiredness or sleepiness. This can last as long as the first 2–4 weeks after a child begins the medicine. During this period the child may take frequent catnaps, especially during boring activities. In some children, perhaps 15%, this sleepiness or fatigue may last longer and be troublesome enough to warrant stopping the medicine.

There may be a mild drop in your child's blood pressure after starting this medication, but this is rarely significant. There may also be a slight decrease in heart rate, but again this is rarely serious. Headaches or dizziness may be noted in some children, again typically within the first 4 weeks of starting the medicine. Some children have complained of nausea, stomachaches, and even vomiting, but these are also usually limited to the first few weeks of starting the medicine. Constipation and dryness of the mouth may also be seen in some children. Much less likely to occur are depression, erratic changes in heartbeat or rhythm, nightmares or disrupted sleep, increased appetite, or increases or decreases in weight. Rarely, problems with increased anxiety, a sensation of coldness in the fingers or toes (known as *Raynaud syndrome*), or water retention may be seen.

The medicine should never be stopped abruptly. If it is, a child may experience a rapid rise in blood pressure, show agitation, and/or become anxious; complain of chest pain or fast and irregular heartbeat; and develop headaches, stomachaches, nausea, or sleep problems.

Clonidine can also interact with other drugs to create problems for a child, so you should advise your physician of any medication a child is on before clonidine is prescribed, or of any new medications being considered for the child while clonidine is being taken.

How Is Clonidine Used with Children?

Before starting this medicine, your physician may want to conduct a complete physical examination of your child, including an EKG and some blood work. Dr. Hunt recommends that children with ADHD be placed on doses of 0.15–0.30 mg/day. The drug is usually begun at much lower doses (0.05 mg given at night). The dose is then gradually increased every few days or less often by adding doses of 0.05 mg given at different times of the day until a child is taking this dose four times a day. At this time it may be necessary to increase the dose from 0.5 to 1.0 mg for one of the four doses each day. These increases can continue until some benefit has been noticed from the medicine or the side effects become a problem for the child. The drug is usually taken orally three to four times a day (commonly at mealtimes and bedtime). Although some improvement in behavior may be seen in the first 2–4 weeks, it can usually take 2–4 months before the full benefit of the medicine is noticed.

A skin patch of clonidine, named Catapres-TTS, is available. It is worn like an adhesive bandage and should be placed on a clean, relatively hairless patch of skin out of easy reach of the child's hands (usually the lower back or over the back of the hips). Each patch can be worn for about 5 days. Children can take baths or showers with the patch on, but after swimming or heavy sweating the patch may need to be replaced. Dr. Hunt recommends that children be started on oral clonidine until the proper dose is determined. They can then be switched to the skin patch, which avoids the problems of taking oral medication at school, if desired.

Any child taking clonidine should be followed by the physician weekly while the different doses are being tried, and then every 4–6 weeks once a stable dose has been reached. Blood pressure, heart rate, and growth should be monitored at these regular visits.

If your physician is not familiar with clonidine or you would like to read more about it yourself, you may wish to consult *Straight Talk about Psychiatric Medications for Kids* by Dr. Timothy E. Wilens (see "Suggested Reading and Videos" at the end of this book).

Support Services for Parents

A large number of parent support associations for ADHD exist throughout the United States and Canada. In addition, there are a number of smaller local or regional groups. Since the contacts for these groups change so frequently, I suggest that you start by contacting one of the national organizations, which maintain current records of all the various support groups. They will be glad to refer you to the group closest to your home. Parents should be aware of the fact that the fast-changing nature of the Internet may mean that some of the Internet addresses listed here are no longer in existence by the time they read this book. Also, others may have changed their Internet site address, requiring some extra effort in searching the Internet for their actual website. I regret any inconvenience such changes may create.

The largest national association is **Children and Adults with Attention-Deficit/Hyperactivity Disorder (CHADD),** which has more than 500 such support associations affiliated with it from almost every state and province. To find the support group nearest you, visit CHADD's website:

www.chadd.org or *www.help4adhd.org*

Another national parent support association is the **Attention Deficit Disorder Association (ADDA).** Visit ADDA's website:

www.add.org

ADHD-Europe is a joint effort among national and regional ADHD organizations in Europe to promote the dissemination of information and support to those who live or are in contact with persons who have ADHD. The organization advocates with the European institutions and community for its members on the topic of ADHD, with a view to affecting policy and improving existing legislation on issues connected to ADHD. More information can be found at their website:

www.adhdeurope.eu/home.html

The national support group for ADHD in Canada is the **Centre for ADHD Awareness, Canada (CADDAC).**

www.caddac.ca

Some support groups serving the United Kingdom and Europe should also be mentioned here. **ADDers.org** is a group that promotes awareness of ADHD in both children and adults with practical suggestions for families in the United Kingdom and elsewhere.

www.adders.org

Newsletters on ADHD can be obtained from CHADD and ADDA, as well as from several other sources. See the "Periodicals" section of "Suggested Reading and Videos" for a list of newsletters.

As I have noted in the Preface to this book, the rapidly increasing availability of the personal computer and the astonishing growth of the Internet have created an explosion of information on every conceivable topic in recent years, and ADHD is no exception. As I have also noted in the Preface, however, considerable caution about the quality of what is available via this new medium is in order. Please be careful about the information about ADHD you receive over the Internet in bulletin boards, chat rooms, and even many websites (especially commercial ones). The "facts" about ADHD that can be found in many of these locations are often unscientific, inaccurate, sensationalized, or merely thinly veiled sales pitches for various unproven remedies for ADHD. Having said this, I do recommend some Internet resources here for you to pursue.

A group called **Attention Deficit Disorder in Europe** provides useful information on ADHD in a number of different languages at its website:

www.pavilion.co.uk/add

ADHD Information Services (ADDISS) provides information, support, and training resources on ADHD in the United Kingdom:

www.addiss.co.uk

Suggested Reading and Videos

Books for Parents and Teachers

American Academy of Pediatrics (2011). *ADHD: What every parent needs to know.* Elk Grove, IL: Author.

Based on the Academy's current clinical practice guidelines, this book gives a broad range of scientifically founded, up-to-date information on diagnosis and treatment; debunks myths; and offers parenting strategies and information on the course of the disorder.

Ashley, S. (2005). *The ADD & ADHD answer book: Professional answers to 275 of the top questions parents ask.* Naperville, IL: Sourcebooks.

Easy to use as a reference, organized by questions with succinct, informative answers on all aspects of ADHD.

Barkley, R. A., & Benton, C. M. (2013). *Your defiant child: Eight steps to better behavior* (2nd ed.). New York: Guilford Press.

An adaptation for parents of the widely used professional textbook *Defiant Children* (see "Professional Publications"). Describes a highly useful eight-step program for improving child behavior and reducing family conflicts.

Barkley, R. A., Robin, A. R., & Benton, C. (2013). *Your defiant teen: 10 steps to resolve conflict and rebuild your relationship* (2nd ed.). New York: Guilford Press.

An adaptation of the professional textbook *Defiant Teens* (see "Professional Publications"), this book explains how ADHD intersects with adolescent development and shows how to adapt the eight-step behavior management program successfully for teenagers, relying heavily on problem solving and communication that supports teenagers' striving for independence.

Beyer, W., & Hunt, R. D. (1999). *Born to be wild: Attention deficit hyperactivity disorder, alcoholism, and addiction*. Midlothian, VA: Judy Wood.

A guide for parents on ADHD and the potential relationship between ADHD and substance abuse/addictions. Includes instructions on educational, medical, and family management.

Bramer, J. S. (1996). *Succeeding in college with attention deficit hyperactivity disorders: Issues and strategies for students, counselors, and educators*. Plantation, FL: Specialty Press.

A fine resource for assisting teens and young adults with ADHD in adjusting to college life and getting the assistance they may require.

Brown, T. (2014). *Smart but stuck: Emotions in teens and adults with ADHD.* San Francisco, CA: Jossey-Bass.

The only book of which I am aware that focuses on the significant problems ADHD poses for emotional self-regulation and the damage it can do in relationships and various other domains of major life activities. The book also contains numerous suggestions for managing these emotion regulation difficulties.

Children and Adults with Attention-Deficit/Hyperactivity Disorder. (2006). *The new CHADD information and resource guide to AD/HD.* Landover, MD: Author.

A useful compendium of resources for families raising a child with ADHD.

Cooper-Kahn, J. & Dietzel, L. (2008). *Late, lost, and unprepared: A parents' guide to helping children with executive functioning.* Bethesda, MD: Woodbine House.

Advice for helping children and adolescents manage demands on them despite weak executive skills and also develop self-management skills as they mature.

Dawson, P., & Guare, R. (2008). *Smart but scattered: The revolutionary executive skills approach to helping kids reach their potential.* New York: Guilford Press.

A very practical guide for assessing executive skills in children ages 4–14 and then using a variety of ways to compensate for deficits, build lagging skills, and manage all the domains of life, from home to school.

Dendy, C. A. Z. (2006). *CHADD educators manual* (2nd ed.). Landover, MD: CHADD.

A terrific review of important information for teachers on ADHD and its management from one of the founding parents of the CHADD organization, who has become an expert on educational advocacy for children with ADHD.

Dendy, C. A. Z. (2007). *Teenagers with ADD and ADHD: A guide for parents and professionals.* Bethesda, MD: Woodbine House.

Information and advice for parents about helping and advocating for their teens with ADHD, with quotes from teens and a focus on executive skills.

Dendy, C. A. Z. (2011). *Teaching teens with ADD, ADHD, and executive function deficits: A quick reference guide for teachers and parents* (2nd ed.). Bethesda, MD: Woodbine House.

This is a marvelously written, easily read, and richly informative book on understanding and managing the executive, organization, attention, and other deficits associated with ADHD/ADD in children and adolescents.

Fowler, M. C. (2000). *Maybe you know my kid: A parent's guide to identifying, understanding, and helping your child with attention-deficit hyperactivity disorder* (3rd ed.). New York: Broadway Books.

One of the few books for parents on the subject of ADHD written by a parent, and one of the best. The author has become a lay expert on the subject of ADHD through her extensive work on the national level with CHADD.

Fowler, M. C. (2001). *Maybe you know my teen: A parent's guide to adolescents with attention-deficit hyperactivity disorder.* New York: Broadway Books.

Fowler, M. C. (2007). *20 questions to ask if your child has ADHD.* Franklin Lakes, NJ: Career Books.

Widely read books by a parent whose first book was about raising her son with ADHD, second book was on the new challenges of adolescence, and third book distills the important issues for easy reference.

Goldstein, S., & Goldstein, M. (1992). *Hyperactivity: Why won't my child pay attention?* Salt Lake City, UT: Neurology, Learning and Behavior Center.

A well-written, informative book for parents on hyperactivity (that is, ADHD) and its management by two clinical experts in the subject.

Guare, R., Dawson, P., & Guare, C. (2013). *Smart but scattered teens: The "executive skills" program for helping teens reach their potential.* New York: Guilford Press.

Hallowell, E. M., & Jensen, P. S. (2010). *Superparenting for ADD: An innovative approach to raising your distracted child*. New York: Ballantine Books.

Shows parents how to focus on the positives in helping their children with ADHD, mirror strengths for ADHD weaknesses, active steps to encourage excellence, and unconditional love.

Hanna, M. (2006). *Making the connection: A parent's guide to medication in AD/HD.* Washington, DC: Ladner-Drysdale.

A very useful guide to all questions regarding medication for children with ADHD.

Hinshaw, S. P., & Scheffler, R. M. (2014). *The ADHD explosion: Myths, medication, money, and today's push for performance.* New York: Oxford University Press.

A very timely review of the history and sociology of the diagnosis of ADHD as well as of the misconceptions held by the public and often noted in the trade media about ADHD and its treatment with medication. This book also covers the issues of over-medication of children as well as the diversion or use of medication by individuals without ADHD to enhance their performance in school or work settings.

Iseman, J. S., Silverman, S. M., & Jeweler, S. (2010). *101 school success tools for students with ADHD*. Waco, TX: Prufrock Press.

Field-tested methods that teachers can use in the classroom and parents can use at home.

Jensen, P. S. (2004). *Making the system work for your child with ADHD*. New York: Guilford Press.

A wonderful guide for helping families negotiate the educational and medical systems to get the maximum assistance for their child with ADHD.

Kutscher, M. (2002). *ADHD Book: Living right now!* White Plains, NY: Neurology Press.

Centered on similar principles to Kutscher's later book, this one includes a valuable chapter for children.

Kutscher, M. (2009). *ADHD: Living without brakes*. Philadelphia: Jessica Kingsley.

Inspiring and practical advice to follow four rules: keep it positive, keep it calm, keep it organized, and keep it going.

Langberg, J. M. (2011). *Homework, organization, and planning skills (HOPS) interventions*. Bethesda, MD: National Association of School Psychologists.

Evidence-based interventions, session-by-session instructions, and a CD-ROM with printable forms.

Latham, P., & Latham, P. (1993). *ADD and the law*. Washington, DC: JKL.

The only book that summarizes the rights of those with ADHD, as well as legal rulings pertaining to those rights, written by two of the best disability-rights attorneys in the business.

Meltzer, L. (2010). *Promoting executive function in the classroom*. New York: Guilford Press.

Helps teachers incorporate executive skill processes into the classroom to boost what students learn by improving how they learn.

Monastra, V. J. (2005). *Parenting children with ADHD: 10 lessons that medicine cannot teach*. Washington, DC: American Psychological Association.

Award-winning book from a clinical psychologist who has studied thousands of individuals with attention and behavior disorders.

Nadeau, K. G., Littman, E. B., & Quinn, P. O. (2000). *Understanding girls with AD/HD*. Silver Spring, MD: Advantage Books.

Helps parents understand how girls with ADHD differ from boys with ADHD, from diagnosis to symptoms.

Parker, H. C. (1999). *Put yourself in their shoes: Understanding teenagers with attention deficit hyperactivity disorder.* Plantation, FL: Specialty Press.

Clinical psychologist, cofounder of CHADD, and author of many publications on ADHD offers an extremely useful guide to help teens succeed during adolescence and beyond, including information on their legal rights.

Pfiffner, L. (2011) *All about ADHD: The complete practical guide for classroom teachers*. New York: Teaching Resources.

Research-based and classroom-tested, this book comes from one of the leading experts on teaching children with ADHD in the mainstream classroom.

Reiff, M. I. (2004). *ADHD: A complete authoritative guide*. Elk Grove, IL: American Academy of Pediatrics.

A fine introduction to the disorder and its management.

Rief, S. F. (2005). *How to reach and teach children with ADD/ADHD: Practice techniques, strategies, and interventions* (2nd ed.). San Francisco: Jossey-Bass.

Describes a wide variety of student intervention plans to engage students' attention, keep them on-task, and minimize behavior problems, while customizing plans for diverse children.

Richfield, S. (2008). *Parent coaching cards: Social and emotional tools for children*. Available from Parent Coaching Cards, Inc., P. O. Box 573, Plymouth Meeting, PA 19462; *www.parentcoachcards.com.*

Handy cards parents can pull out during challenging moments to remind them of something constructive to say and to offer tools for both parents and their children with ADHD to use to handle problems.

Sarkis, S. M. (2008). *Making the grade with ADD: A student's guide to succeeding in college with attention deficit disorder.* Oakland, CA: New Harbinger.

Practical advice for meeting academic challenges, handling social issues, and adopting a healthy lifestyle in college.

Sarkis, S. M., & Klein, K. (2009). *ADD and your money*. Oakland, CA: New Harbinger.

Great ideas for managing bills, staying out of debt, and budgeting.

Silverman, S. M., Iseman, J. S., & Jeweler, S. (2009). *School success for kids with ADHD.* Waco, TX: Prufrock Press.

Tested teaching and coaching methods, information on the role of technology, and a 12-point multimodal action plan.

Tuckman, A. (2009). *More attention, less deficit: Success strategies for adults with ADHD*. Plantation, FL: Specialty Press.

Before getting into practical strategies for managing the demands of adult life with ADHD, this book explains how ADHD affects the brain, how to get diagnosed, and how to choose among medication, therapy, and coaching as treatments.

Wilens, T. (2008). *Straight talk about psychiatric medications for kids* (3rd ed.). New York: Guilford Press.

Clearly the best book written for parents on this topic, with the most up-to-date information on psychiatric medications most likely to be used in the treatment of children's psychological and psychiatric disorders. The author is a nationally known expert in this field.

Zentall, S. S., & Goldstein, S. (1999). *Seven steps to homework success*. Plantation, FL: Specialty Press.

A detailed guide to a variety of strategies proven to improve homework time at home. Truly a family guide to solving common homework problems.

Books for Kids about ADHD

Corman, C., & Trevino, E. (1995). *Eulcee the jumpy jumpy elephant*. Plantation, FL: Specialty Press.

An imaginative story conveying information on ADHD for young children.

Dendy, C. A. Z., & Zeigler, A. (2003). *A bird's-eye view of life with ADD and ADHD: Advice from young survivors* (2nd ed.). Available from Chris A. Zeigler Dendy Consulting LLC, P.O. Box 189, Cedar Bluff, AL 35959; *www.chrisdendy.com*.

Among the few books written about teens with ADHD by teens with ADHD with help from a parent and educator, presenting stories from 12 individuals ages 12–18.

Galvin, M. (1995). *Otto learns about his medicine: A story about medication for children* (rev. ed.). Washington, DC: American Psychological Association.

A great illustrated book for kids with ADHD on the subject of taking medication for the management of hyperactivity.

Gordon, M. (1992). *I would if I could*. DeWitt, NY: Gordon Systems.

A fine, brief book about ADHD written from a child's perspective, showing both humor and sensitivity.

Gordon, M. (1992). *My brother's a world class pain*. DeWitt, NY: Gordon Systems.

Told from the point of view of a fictional big sister, this book uses child-friendly language to explain what ADHD is, how her family manages it, and how it affects her life.

Krauss, J. (2005). *Cory stories: A kid's book about living with ADHD*. Washington, DC: Magination Press.

An empathetic story told from the point of view of a young boy with ADHD.

Moss, D. (1989). *Shelly the hyperactive turtle*. Rockville, MD: Woodbine House.

This short illustrated story was one of the first to explain ADHD (hyperactivity) to children. It remains useful in this regard, despite the change in terminology from hyperactivity to ADHD.

Nadeau, K. G. (2006). *Survival guide for college students with ADD or LD*. Washington, DC: American Psychological Association.

A highly useful manual for young adults with ADHD or learning disabilities who are heading off to college, as well as for their parents. Filled with lots of tips for success in the college setting, which can often prove daunting to those with ADHD.

Nadeau, K. G. (2006). *Help4ADD@HighSchool*. Bethesda, MD: Advantage Books.

Designed as a website that readers can surf, with illustrations by a 16-year-old artist.

Nadeau, K. G., & Dixon, E. B. (2004). *Learning to slow down and pay attention: A book for kids about ADHD*.

Includes useful checklists for managing time and tasks, for ages 6 and up.

Parker, R. (1992). *Making the grade*. Plantation, FL: Specialty Press.

A brief, warm, sensitive story about the impact of ADHD on school success and self-esteem, told from an older child's perspective.

Quinn, P. (1994). *ADD and the college student*. Washington, DC: American Psychological Association.

A most informative text for parents of college students with ADHD, and for the students themselves, on surviving in the university environment with ADHD.

Quinn, P., & Stern, J. (1991). *Putting on the brakes: Young people's guide to understanding attention deficit hyperactivity disorder*. Washington, DC: American Psychological Association.

Written expressly for children entering adolescence (or older); renders the information about ADHD in a thoughtful, caring, and upbeat manner.

Shapiro, L. E. (2010). *The ADHD workbook for kids*. Oakland, CA: Instant Help Books.

Includes 40 activities that can be done in just 10 minutes a day.

Taylor, J. T. (2006). *Survival guide for kids with ADD or ADHD*. Minneapolis, MN: Free Spirit Publishing.

A positive, lively guide for children in grades three through five.

Books for Adults with ADHD

Adler, L. (2006). *Scattered minds: Hope and help for adults with attention deficit hyperactivity disorders*. New York: Putnam.

Helps adults see hidden signs of ADHD, debunks misconceptions, and explains diagnosis and treatment options.

Barkley, R.A., & Benton, C. M. (2010). *Taking charge of adult ADHD*. New York: Guilford Press.

A new volume packed with practical strategies for managing symptoms, information on medication, answers to frequently asked questions, and skills-building exercises.

Hallowell, E. M., & Ratey, J. J. (2005). *Delivered from distraction: Getting the most out of life with attention deficit disorder*. New York: Ballantine Books.

Follow-up to Hallowell and Ratey's first book, written by authors with adult ADHD.

Hallowell, E. M., & Ratey, J. J. (2010). *Answers to distraction*. New York: First Anchor Books.

Up-to-date information in convenient question-and-answer format.

Hallowell, E. M., & Ratey, J. J. (2011). *Driven to distraction* (rev. ed.). New York: Anchor Books.

A bestseller on ADHD in adults, written by two psychiatrists who profess to have ADHD themselves. Well-written, thoughtful, and filled with numerous informative case vignettes from their adult clients with ADHD, as well as with many useful tips on coping with the disorder.

Kolberg, J., & Nadeau, K. G. (2002). *ADD-friendly ways to organize your life*. New York: Routledge.

Specific advice for getting organized based on the needs of those with ADHD.

Matlen, T. (2005). *Survival tips for women with AD/HD: Beyond piles, palms, & post-its*. Plantation, FL: Specialty Press.

Practical advice divided by tasks and life domains for easy reference.

Nadeau, K. G. (1997). *ADD in the workplace: Choices, changes, and challenges*. Philadelphia: Brunner/Mazel.

Advice on finding the best work environment, obtaining reasonable accommodations in the workplace, and more tips for success.

Nadeau, K. G., & Quinn, P. O. (2002). *Understanding women with AD/HD*. Silver Spring, MD: Advantage Books.

Issues and advice pertinent to women across the lifespan.

Orlov, M. (2010). *The ADHD effect on marriage: Understand and rebuild your relationship in six steps*. Plantation, FL: Specialty Press.

Help for couples struggling with their personal relationship when one of them has ADHD, including illustrations of struggles from actual marriages.

Pera, G. (2008). *Is it you, me, or adult ADHD?* San Francisco: 1201 Alarm Press.

How to recognize hidden signs of ADHD, particularly for couples, with practical solutions.

Pinsky, S. C. (2006). *Organizing solutions for people with attention deficit disorder*. Gloucester, MA: Fair Winds Press.

Practical suggestions for organizing life at work, with kids, at home, and in personal life.

Quinn, P. O. (2005). *When moms and kids have ADD*. Washington, DC: Advantage Books.

Encourages mothers to get help for their own ADHD before trying to help their children.

Kelly, K., & Ramundo, P. (2006). *You mean I'm not lazy, stupid, or crazy?!: The classic self-help book for adults with attention deficit disorder*. New York: Scribner.

A fine introduction to the nature and treatment of ADHD in adults.

Ratey, N. A. (2008). *The disorganized mind: Coaching your ADHD brain to take control of your time, tasks, & talents*. New York: St. Martins Press.

Broad-ranging book for adults with information on how ADHD affects men and women differently, its effects on sexuality, and information on diagnosis, plus more.

Videos for Parents, Teachers, and Kids

ADHD—What do we know?, *ADHD—What can we do?*, *ADHD in the classroom*, and *ADHD in adults*, by R. A. Barkley. The Guilford Press, 72 Spring Street, New York, NY 10012; (800) 365-7006; *www.guilford.com*.

Four award-winning DVDs on ADHD spanning a variety of topics and using children and adults with ADHD who tell their own stories about living with ADHD.

All about attention deficit disorder, by T. Phelan. ParentMagic, Inc., 800 Roosevelt Road, B-309, Glen Ellyn, IL 60137; (800) 442-4453; *www.parentmagic.com*.

A good review of the disorder for parents and teachers, from a popular clinical professional whose videotape *3–2–1 Magic* has been widely acclaimed for its help in managing noncompliant child behavior.

Classroom interventions for ADHD, by G. J. DuPaul & G. Stoner. The Guilford Press, 72 Spring Street, New York, NY 10012; (800) 365-7006; *www.guilford.com*.

An excellent video for school professionals on the specific methods recommended for school-based assessment of children with ADHD and specific methods on classroom management for such children.

It's just an attention disorder, *Why won't my child pay attention?*, and *Educating inattentive children*, by S. Goldstein & M. Goldstein. Neurology, Learning and Behavior Center, 230 South 500 East, Suite 100, Salt Lake City, UT 84102; (801) 532-1484; *www.samgoldstein.com*.

The first video is an excellent introduction to ADHD, intended for older children and teens with ADHD. It has a fast-paced format and uses comments from teens with ADHD about coping with their disorder. The second and third videos are intended for viewing by parents and teachers, respectively, and provide a fine overview of the disorder and its management at home and school.

Jumping Johnny, get back to work!: The video, by M. Gordon. Gordon Systems, Inc., P.O. Box 746, DeWitt, NY 13214; (315) 446-4849; *www.gsi-add.com.*

An excellent animated video for children with ADHD that discusses the disorder and its treatment from a child's perspective.

A new look at ADHD: Inhibition, time, and self-control, by R. A. Barkley. The Guilford Press, 72 Spring Street, New York, NY 10012; (800) 365-7006; *www.guilford.com.*

A video providing a clear framework in which to understand the theory of ADHD described in the present book, as well as its implications for the clinical management of the disorder.

Restless minds, restless kids: Attention-deficit/hyperactivity disorder in children and adolescents, by C. K. Conners & J. S. March. Multi-Health Systems, North Tonawanda, NY, 14120-2060; (800) 456-3003; *www.mhs.com.*

A very informative overview of ADHD.

Teens and ADHD, by the Hazelden Foundation. Hazelden Publishing, 15251 Pleasant Valley Road, Center City, MN 55012-0176; (800) 328-9000; *www.hazelden.org.*

This video features students with ADHD discussing how it affects their lives and how they have tried to cope with it.

Understanding the defiant child and *Managing the defiant child,* by R. A. Barkley. The Guilford Press, 72 Spring Street, New York, NY 10012; (800) 365-7006; *www.guilford.com.*

These two videos complement the parent training program described in *Defiant Children* (see "Professional Publications") and *Your Defiant Child* (see "Books for Parents and Teachers"). They provide a clear, concise understanding of the factors that contribute to defiance in children, and specific methods parents can employ to reduce it and improve parent–child relationships.

Professional Publications

Accardo, P. J., Blondis, T. A., Whitman, B. Y., & Stein, M. A. (1999). *Attention deficits and hyperactivity in children and adults: Diagnosis, treatment, management* (2nd ed.). New York: Marcel Dekker.

An edited collection of scholarly reviews concerning the nature, causes, associated disorders, and therapies for ADHD.

American Academy of Child and Adolescent Psychiatry. (2002, February). Practice parameter for the use of stimulant medications in the treatment of children, adolescents, and adults. *Journal of the American Academy of Child and Adolescent Psychiatry, 41*(2 Suppl.), 26S–49S.

Describes treatment with methylphenidate, dextroamphetamine, mixed-salts amphetamine, and pemoline; the parameter uses an evidence-based medicine approach derived from a detailed literature review and expert consultation.

American Psychiatric Association. (2013). *Diagnostic and statistical manual of mental disorders* (5th ed.). Washington, DC: Author.

This is a manual for professionals that sets forth the criteria to be used for diagnosing mental disorders (within the United States). It includes the most recent criteria for ADHD and related disorders.

Barkley, R. A. (1997). *ADHD and the nature of self-control*. New York: Guilford Press.

A scholarly scientific textbook for professionals detailing the theory of ADHD described in the present book, and describing the research behind it.

Barkley, R. A. (2013). *Defiant children: A clinician's manual for assessment and parent training* (3rd ed.). New York: Guilford Press.

A manual intended to instruct professionals step by step in conducting a 10-session training program for parents of children (between 2 and 12 years old) with ADHD and/or oppositional defiant disorder.

Barkley, R. A. (2014). *Attention-deficit hyperactivity disorder: A handbook for diagnosis and treatment* (4th ed.). New York: Guilford Press.

A highly detailed professional textbook intended to serve as a handbook for clinicians who provide diagnosis, assessment, and treatment services for children and adults with ADHD, including parent training, classroom management, family therapy, and medications for ADHD.

Barkley, R. A. (2012). *Executive functions: What they are, how they work, and why they evolved*. New York: Guilford Press.

Presents a model of executive functions that is rooted in meaningful activities of daily life and may support much-needed advances in assessment and treatment. The book describes how abilities such as emotion regulation, self-motivation, planning, and working memory enable people to pursue both personal and collective goals that are critical to survival. Key stages of executive function development are identified and the far-reaching individual and social costs of executive function deficits detailed.

Barkley, R. A., & Robin, A. R. (2014). *Defiant teens: A clinician's manual for assessment and family intervention* (2nd ed.). New York: Guilford Press.

A step-by-step manual for clinical professionals on conducting an 18-session family therapy program based on sound behavioral principles and cognitive therapy (problem-solving) strategies. Also contains useful assessment instruments for the clinical evaluation of defiant teens.

Barkley, R. A., & Murphy, K. R. (2006). *Attention-deficit hyperactivity disorder: A clinical workbook* (3rd ed.). New York: Guilford Press.

A compendium of useful tools for professionals for the assessment of children and adults with ADHD.

Barkley, R. A., Murphy, K. R., & Fischer, M. (2008). *ADHD in adults: What the science says*. New York: Guilford Press.

Provides specific chapters on each impairment likely to coexist with ADHD and discusses how this might affect clinical decision making about patients with ADHD. An excellent starting point for information on the risks in ADHD.

Brown, T. (2008). *Attention deficit disorder and comorbidities in children, adolescents, and adults* (2nd ed.). Washington, DC: American Psychiatric Press.

Twenty-five leading researchers discuss how ADHD and common comorbid disorders interact and how to treat both.

Buell, J. (2003). *Closing the book on homework*. Philadelphia: Temple University Press.

Makes a case for the idea that, in robbing children of unstructured play time, homework hinders instead of enhances emotional and intellectual development and offers an alternative roadmap for learning.

Buitelaar, J. K., Kan, C. C., & Asherson, P. (2011). *ADHD in adults: Characterization, diagnosis, and treatment*. New York: Cambridge University Press.

Reviews our growing knowledge of adult ADHD and presents a transatlantic perspective on the identification, assessment, and treatment of the disorder.

Dawson, P., & Guare, R. (2010). *Executive skills in children and adolescents* (2nd ed.): A practical guide to assessment and intervention. New York: Guilford Press.

Describes assessment measures, links assessment to intervention, and presents strategies for promoting executive skills, environmentally, through coaching, in the classroom, and for specific populations.

DuPaul, G. J., & Stoner, G. (2003). *ADHD in the schools* (2nd ed.): *Assessment and intervention strategies*. New York: Guilford Press.

A comprehensive guide for school-based professionals concerning the assessment and management of ADHD in the schools.

Goldstein, S., & Ellison, A. T. (2002). *Clinician's guide to adult ADHD: Assessment and intervention*. New York: Academic Press.

A fine introduction to the clinical diagnosis and management of ADHD in adults.

Goldstein, S., & Goldstein, M. (1998). *Managing attention deficit hyperactivity disorder in children* (2nd ed.). New York: Wiley.

A thorough review of the clinical literature concerning the diagnosis and treatment of ADHD in children.

Gordon, M., & Keiser, S. (1998). *Accommodations in higher education under the Americans with Disabilities Act: A no-nonsense guide for clinicians, educators, administrators, and lawyers*. New York: Guilford Press.

One of the best texts on how the Americans with Disabilities Act applies to a wide range of disorders, including ADHD, and the types of guidelines that apply to requesting such accommodations in college settings.

Gordon, M., & McClure, D. (2008). *The down and dirty guide to adult ADHD*. DeWitt, NY: Gordon Systems.

A witty, incisive, and cleverly presented guide to the clinical evaluation and treatment of ADHD in adults.

Gregg, N. (2009). *Adolescents and adults with learning disabilities and ADHD: Assessment and accommodation*. New York: Guilford Press.

Helps educators and clinicians navigate the maze of laws, policies, and scientific research relating to diagnostic and intervention decision making for adolescents and adults. Provides guidance on how to conduct and document evidence-based assessments and select appropriate instructional and testing accommodations.

Kralovec, E., & Buell, J. (2000). *The end of homework: How homework disrupts families, overburdens children, and limits learning*. Boston: Beacon Press.

One of the first books to look at school reform in terms of reducing the reliance on homework.

Mapou, R. (2009). *Adult learning disabilities and ADHD: Research informed assessment*. New York: Oxford University Press.

Based on the author's popular workshop, this concise volume provides scientific and practical guidance on assessing learning disabilities and ADHD in adults.

Mash, E. J., & Barkley, R. A. (Eds.). (2014). *Child psychopathology* (3rd ed.). New York: Guilford Press.

Integrates state-of-the-art theory and empirical research on a wide range of child and adolescent disorders, with contributions from leading scholars and clinicians. Offers comprehensive coverage of the biological, psychological, and social-contextual determinants of childhood problems.

Mash, E. J., & Barkley, R. A. (Eds.). (2005). *Treatment of childhood disorders* (3rd ed.). New York: Guilford Press.

Leading contributors offer an authoritative review of evidence-based treatments for the most prevalent child and adolescent problems.

Mash, E. J., & Barkley, R. A. (Eds.). (2007). *Assessment of childhood disorders* (4th ed.). New York: Guilford Press.

Offers best-practice recommendations for assessing a comprehensive array of child and adolescent mental health problems and health risks.

Nigg, J. (2006). *What causes ADHD? Understanding what goes wrong and why*. New York: Guilford Press.

Traces the intersecting causal influences of genetic, neural, and environmental factors, confronting enduring controversies such as the validity of ADHD as a clinical construct. Specific suggestions are provided for studies that might further refine the conceptualization of the disorder, with significant potential benefits for treatment and prevention.

Phelps, L., Brown, R. T., & Power, T. J. (2001). *Pediatric psychopharmacology: Combining medical and psychosocial interventions*. Washington, DC: American Psychological Association.

Informs practitioners about integrating medications proven effective in the treatment of children and adolescents via double-blind studies and nonpharmacological interventions that have empirical support.

Robin, A. L. (1998). *ADHD in adolescents: Diagnosis and treatment*. New York: Guilford Press.

A comprehensive textbook for professionals on the nature, diagnosis, assessment, and management of ADHD in teenagers.

Pliszka, S. R. (2009). *Treating ADHD and comorbid disorders: Psychosocial and psychopharmacological interventions*. New York: Guilford Press.

Organized around detailed case presentations, this book helps clinicians make sound decisions when assessing and treating the full range of ADHD comorbidities—how to avoid common diagnostic errors, develop an individualized medication regimen, minimize health risks and side effects, collaborate successfully with parents, and tailor psychosocial treatments to each family's needs.

Ramsay, J. R. (2009). *Nonmedication treatments for adult ADHD: Evaluating impact on daily functioning and well-being.* Washington, DC: American Psychological Association.

A comprehensive review of the current status of nonmedication interventions available for adults with ADHD, from psychosocial treatment to academic support and accommodations for postsecondary students, career counseling and workplace support, relationships and social functioning, neurofeedback and neurocognitive training, and complementary and alternative treatments.

Ramsay, J. R., & Rostain, A. L. (2008). *Cognitive-behavioral therapy for adult ADHD: An integrative psychosocial and medical approach.* New York: Taylor & Francis.

Discusses the factors involved in treatment, relapse prevention, and long-term management of adult ADHD, using a combined biological and psychosocial treatment approach.

Rapoport, E. M. (2009). *ADHD and social skills: A step-by-step guide for teachers and parents*. Lanham, MD: Rowman & Littlefield.

Innovative techniques that teachers can use at school and parents can use at home to help children with ADHD improve their behavior and their understanding of social cues to improve their peer relationships.

Safren, S. A., Sprich, S., Perlman, C., & Otto, M. (2005). *Mastery of your adult ADHD: A cognitive behavioral treatment program*. New York: Oxford University Press.

A session-by-session guide to conducting outpatient cognitive-behavioral treatment for adults with ADHD. A client workbook is also available.

Sleeper-Triplett, J. (2010). *Empowering youth with ADHD: Your guide to coaching adolescents and young adults for coaches, parents, and professionals*. Plantation, FL: Specialty Press.

Complete instructions for professionals and parents on what ADHD coaching for young people is and how it can dramatically improve their lives.

Solanto, M. (2011). *Cognitive-behavioral therapy for adult ADHD: Targeting executive dysfunction*. New York: Guilford Press.

Describes effective cognitive-behavioral strategies for helping clients improve key time management, organizational, and planning abilities that are typically impaired in ADHD. Each of the 12 group sessions—which can also be adapted for individual therapy—is reviewed in step-by-step detail.

Teeter, P. A. (1998). *Interventions for ADHD: Treatment in developmental context*. New York: Guilford Press.

An important lifespan view of ADHD and its management. The author reviews various treatment interventions and the specific challenges that arise in various stages of development.

Triolo, S. J. (1999). *Attention deficit hyperactivity disorder in adulthood: A practitioner's handbook*. Philadelphia: Brunner/Mazel.

An in-depth discussion of the theory, assessment, and management of ADHD in adults.

Tuckman, A. (2007). *Integrative treatment for adult ADHD: A practical, easy-to-use guide for clinicians*. Oakland, CA: New Harbinger.

Describes a treatment model that integrates education, medication, coaching, and cognitive-behavioral therapy.

Wasserstein, J., Wolf, L., & Lefever, F. (Eds.). (2001). *Adult attention deficit disorder: Brain mechanisms and life outcomes* (Annals of the New York Academy of Sciences, Vol. 931). New York: New York Academy of Sciences.

Includes current and historical thinking by world-renowned researchers and clinicians when adult ADHD was a relatively recent and still controversial diagnosis. Comprehensive coverage of biological theories and research findings, clinical assessment, executive dysfunction, overlapping conditions, and modalities of treatment.

Weiss, M., Hechtman, L., & Weiss, G. (1999). *ADHD in adulthood: A guide to current theory, diagnosis, and treatment*. Baltimore: Johns Hopkins University Press.

Among the best clinical guides for professionals regarding the nature of ADHD in adults and its assessment and management.

Young, J. (2007). *ADHD grown up: A guide to adolescent and adult ADHD*. New York: Norton.

Concise but comprehensive overview of adult ADHD, including the different subtypes.

Periodicals

ADDA E-News, ADDA, P. O. Box 7557, Wilmington, DE 19083-9997; (800) 939-1019; *www.add.org.*

The newsletter for ADDA members.

ADDitude: The Happy Healthy Lifestyle Magazine for People with ADD (online and print periodical), 39 West 37th Street, 15th floor, New York, NY 10018; (888) 762-8475; *www.additudemag.com.*

A highly informative and reasonably accurate magazine and website for obtaining information about ADHD. The graphics at the website are excellent and it is easy to explore. The information each issue provides is quite current. Many different topics are covered. A subscription (either online or in print) is required to obtain the full content of each issue. Although the magazine's content appears to be scientically based in many respects, this is not to be taken as an endorsement of those advertising in either the print or online versions of this periodical.

ADDvice for ADD-Friendly Living, The National Center for Girls and Women with ADHD, 3268 Arcadia Place NW, Washington, DC 20015; *http://ncgiadd.org.*

An innovative new monthly e-newsletter focusing on women and girls with ADHD.

The ADHD Report, edited by R. A. Barkley, The Guilford Press, 72 Spring Street, New York, NY 10012; (800) 365-7006; *www.guilford.com.*

The only newsletter specifically dedicated to practicing clinicians who want to remain current on the extensive and rapidly changing scientific and clinical literature on ADHD. Parents of children with ADHD, as well as adults with ADHD, may also find the contents useful for staying current on controversial issues and research reports as well.

Attention! Magazine, CHADD National Headquarters, 8181 Professional Place, Suite 150, Landover, MD 20785; (800) 233-4050; *www.chadd.org.*

A flashy, entertaining, and informative magazine on ADHD created by the largest national support organization for ADHD (CHADD) and dedicated to keeping parents (as well as adults with ADHD) informed about the numerous issues related to ADHD.

CHADD Newsletter, CHADD National Headquarters, 8181 Professional Place, Suite 150, Landover, MD 20785; (800) 233-4050; *www.chadd.org.*

A newsletter for parents of children with ADHD and adults with ADHD who are members of CHADD.

Suppliers

ADD Warehouse
300 Northwest 70th Avenue, Suite 102
Plantation, FL 33317
(800) 233-9273
www.addwarehouse.com

Childswork Childsplay
P. O. Box 1246
Wilkes-Barres, PA 18703-1246
(800) 962-1141
childswork.com

References

A number of published studies have been referenced throughout this book and are listed here for the interested reader. Citations for many other references to research can be found in my 2006 book and at my website, *www.russellbarkley.org.*

Abikoff, H., Courtney, M. E., Szeibel, P. J., & Koplewicz, H. S. (1996). The effects of auditory stimulant on the arithmetic performance of children with ADHD and nondisabled children. *Journal of Learning Disabilities, 29,* 238–246.

American Psychiatric Association. (2013). *Diagnostic and statistical manual of mental disorders* (5th ed.). Washington, DC: Author.

Barkley, R. A. (1981). *Hyperactive children: A handbook for diagnosis and treatment.* New York: Guilford Press.

Barkley, R. A. (2006). *Attention-deficit hyperactivity disorder: A handbook for diagnosis and treatment* (3rd ed.). New York: Guilford Press.

Barkley, R. A. (2012). *Executive functions: What they are, how they work, and why they evolved.* New York: Guilford Press.

Barkley, R. A. (in press). Children and adolescents with sluggish cognitive tempo versus attention-deficit/hyperactivity disorder: Executive functioning, impairment, and comorbidity. *Journal of Clinical Child and Adolescent Psychology.*

Barkley, R. A., & Benton, C. (in press). *Your defiant child: Eight steps to better behavior.* New York: Guilford Press.

Barkley, R. A., & Cox, D. J. (2007). A review of driving risks and impairments associated with attention-deficit/hyperactivity disorder and the effects of stimulant medication on driving performance. *Journal of Safety Research, 38,* 113–128.

Barkley, R. A., Cunningham, C., & Karlsson, J. (1983). The speech of hyperactive children and their mothers: Comparisons with normal children and stimulant drug effects. *Journal of Learning Disabilities, 16,* 105–110.

Barkley, R. A., Edwards, G., Laneri, M., Fletcher, K., & Metevia, L. (2001). Executive functioning, temporal discounting, and sense of time in adolescents with attention deficit hyperactivity disorder and oppositional defiant disorder. *Journal of Abnormal Child Psychology, 29,* 541–556.

Barkley, R. A., Fischer, M., Smallish, L., & Fletcher, K. (2003). Does the treatment of ADHD with stimulant medication contribute to illicit drug use and abuse in adulthood? Results from a 15–year prospective study. *Pediatrics, 111,* 109–121.

Barkley, R. A., Fischer, M., Smallish, L., & Fletcher, K. (2006). Young adult follow-up of hyperactive children: Adaptive functioning in major life activities. *Journal of the American Academy of Child and Adolescent Psychiatry, 45,* 192–202.

Barkley, R. A., Guevremont, D. G., Anastopoulos, A. D., DuPaul, G. J., & Shelton, T. L. (1993). Driving-related risks and outcomes of attention deficit hyperactivity disorder in adolescents and young adults: A 3–5 year follow-up survey. *Pediatrics, 92,* 212–218.

Barkley, R. A., McMurray, M. B., Edelbrock, C. S., & Robbins, K. (1990). The side effects of Ritalin in ADHD children: A systematic, placebo controlled evaluation. *Pediatrics, 86,* 184–192.

Barkley, R. A., Murphy, K. R., & Fischer, M. (2008). *ADHD in adults: What the science says.* New York: Guilford Press.

Barkley, R. A., & Peters, H. (2012). The earliest reference to ADHD in the medical literature? Melchior Adam Weikard's description in 1775 of "Attention Deficit" (Mangel der Aufmerksamkeit, attentio volubilis). *Journal of Attention Disorders,* published online first, DOI 10.1177/1087054711432309.

Barkley, R. A., & Ullman, D. G. (1975). A comparison of objective measures of activity and distractibility in hyperactive and non-hyperactive children. *Journal of Abnormal Child Psychology, 3,* 213–244.

Bauermeister, J. J., Matos, M., Reina, G., Salas, C. C., Martínez, J. V., Cumba, E., & Barkley, R. (2005). Comparison of the DSM-IV combined and inattentive types of ADHD in a school-based sample of Latino/Hispanic children. *Journal of Child Psychology and Psychiatry, 46,* 166–179.

Biederman, J., Faraone, S. V., Keenan, K., Knee, D., & Tsuang, M. T. (1990). Family–genetic and psychosocial risk factors in DSM-III attention deficit disorder. *Journal of the American Academy of Child and Adolescent Psychiatry, 29,* 526–533.

Bremer, D. A., & Stern, J. A. (1976). Attention and distractibility during reading in hyperactive boys. *Journal of Abnormal Child Psychology, 4,* 381–387.

Bridge, J. A., Iyengar, S., Salary, C. B., Barbe, R. P., Birmaher, B., Pincus, H. A., Ren, L., & Brent, D. A. (2007). Clinical response and risk for reported ideation and suicide attempts in pediatric antidepressant treatment. A meta-analysis of randomized controlled trials. *Journal of the American Medical Association, 297,* 1683–1696.

Bronowski, J. (1977). Human and animal languages. In *A sense of the future* (pp. 104–131). Cambridge, MA: MIT Press.

Buchsbaum, M., & Wender, P. (1973). Averaged evoked responses in normal and minimally brain dysfunctioned children treated with amphetamine: a preliminary report. *Archives of General Psychiatry, 29,* 764–770.

Campbell, S. B. (1975). Mother–child interactions: A comparison of hyperactive, learning disabled, and normal boys. *American Journal of Orthopsychiatry, 45,* 51–57.

Campbell, S. B., & Ewing, L. J. (1990). Follow-up of hard to manage preschoolers: Adjustment at age 9 and predictors of continuing symptoms. *Journal of Child Psychology and Psychiatry, 31,* 871–889.

Campbell, S. B., Szumowski, E. K., Ewing, L. J., Gluck, D. S., & Breaux, A. M. (1982). A multidimensional assessment of parent-identified behavior problem toddlers. *Journal of Abnormal Child Psychology, 10,* 569–592.

Cantwell, D. (1975). *The hyperactive child*. New York: Spectrum.

Chilcoat, H. D., & Breslau, N. (1999). Pathways from ADHD to early drug use. *Journal of the American Academy of Child and Adolescent Psychiatry, 38,* 1347–1354.

Cooper, W. O., Habel, L. A., Sox, C. M., Chan, L. A., Arbogast, P. G., Cheetham, T. C., et al. (2011). ADHD drugs and serious cardiovascular events in children and young adults. *New England Journal of Medicine, 365*, 1896–1904.

Covey, S. R. (1989). *The seven habits of highly effective people: Restoring the character ethic*. New York: Simon & Schuster.

Crichton, A. (1798). *An inquiry into the nature and origin of mental derangement: Comprehending a concise system of the physiology and pathology of the human mind and a history of the passions and their effects*. London: T. Cadell Hr. & W. Davies. (Reprinted by AMS Press, New York, 1976)

Crook, W. G. (1986). *The yeast connection: A medical breakthrough.* New York: Vintage Books.

Cunningham, C., & Barkley, R. (1979). The interactions of hyperactive and normal children with their mothers during free play and structured tasks. *Child Development, 50*, 217–224.

Demaray, M., & Jenkins, L. N. (2011). Relations among academic enablers and academic achievement in children with and without high levels of parent-rated symptoms of inattention, impulsivity, and hyperactivity. *Psychology in the Schools, 48*, 573–586.

Diener, M. B., & Milich, R. (1997). Effects of positive feedback on the social interactions of boys with attention deficit hyperactivity disorder: A test of the self-protective hypothesis. *Journal of Clinical Child Psychology, 26,* 256–265.

Dimond, S. J. (1980). *Neuropsychology: A textbook of systems and psychological functions of the human brain.* London: Butterworth.

Douglas, V. I. (1980). Treatment and training approaches to hyperactivity: Establishing internal or external control. In C. Whalen & B. Henker (Eds.), *Hyperactive children: The social ecology of identification and treatment* (pp. 283–318). New York: Academic Press.

Dunnick, J. K., & Hailey, J. R. (1995). Experimental studies on the long-term effects of methylphenidate hypdrochloride. *Toxicology, 103*, 77–84.

El-Zein, R. A., Abdel-Rahman, A., Hay, M. J., Lopez, M. S., Bondy, M. L., Morris, D. L., et al. (2005). Cytogentic effects in children treated with methylphenidate. *Cancer Letters, 230,* 284–291.

Erchul, W. P., DuPaul, G. J., Bennett, M. S., Grissom, P. F., Jitendra, A. K., Tresco, K. E., et al. (2009). A follow-up study of relational processes and consultation outcomes for students with attention deficit hyperactivity disorder. *School Psychology Review, 38*, 28–37.

Feingold, B. F. (1975). *Why your child is hyperactive*. New York: Random House.

Fiedler, N. L., & Ullman, D. G. (1983). The effects of stimulant drugs on the curiosity behaviors of hyperactive children. *Journal of Abnormal Child Psychology, 11*, 193–206.

Fischer, M., Barkley, R. A., Edelbrock, K., & Smallish, L. (1990). The adolescent outcome of hyperactive children diagnosed by research criteria: II. Academic, attentional, and neuropsychological status. *Journal of Consulting and Clinical Psychology, 58*, 580–588.

Fuster, J. M. (1989). *The prefrontal cortex*. New York: Raven Press.

Gillis, J. J., Gilger, J. W., Pennington, B. F., & DeFries, J. C. (1992). Attention deficit disorder in reading-disabled twins: Evidence for a genetic etiology. *Journal of Abnormal Child Psychology, 20,* 303–315.

Gordon, M. (1979). The assessment of impulsivity and mediating behaviors in hyperactive and non-hyperactive children. *Journal of Abnormal Child Psychology, 7,* 317–326.

Hartsough, C. S., & Lambert, N. M. (1985). Medical factors in hyperactive and normal children: Prenatal, developmental, and health history findings. *American Journal of Orthopsychiatry, 55,* 190–210.

Hauser, P., Zametkin, A. J., Martinex, P., Vitiello, B., Matochik, J. A., Mixson, A. J., et al. (1993). Attention deficit-hyperactivity disorder in people with generalized resistance to thyroid hormone. *New England Journal of Medicine, 328,* 997–1001.

Hayes, S. C. (1989). *Rule-governed behavior: Cognition, contingencies, and instructional control.* New York: Plenum.

Hoover, D. W., & Milich, R. (1994). Effects of sugar ingestion expectancies on mother–child interactions. *Journal of Abnormal Child Psychology, 22,* 501–515.

Hunt, R. D., Capper, L., & O'Connell, P. (1990). Clonidine in child and adolescent psychiatry. *Journal of Child and Adolescent Psychopharmacology, 1,* 87–102.

Ingersoll, B., & Goldstein, S. (1993). *Attention deficit disorder and learning disabilities: Realities, myths, and controversial treatments.* New York: Main Street Books.

Jacob, R. G., O'Leary, K. D., & Rosenblad, C. (1978). Formal and informal classroom settings: Effects on hyperactivity. *Journal of Abnormal Child Psychology, 6,* 47–59.

Jensen, P. S., Shervette, R. E., Xenakis, S. N., & Bain, M. W. (1988). Psychosocial and medical histories of stimulant-treated children. *Journal of the American Academy of Child and Adolescent Psychiatry, 27,* 798–801.

Kabat-Zin, J. (2005). *Wherever you go, there you are.* New York: Hyperion.

Kavale, K. A., & Forness, S. R. (1983). Hyperactivity and diet treatment: A meta-analysis of the Feingold hypothesis. *Journal of Learning Disabilities, 16,* 324–330.

Kessler, R. C., Adler, L., Barkley, R. A., Biederman, J., Conners, C. K., Demler, O., et al. (2006). The prevalence and correlates of adult ADHD in the United States: Results from the National Comorbidity Survey Replication. *American Journal of Psychiatry, 163,* 716–723.

Klorman, R., Brumaghim, J. T., Coons, H. W., Peloquin, L., Strauss, J., Lewine, J. D., Borgstedt, A. D., & Goldstein, M. G. (1988). The contributions of event-related potentials to understanding effects of stimulants on information processing in attention deficit disorder. In L. M. Bloomingdale & J. A. Sergeant (Eds.), *Attention deficit disorder: Criteria, cognition, intervention* (pp. 199–218). London: Pergamon Press.

Landau, S., Lorch, E. P., & Milich, R. (1992). Visual attention to and comprehension of television in attention deficit hyperactivity disordered and normal boys. *Child Development, 63,* 928–937.

Levinson, H. (1992). *Total concentration: How to understand attention deficit disorders.* New York: Evans.

Lezak, M. D. (2004). *Neuropsychological assessment* (4th ed.). New York: Oxford University Press.

Lofthouse, N., Arnold, L. E., & Hurt, E. (2012). Current status of neurofeedback for attention-deficit/hyperactivity disorder. *Current Psychiatry Reports,* published online first, DOI 10.1007/s11920–012–0301–z.

Loo, S. K., & Barkley, R. A. (2005). Clinical utility of EEG in attention deficit hyperactivity disorder. *Applied Developmental Neuropsychology, 12,* 64–76.

Lou, H. C., Henriksen, L., & Bruhn, P. (1984). Focal cerebral hypoperfusion in children with dysphasia and/or attention deficit disorder. *Archives of Neurology, 41,* 825–829.

Milberger, S., Biederman, J., Faraone, S. V., Chen, L., & Jones, J. (1996). Is maternal smoking during pregnancy a risk factor for attention deficit hyperactivity disorder in children? *American Journal of Psychiatry, 153,* 1138–1142.

Milich, R., Kern, M. H., & Scrambler, D. J. (1996). Coping with childhood teasing. *ADHD Report, 4*(5), 9–12.

Milich, R., & Pelham, W. E. (1986). Effects of sugar ingestion on the classroom and playground behavior of attention deficit disordered boys. *Journal of Consulting and Clinical Psychology, 54,* 714–718.

Milich, R., Wolraich, M., & Lindgren, S. (1986). Sugar and hyperactivity: A critical review of empirical findings. *Clinical Psychology Review, 6,* 493–513.

Morrison, J., & Stewart, M. (1973). The psychiatric status of the legal families of adopted hyperactive children. *Archives of General Psychiatry, 28,* 888–891.

Multimodal Treatment of ADHD Group. (1999). Moderators and mediators of treatment response for children with attention-deficit/hyperactivity disorder: The Multimodal Treatment Study of children with attention-deficit/hyperactivity disorder. *Archives of General Psychiatry, 56*(12), 1088–1096.

Murphy, K., & Barkley, R. A. (1996). Prevalence of DSM-IV ADHD symtoms in adult licensed drivers. *Journal of Attention Disorders, 1,* 147–161.

Nakao, T., Radua, J., Rubia, K., & Mataix-Cols, D. (2011). Gray matter volume abnormalities in ADHD: Voxel-based meta-analysis exploring effects of age and stimulant medication. *American Journal of Psychiatry, 168,* 1154–1163.

Neuman, R. J., Lobos, E., Reich, W., Henderson, C. A., Sun, L. W., & Todd, R. D. (2007). Smoking exposure and dopaminergic genotypes interact to cause a severe ADHD subtype. *Biological Psychiatry, 61,* 1320–1328.

Nichols, P. L., & Chen, T. C. (1981). *Minimal brain dysfunction: A prospective study.* Hillsdale, NJ: Erlbaum.

Nigg, J. T. (2006). *What causes ADHD?: Understanding what goes wrong and why.* New York: Guilford Press.

Nigg, J. T., Lewis, K., Edlinger, T., & Falk, M. (2012). Meta-analysis of attention-deficit/hyperactivity disorder or attention-deficit/hyperactivity disorder symptoms, restriction diet, and synthetic food color additives. *Journal of the American Academy of Child and Adolescent Psychiatry, 51,* 86–97.

Pagani, L., Tremblay, R. E., Vitaro, F., Boulderice, B., & McDuff, P. (2001). Effects of grade retention on academic performance and behavioral development. *Development and Psychopathology, 13,* 297–315.

Paloyelis, Y., Mehta, M. A., Kuntsi, J., & Asherson, P. (2007). Functional MRI in ADHD: A systematic literature review. *Expert Reviews in Neurotherapeutics, 7,* 1337–1356.

Pelham, W. E., & Bender, M. E. (1982). Peer relationships in hyperactive children: Description and treatment. In K. D. Gadow & I. Bialer (Eds.), *Advances in learning and behavioral disabilities* (Vol. 1, pp. 365–436). Greenwich, CT: JAI Press.

Pelsser, L. M., Frankena, K., Toorman, J., Savelkoul, H. F., DuBois, A. E., Periera, R. R., Haagen, T. A., Rommelse, N. N., & Buitelaar, J. K. (2011). Effects of a restricted elimination diet on the behavior of children with attention-deficit hyperactivity disorder (INCA study): A randomized controlled trial. *Lancet, 377,* 494–503.

Porrino, L. J., Rapoport, J. L., Behar, D., Sceery, W., Ismond, D. R., & Bunney, W. E. Jr. (1983). A naturalistic assessment of the motor activity of hyperactive boys. *Archives of General Psychiatry, 40,* 681–687.

Rapport, M. D., Tucker, S. B., DuPaul, G. J., Merlo, M., & Stoner, G. (1986). Hyperactivity and frustration: The influence of control over and size of rewards in delaying gratification. *Journal of Abnormal Child Psychology, 14,* 181–204.

Richards, T. L., Deffenbacher, J. L., Rosen, L. A., Barkley, R. A., & Rodricks, T. (2006). Driving anger and driving behavior in adults with ADHD. *Journal of Attention Disorders, 10,* 54–64.

Rosemond, J. (2009). *The well-behaved child: Discipline that really works.* Nashville, TN: Thomas Nelson.

Rosen, L. A., Booth, S. R., Bender, M. E., McGrath, M. L., Sorrell, S., & Drabman, R. S. (1988). Effects of sugar (sucrose) on children's behavior. *Journal of Consulting and Clinical Psychology, 56,* 583–589.

Rosen, L. A., O'Leary, S. G., Joyce, S. A., Conway, C., & Pfiffner, L. J. (1984). The importance of prudent negative consequences for maintaining the appropriate behavior of hyperactive children. *Journal of Abnormal Child Psychology, 12,* 581–604.

Rosenthal, R. H., & Allen, T. W. (1980). Intratask distractibility in hyperkinetic and nonhyperkinetic children. *Journal of Abnormal Child Psychology, 8,* 175–187.

Rubia, K., Smith, A. B., Hafari, R., Matsukura, F., Mohammad, M., Taylor, E., et al. (2009). Disorder-specific dissociation of orbitofrontal dysfunction in boys with pure conduct disorder during reward and ventrolateral prefrontal dysfunction in boys with pure ADHD during sustained attention. *American Journal of Psychiatry, 166,* 83–94.

Shaw, G. A., & Giambra, L. M. (1993). Task-unrelated thoughts of college students diagnosed as hyperactive in childhood. *Developmental Neuropsychology, 9,* 17–30.

Shaw, P., Eckstrand, K., Sharp, W., Blumenthal, J., Lorch, L. P., Greenstein, D., et al. (2007). Attention-deficit/hyperactivity disorder is characterized by a delay in cortical maturation. *Proceedings of the National Academy of Sciences, 104,* 19649–19654.

Shelton, T. L., Barkley, R. A., Crosswait, C., Moorehouse, M., Fletcher, K., Barrett, S., et al. (1998). Psychiatric and psychological morbidity as a function of adaptive disability in preschool children with high levels of aggressive and hyperactive-impulsive-inattentive behavior. *Journal of Abnormal Child Psychology, 26,* 475–494.

Sieg, K. G., Gaffney, G. R., Preston, D. F., & Hellings, J. A. (1995). SPECT brain imaging abnormalities in attention deficit hyperactivity disorder. *Clinical Nuclear Medicine, 20,* 55–60.

Stein, M. A., Szumowski, E., Blondis, T. A., & Roizen, N. J. (1995). Adaptive skills dysfunction in ADD and ADHD children. *Journal of Child Psychology and Psychiatry, 36,* 663–670.

Stewart, M. A., Thach, B. T., & Friedin, M. R. (1970). Accidental poisoning and the hyperactive child syndrome. *Disease of the Nervous System, 31,* 403–407.

Still, G. F. (1902). Some abnormal psychical conditions in children. *Lancet, 1,* 1008–1012, 1077–1082, 1163–1168.

Tallmadge, J., & Barkley, R. A. (1983). The interactions of hyperactive and normal boys with their mothers and fathers. *Journal of Abnormal Child Psychology, 11,* 565–579.

Tannock, R. (1997). Television, videogames, and ADHD: Challenging a popular belief. *ADHD Report, 5*(3), 3–7.

Tucker, J. D., Suter, W., Petibone, D. M., Thomas, R. A., Bailey, N. L., Zhou, Y., et al. (2009). Cytogenetic assessment of methylphenidate treatment in patients treated for attention deficit hyperactivity disorder. *Mutation Research/Genetic Toxicology and Environmental Mutagenesis, 677,* 53–58.

Valera, E. M., Faraone, S. V., Murray, K. E., & Seidman, L. J. (2007). Meta-analysis of structural imaging findings in attention-deficit/hyperactivity disorder. *Biological Psychiatry, 61,* 1361–1369.

Warner, J. (2011). *We've got issues: Children and parents in the age of medication*. New York: Riverhead Trade.

Weiss, G., & Hechtman, L. T. (1993). *Hyperactive children grown up* (2nd ed.): *ADHD in children, adolescents, and adults.* New York: Guilford Press.

Whalen, C. K., Henker, B., Collins, B. E., McAuliffe, S., & Vaux, A. (1979). Peer interaction in structured communication task: Comparisons of normal and hyperactive boys and of methylphenidate (Ritalin) and placebo effects. *Child Development, 50,* 388–401.

Wilens, T. E., Faraone, S. V., Biederman, J., & Gunawardene, S. (2003). Does stimulant therapy of attention deficit/hyperactivity disorder beget later substance abuse? A meta-analytic review of the literature. *Pediatrics, 11*(1), 179–185.

Wolraich, M., Millich, R., Stumbo, P., & Schultz, F. (1985). The effects of sucrose ingestion on the behavior of hyperactive boys. *Pediatrics, 106,* 657–682.

Zametkin, A. J., Nordahl, T. E., Gross, M., King, A. C., Semple, W. E., Rumsey, J., et al. (1990). Cerebral glucose metabolism in adults with hyperactivity of childhood onset. *New England Journal of Medicine, 323,* 1361–1366.

Zentall, S. S., Falkenberg, S. D., & Smith, L. B. (1985). Effects of color stimulation and information on the copying performance of attention-problem adolescents. *Journal of Abnormal Child Psychology, 13,* 501–511.

Zentall, S. S., & Smith, Y. S. (1993). Mathematical performance and behavior of children with hyperactivity with and without coexisting aggression. *Behaviour Research and Therapy, 31,* 701–710.

Index

Academic achievement. *See also* School functioning
- adolescents and, 280–283
- diagnosis of ADHD and, 21
- medication and, 302
- other problems associated with ADHD and, 112–114
- stimulant treatment and, 298

Accepting a diagnosis, 153–154, 157
Activities, extracurricular, 222–223
Activity levels, 36, 45–48. *See also* Hyperactivity
Adaptive functioning, 117
Adderall. *See* Medication
Adderall XR. *See* Medication
ADDers.org, 328
Addiction, stimulant treatment and, 296–297
ADHD in general. *See also* Causes of ADHD; Diagnosis; Evaluating for ADHD; Information regarding ADHD
- activity level and, 45–48
- adolescent development and, 228–229
- challenges in parenting and, 5–6
- distractibility, 38–41
- executive functions and, 54–65
- facts versus fiction regarding, 22–25
- filtering information, 38
- following instructions, 48–51
- guiding principles for raising a child with ADHD, 158–168
- how many children have, 101–103
- impulse control and, 41–45
- inconsistent work performance, 51–52
- new view of ADHD, 52
- in other countries, 100–101
- other problems associated with ADHD, 112–118
- overview, 19–21, 34–52, 53–54, 119
- perspectives of ADHD and, 25–26
- sustaining attention, 36–38
- symptoms changing with the situation and, 108–112, 109*t*, 110*t*
- types of, 150–151

ADHD Information Services (ADDISS), 328
ADHD—predominantly inattentive type, 35–36, 150–151. *See also* Sluggish cognitive tempo (SCT)
Adolescents. *See also* Developmental processes
- ADHD changes with development and, 106
- communication with, 237–238, 238*t*
- coping attitudes and, 229–233, 231*t*
- "golden rules" for survival and, 227–228
- managing academic problems, 280–283
- medication and, 312
- overview, 226–227
- problem solving and, 238–243, 240*t*, 244
- rules and, 233–237
- stimulant treatment and, 297–298

Adults with ADHD, 107–108
Advocating for your child, 10–12. *See also* Communicating with schools and service providers
Aggression, 183–184, 221–222, 270
Alcohol use, 81–82, 128, 177
Allergies, myths regarding causes of ADHD and, 88–89
Amniotic fluid, 96
Anger, 153, 183–184
Animal studies, causes of ADHD and, 73–74
Anterior cingulate cortex, 80. *See also* Brain structure
Anticipation, 214–215, 264–265
Antidepressants, 293, 319–322, 322–323. *See also* Medication

Antihypertensive drugs, 316–318, 323–326. *See also* Medication
Anxiety, 311, 319–320, 325
Apologizing, principle-centered approach to parenting and, 9
Appearance, 116
Appetite, 305
Assignments. *See also* School functioning
  family relationships and, 286–287
  managing academic problems of adolescents and, 282–283
  priorities for parents and, 289–290
  school functioning and, 257–258
Attention, positive, 185–189, 190–191, 194–195
Attention Deficit Disorder in Europe, 328
Attention Deficit Disorders Association (ADDA)
  becoming a scientific parent and, 13
  educating yourself following a diagnosis, 156–157
  overview, 327
  school placement considerations and, 259
Attentional functioning, 36–38, 53–54, 56
Attitudes, 229–233, 231*t*
Attributions, 230, 231*t*
Authority, rules for adolescents and, 236
Awareness of moments, 175–176

B

Basal ganglia, 74, 77. *See also* Brain structure
Behavior improvement program. *See also* Behavioral problems; Parenting
  commands and, 191–193
  expanding your use of time outs step, 203–204
  future behavior problems and, 207–208
  give positive attention step, 185–189
  home token system, 195–198, 197*t*
  managing your child in public step, 204–208
  overview, 208–209
  punishing misbehavior constructively step, 198–203
  steps to better behavior, 181–184
  teaching your child not to interrupt your activities step, 193–195
  time-outs and, 200–204
  using attention to gain compliance step, 190–191
Behavior management, 265–273
Behavior rating cards in school, 224
Behavioral contracts, 244
Behavioral inhibition, 25, 60–62
Behavioral problems. *See also* Behavior improvement program
  choosing a teacher and, 254–256
  classroom and curriculum considerations and, 256–258
  guiding principles for raising a child with ADHD and, 158–168
  medication and, 302, 311
  other problems associated with ADHD and, 118
  responding to, 125–126
  school functioning and, 252
  steps to better behavior, 181–209
Behavioral report cards, 274–279, 282
Best or Worst Supervisor activity, 187
Biofeedback, 78
Birth complications, 95–96. *See also* Pregnancy
Blood pressure, 305
Boredom, 38, 40–41, 42
Brain activity, 76–80. *See also* Brain structure
Brain chemistry, 75–76. *See also* Brain structure
Brain electrical activity, 305–306
Brain injuries, 73–74, 310
Brain structure. *See also* Neurological factors
  brain development, 74–86
  brain injuries, 73–74, 310
  causes of ADHD and, 72–86, 98–99
  development of executive functions and, 69–70
  environmental agents and, 81–82
  how stimulants work, 300–304
  overview, 74–81
Brainstorming solutions, 211–212

C

Caffeine, 177
Candida albicans, 90–91
Careers. *See* Employment functioning
Caudate nucleus, 74, 77, 84–85. *See also* Brain structure
Causes of ADHD. *See also* ADHD in general
  brain development, 74–86
  brain injuries and, 73–74
  current evidence, 72–86
  environmental agents, 81–82
  facts versus fiction regarding, 22–23
  heredity, 83–86
  myths regarding, 86–94
  overview, 71–72, 98–99
  risk for developing ADHD and, 94–98
Centre for ADHD Awareness, Canada (CADDAC), 327
Cerebellum, 74. *See also* Brain structure

Checkup mode of treatment, 243
Chemical food additives, 86–87
Chemical substances, 177
Children and Adults with Attention-Deficit/ Hyperactivity Disorder (CHADD)
  becoming a scientific parent and, 13
  diagnosis of ADHD and, 21
  educating yourself following a diagnosis, 156–157
  overview, 327
  school placement considerations and, 259
Chore cards, 193
Classroom environments. *See also* School environment
  behavior management and, 265–273
  home-based reward programs and, 274–279
  overview, 256–258
  priorities for parents and, 289
  retaining children in their grade and, 262
  school management and, 263–265
Clonidine, 293, 323–326. *See also* Medication
Coaching, 282
Commands, 190–193
Communicating with schools and service providers, 10–12. *See also* Home–school communication; Professionals, working with
Communication, adolescents and, 227, 237–238, 238*t*
Communication skills
  adolescents and, 237–238, 238–243, 238*t*, 240*t*
  executive functions and, 65–68
  problem solving and, 238–243, 240*t*
  self-directed mental play and, 64–65
  self-directed speech and, 60–62
Community, 222–223, 233–237, 288
Compliance, 190–193, 204–205
Concentrating, 36–38, 53–54, 56
Concerta. *See* Medication
Conflict
  ADHD changes with development and, 105–106
  adolescents and, 227, 229–233, 231*t*, 238–243, 240*t*
  the affect ADHD has on parent–child interactions, 124–125
  improving behavior and, 181
  responding to misconduct and, 125–126
Congenital problems. *See* Medical problems
Consequences
  behavior management methods for the classroom and, 265–273
  guiding principles for raising a child with ADHD and, 159, 160–161
  home-based reward programs and, 275
  punishing misbehavior constructively step, 198–203
  rules for adolescents and, 236
  school management and, 264
  when/then strategies, 214–215
Consistency, 164–165, 264–265
Cooperation, 9–10, 68
Coping, 171–172
Corpus collosum, 74. *See also* Brain structure
Costs of professional help, 135
Counselors, 134, 280–281. *See also* Professionals, working with
Court system, 237
Covey, Dr. Stephen R., 6–10
Criticism, 186, 224, 272
Cultural factors, 23–24, 100–103
Curiosity, 39–40
Curriculum, 256–258, 262
Cylert, 304. *See also* Medication

D

D4RD gene, 85. *See also* Genetic factors
Dangerous behavior, 43–44, 229. *See also* Safety
DAT1 gene, 85. *See also* Genetic factors
Daytrana skin patch. *See* Medication
Deadlines, giving more effective commands and, 193
Deferred gratification, 40–41, 42
Defiance, 183–184
Demands, 229–230
Denial, 152–153
Depression, medication and, 319–320
Developmental processes
  ADHD changes with, 103–108
  adolescents and, 106, 228–229
  adults, 107–108
  brain development, 74–86
  evaluating for ADHD and, 132
  executive functions and, 68–70
  improving behavior and, 182, 184
  other problems associated with ADHD and, 114–115
  prenatal exposure to environmental agents and, 81–82
  preschool children, 103–104
  priorities and, 288–289
  retaining children in their grade, 260–262
  risk for developing ADHD and, 94–98
  school-age children, 104–106
  symptoms changing with the situation and, 110*t*

Dexedrine. *See* Medication
Diagnosis. *See also* Evaluating for ADHD
adults with ADHD and, 108
coping with, 152–157
educating yourself following a diagnosis, 155–157
facts versus fiction regarding, 22–25
how many children have ADHD, 101–103
improving behavior and, 184
medication and, 309–312
overview, 20–21, 148–151
sluggish cognitive tempo (SCT) and, 150–151
symptoms changing with the situation and, 108–112, 109*t*, 110*t*
treatment options and, 154–155
Diagnostic and Statistical Manual of Mental Disorders (5th ed.; DSM-5), 102–103, 135, 148–149
Dietary considerations, 86–89
Differential diagnosis, 148. *See also* Diagnosis
Direct instruction, 258
Disability
ADHD as, 19–20, 24–25
costs of professional help and, 135
guiding principles for raising a child with ADHD and, 166
Discipline, 198–203, 233–237. *See also* Consequences; Punishment
Distractibility, 36, 38–41. *See also* Attentional functioning; Sustaining attention
Doctors. *See* Physicans
Dopamine transporter mechanism, 76, 85. *See also* Brain structure
Driving safety
adolescents and, 106
diagnosis of ADHD and, 21
impulse control and, 43–44
self-directed imagery and, 59–60
Dropping out of school, 21, 49–50
Drug abuse, stimulant treatment and, 296–297

E

EEG (electroencephalography), 76–80, 78
Elavil. *See* Medication
Emotional problems, 118
Emotions, 62–64, 261–262, 302
Empathy, 157
Employment functioning, 49–50, 51–52, 107–108
Engagement in learning, 246
Environmental factors. *See also* Classroom environments; Family; School environment
causes of ADHD and, 81–82, 84, 91–94
symptoms changing with the situation and, 111
Evaluating for ADHD. *See also* Diagnosis; Treatment
costs of professional help, 135
making the diagnosis, 148–151
medical examination, 147–148
overview, 131, 138
preparing for, 139–151
seeking out professionals for, 133–138
what to expect from the evaluation, 142–147
when to seek out, 131–133
Executive functions
adolescent development and, 228
development of, 68–70
levels of, 65–68
other problems associated with ADHD and, 114
overview, 25–26, 36, 54–65
self-directed attention, 56
self-directed emotions, 62–64
self-directed imagery, 56–60
self-directed inhibition, 55–56
self-directed mental play, 64–65
self-directed speech, 50–51, 60–62
social purposes of, 65–68
Executive parenting, 10–12. *See also* Parenting
Exercise, 177
Expectations, 229–230, 229–233, 231*t*

F

Family. *See also* Interacting with your child; Parenting; Relationship with your child
ADHD changes with development and, 105
the affect ADHD has on parent–child interactions, 124–125
challenges in, 5–6
fathers and their interactions with children with ADHD and, 124
improving behavior and, 181
lessons in family life, 286–287
mothers and their interactions with children with ADHD and, 122–124
myths regarding causes of ADHD and, 91–94
overview, 120–122, 128
parental mental health, 126–128
priorities and, 288–290
responding to misconduct and, 125–126
risk for developing ADHD and, 94–95

Fearfulness, 311
Fears of parents, 230, 231*t*
Feedback
behavior management methods for the classroom and, 265–273
guiding principles for raising a child with ADHD and, 159–160
school management and, 264
Fetch commands, 190–191. *See also* Commands
Filtering information, 38
Financial difficulties, 44
Fining your child, 199–200, 269–270. *See also* Consequences; Punishment
FMRI (functional magnetic resonance imaging), 79
Focalin. *See* Medication
Following instructions, 48–51. *See also* Commands
Food allergies, 88–89
Foresight
development of, 69
other problems associated with ADHD and, 114
overview, 25
self-directed imagery, 57, 58
Forgiveness, 167–168
Friendships, 118–119, 220–222. *See also* Peer relationships; Social skills
Frontal regions of the brain, 74. *See also* Brain structure
Future, fear of, 58

G

Gender, 94–95, 102–103
Genetic factors, 83–86, 147. *See also* Causes of ADHD
Goals, 7, 268
Graduating high school, 21, 49–50. *See also* School functioning
Grandma's rule, 214–215
Gratification delay. *See* Deferred gratification
Grief, coping with a diagnosis and, 153
Group programs, behavior management methods for the classroom and, 267–268

H

Health
diagnosis of ADHD and, 21
medical examination and, 147–148
other problems associated with ADHD and, 115, 116–117
priorities and, 288–289
stimulant treatment and, 298–299
symptoms changing with the situation and, 110*t*
Hearing, 115
Heart rate, 305, 320–321, 324–325
Heredity, 83–86, 147. *See also* Causes of ADHD
Hindsight, 36, 58, 114
History of ADHD, 27–36
Hobbies, self-care for parents and, 174
Home point system, 196–198, 218–219, 236
Home Situations Questionnaire, 140, 141*f*
Home-based reward programs, 274–279
Home-school communication, 10–12, 252–253, 274–279. *See also* Professionals, working with; School environment
Homework, 282–283, 286–287, 289–290. *See also* Assignments; School functioning
Hormones, myths regarding causes of ADHD and, 89–90
Humiliation, peer relationships and, 224
Hyperactivity, 35–36, 45–48. *See also* Activity levels
Hyperreactivity, 47–48. *See also* Activity levels; Reactiveness
Hypothetical futures, 57. *See also* Imagery

I

Ignoring, behavior management methods for the classroom and, 268–269
Imagery, 56–60
Impulse control, 36, 41–45, 62–64
Impulsivity, 6–10, 35–36, 45, 229
Inattentiveness, 35–36
Incentives. *See also* Reward
behavior management methods for the classroom and, 265–273
guiding principles for raising a child with ADHD and, 161–162
home token/point system and, 195–198, 197*t*
managing your child in public and, 204–205
rules for adolescents and, 236
school management and, 264
social skills and, 218–219
when/then strategies, 214–215
Inconsistent work performance, 51–52
Independence, adolescent development and, 228
Individual attention, 111

Individualized education program (IEP), 253–254
Individuals with Disabilities Education Act (IDEA), 258–260
Infancy, 96. *See also* Developmental processes
Information regarding ADHD. *See also* ADHD in general
- becoming a scientific parent and, 12–14
- choosing a teacher and, 253–254
- educating yourself following a diagnosis, 155–157
- evaluating for ADHD and, 132
- school functioning and, 258–260
- sources for, 327–328

Inhibition
- development of, 68–69, 69–70
- impulse control and, 41
- overview, 36, 53–54
- self-directed imagery and, 58
- self-directed inhibition, 55–56

Insomnia, 306, 317. *See also* Sleeping problems
Instructions, following, 48–51. *See also* Commands
Instrumental/self-directed level of executive functioning, 66–67. *See also* Executive functions
Insurance, 135
Intelligence, 112, 310
Interacting with your child. *See also* Family; Parenting; Relationship with your child
- adolescents and, 227, 229, 237–238, 238*t*
- the affect ADHD has on, 124–125
- challenges in, 100
- fathers and their interactions with children with ADHD and, 124
- following instructions and, 48–51
- improving behavior and, 181
- lessons in family life, 286–287
- mothers and their interactions with children with ADHD and, 122–124
- myths regarding causes of ADHD and, 91–94
- principle-centered approach to parenting and, 8–10
- priorities and, 288–290
- responding to misconduct and, 125–126

Interest levels, 53–54
Internalization, 63–64
Internalized speech. *See* Self-directed speech
Interpersonal skills, 288. *See also* Social skills
Interruptions, 193–195
Intuniv, 316–318. *See also* Medication
Irritability, adolescents and, 229
Isolation, 221–222, 270

K

Khan Academy, 265, 283
Knowledge, becoming a scientific parent and, 12–13

L

Large Time Timer, 162
Lead exposure, 82. *See also* Causes of ADHD
Learning, medication and, 302
Learning disabilities, 113–114, 128, 155
Learning Disabilities Association of American (LDA), 327
"Least restrictive environment," 259–260
Legal rights, 137, 237, 258–260
Listening ability, 48–51
Listening to your child, 9

M

Mannerisms, 306–307
Maturity level
- adolescent development and, 228–229
- deferred gratification and, 40
- following instructions and, 49–50
- retaining children in their grade, 260–262

Medadate CD. *See* Medication
Media, 93–94, 221, 287
Medical examination, 147–148. *See also* Evaluating for ADHD
Medical problems
- diagnosis of ADHD and, 21
- medical examination and, 147–148
- other problems associated with ADHD and, 115, 116–117
- sluggish cognitive tempo (SCT) and, 151
- stimulant treatment and, 298–299
- symptoms changing with the situation and, 110*t*

Medication. *See also* Treatment
- antihypertensive drugs, 316–318
- brain chemistry and, 75–76
- Clonidine, 323–326
- decisions regarding, 309–312
- facts versus fiction regarding, 24–25
- how stimulants are prescribed, 312–314
- how stimulants work, 300–304
- Intuniv, 316–318
- myths regarding, 294–300
- overview, 293
- peer relationships and, 223

seeking out professionals for evaluation and, 133–134
side effects of, 304–309, 320–322, 324–325
stimulants, 293–304
Strattera, 314–316
treatment options and, 154–155
tricyclic antidepressants, 319–322
Wellbutrin, 322–323
what to look for in a school and, 252
when to stop, 314
Meditation, 171, 175–176
Memory
guiding principles for raising a child with ADHD and, 163
other problems associated with ADHD and, 114
self-directed imagery, 56–60
working memory, 36, 57
Mental abilities, 114
Mental health
brain activity in ADHD and, 79–80
other problems associated with ADHD and, 118
of parents, 126–128
treatment options and, 155
Mentors, managing academic problems of adolescents and, 282
Meta-analysis, 74
Military service, 299
Mindfulness meditation, self-care for parents and, 175–176
Money problems, impulse control and, 44
Monitoring, 218–219, 221, 234–237
Mood disorders, 128
Moodiness, adolescents and, 229
Moral development, 288
Motion sickness, myths regarding causes of ADHD and, 90
Motivation
choosing a teacher and, 254
guiding principles for raising a child with ADHD and, 163–164
school functioning and, 246
self-directed emotions and, 63–64
Motor skills, 115–116
Mutualism, 68
Myths regarding ADHD
causes of ADHD and, 86–94
overview, 22–25
stimulant treatment and, 294–300

N

"Nag tapes," 257
Negotiation, 8–9
Nervous tics, 306–307, 322
Neurofeedback, 78
Neurological factors, 69–70. *See also* Brain structure
Neurotransmitters, 75–76. *See also* Brain structure
Nonstimulant medications, 75–76. *See also* Medication
Nonverbal signs of approval, 188. *See also* Positive feedback
Nonverbal working memory, 57. *See also* Memory
Norepinephrine, 76, 314–316. *See also* Brain structure
Norpramin. *See* Medication

O

Obeying, 190–193. *See also* Commands
ODD (oppositional defiant disorder), 27–29, 28, 98, 183
Online sources of information, 13–14, 156, 328. *See also* Information regarding ADHD
Oppositional behavior, 183–184

P

Parenting. *See also* Behavior improvement program; Family; Interacting with your child; Relationship with your child; Self-care for parents
adolescents and, 229–233, 231*t*, 233–237, 238–243, 240*t*
challenges in, 5–6, 100
executive parents, 10–12
guiding principles for, 158–168
improving behavior and, 181–182
lessons in family life, 286–287
myths regarding causes of ADHD and, 91–94
overview, 128
parental mental health, 126–128
principle-centered parents, 6–10
priorities and, 288–290
responding to misconduct and, 125–126
risk for developing ADHD and, 94–95
rules for adolescents and, 233–237
school management and, 265
scientific parents, 12–14
sharing, 145
Paying attention, 36–38, 53–54, 56
Peer relationships. *See also* Friendships; Social skills
behavior management methods for the classroom and, 267–268, 273

Peer relationships (*cont.*)
other problems associated with ADHD and, 118–119
overview, 216–217
positive peer contacts in the community, 222–223
school involvement in, 223–225
setting up positive peer contacts at home, 220–222
social skills and, 217–219
teasing and, 219–220
Penalties, 269–270. *See also* Fining your child
Personality, risk for developing ADHD and, 97
Pertofrane. *See* Medication
PET (positron emission tomography) scans, 79
Physical appearance, 116
Physical development, 114–115. *See also* Developmental processes
Physicians. *See also* Professionals, working with
Clonidine, 325–326
how stimulants are prescribed, 312–314
Intuniv, 317–318
medication and, 295
seeking out professionals for evaluation and, 133–134
Strattera, 315
Physicians' Desk Reference (PDR), 293–294. *See also* Medication
Placement considerations, 258–260. *See also* School functioning; Special education programs
Planning ahead, 165–166
Point of performance, 163–164
Point system
behavior management methods for the classroom and, 265–273
overview, 196–198
rules for adolescents and, 236
social skills and, 218–219
Police, rules for adolescents and, 237
Popularity, 220–222. *See also* Peer relationships
Positive attention, 185–189, 190–191, 194–195
Positive feedback, 159–160, 185–189
Praise
behavior management methods for the classroom and, 265–266
social skills and, 218
steps to better behavior and, 185–189
teaching your child not to interrupt your activities step, 194–195
using attention to gain compliance step, 191
Prefrontal region, 80, 84–85. *See also* Brain structure
Pregnancy, 81–82, 95–96, 115
Premack principle, 214–215
Prenatal development, 81–82, 95–96. *See also* Developmental processes
Preschool years, 97–98, 103–104, 186. *See also* Developmental processes
Preservatives in foods, myths regarding causes of ADHD and, 86–87
Prevalence of ADHD, 101–103. *See also* ADHD in general
Principle-centered approach to parenting. *See also* Parenting
becoming a principle-centered parent, 6–10
evaluating for ADHD and, 149
guiding principles for raising a child with ADHD and, 158–168
self-care for parents and, 173–174
Priorities
principle-centered approach to parenting and, 7–88
self-care for parents and, 173–174
Privileges
home token/point system and, 195–198, 197*t*
when/then strategies, 214–215
Proactiveness, becoming an executive parent and, 11
Problem solving
adolescents and, 227, 238–243, 240*t*, 244
guiding principles for raising a child with ADHD and, 164
overview, 210–213
preparing your child for transitions, 213–214
rules for adolescents and, 233–234
self-directed mental play, 64–65
when/then strategies, 214–215
Productivity, diagnosis of ADHD and, 21
Professionals, working with. *See also* Evaluating for ADHD; Home–school communication; Treatment
adolescents and, 228, 236–237, 243, 281–282
becoming an executive parent and, 10–12
choosing a teacher and, 253–256
Clonidine, 325–326
costs of professional help, 135
how stimulants are prescribed, 312–314
Intuniv, 317–318
medication and, 295
overview, 10–12
seeking out professionals for evaluation, 133–138

Strattera, 315
what to look for in a school and, 252–253
Psychiatric disorders
brain activity in ADHD and, 79–80
improving behavior and, 184
medication and, 311
other problems associated with ADHD and, 118
parental, 126–128
treatment options and, 155
Psychologists, 134. *See also* Professionals, working with
Psychosis, 307, 311, 321
Puberty, 229, 297–298. *See also* Adolescents; Developmental processes
Public areas, 204–208, 214
Punishment. *See also* Consequences
behavior management methods for the classroom and, 265–273
incentives instead of, 161–162
managing your child in public and, 205–207
punishing misbehavior constructively step, 198–203
school management and, 264

R

Reactions to a diagnosis, 152–154
Reactiveness, 7, 47–48, 58. *See also* Activity levels; Hyperreactivity
Reflection, 50–51
Rejection, peer relationships and, 221–222
Relationship with your child. *See also* Family; Interacting with your child; Parenting
challenges in, 100
improving behavior and, 181
lessons in family life, 286–287
myths regarding causes of ADHD and, 91–94
principle-centered approach to parenting and, 8–10
priorities and, 288–290
responding to misconduct and, 125–126
Relationships. *See* Relationship with your child; Relationships with peers; Teacher–student relationship
Relationships with peers. *See also* Social skills
other problems associated with ADHD and, 118–119
overview, 216–217
positive peer contacts in the community, 222–223
school involvement in, 223–225
setting up positive peer contacts at home, 220–222
social skills and, 217–219
teasing and, 219–220
Relaxation, self-care for parents and, 171
Relief, coping with a diagnosis and, 152–153
Reminders, 163
Renewal, 10, 172–174
Reprimands, 269
Resistance, 183–184
Response cost, 269–270. *See also* Fining your child
Response inhibition
development of, 69–70
self-directed emotions, 62–64
self-directed imagery and, 58
self-directed inhibition, 55–56
self-directed speech and, 51
Responsibilities, 8, 224
Reward. *See also* Positive attention
behavior management methods for the classroom and, 265–273
distractibility and, 39
guiding principles for raising a child with ADHD and, 160, 161–162
home token/point system and, 195–198, 197*t*
school management and, 264
social skills and, 218–219
steps to better behavior and, 185–189
when/then strategies, 214–215
Right hemisphere of the brain, 74. *See also* Brain structure
Risk factors, 94–98. *See also* Causes of ADHD
Risk taking, 43–44, 229. *See also* Safety
Ritalin. *See* Medication
Routine, 256–258
Ruination, adolescent "attitudes" and, 230, 231*t*
Rule-governed behavior, 60–62
Rules
adolescents and, 227, 233–237
behavior management methods for the classroom and, 265–273
classroom and curriculum considerations and, 256–258
following instructions and, 48–51
giving more effective commands and, 191–193
guiding principles for raising a child with ADHD and, 166
managing your child in public and, 204
self-directed speech and, 60–62
time-outs and, 271
using attention to gain compliance step, 190–191

S

Safety
  adolescents and, 106, 226–227
  diagnosis of ADHD and, 21
  impulse control and, 43–44
  self-directed imagery and, 59–60
Schedule, classroom and curriculum considerations and, 256–258
School environment. *See also* Professionals, working with; School functioning
  behavior management methods for the classroom and, 265–273
  classroom and curriculum considerations and, 256–258
  evaluating for ADHD and, 136–138
  home-based reward programs and, 274–279
  school management, 263–265
  seeking out professionals for evaluation and, 136–138
  what to look for in a school, 247–253
  working with schools, 10–12
School functioning. *See also* Academic achievement; School environment; Teacher–student relationship
  ADHD changes with development and, 105
  adolescents and, 280–283
  case examples, 27–34
  choosing a teacher and, 253–256
  diagnosis of ADHD and, 21
  family relationships and, 286–287
  following instructions and, 49–50
  home-based reward programs and, 274–279
  inconsistent work performance, 51–52
  managing academic problems, 280–283
  medication and, 302
  other problems associated with ADHD and, 112–114
  overview, 246–247
  peer relationships and, 223–225
  placement considerations, 258–260
  preschool children, 104
  priorities for parents and, 288–290
  retaining children in their grade, 260–262
  school management, 263–265
  self-directed instruction and, 279–280
  symptoms changing with the situation and, 111
  what to look for in a school, 247–253
School-age children, 104–106, 186. *See also* Developmental processes
Scientific parenting, 12–14, 132, 155–157. *See also* Parenting
Scouts, 222–223
Seizures, 321
Self-awareness
  development of, 68–69
  overview, 36
  self-directed attention, 56
  self-directed imagery and, 56–60
  self-directed speech and, 60–62
Self-care for parents. *See also* Parenting
  adolescents and, 244–245
  coping with the inevitable and, 171–172
  overview, 169–177
  personal renewal and, 172–174
  principle-centered approach to parenting and, 10
  stressful events and, 169–172
  time management and, 173–174
Self-care skills, 117
Self-control
  executive functions and, 54–65
  new view of ADHD and, 52
  self-directed emotions and, 63–64
  self-directed inhibition, 55–56
  self-directed instruction and, 279–280
  social purposes of, 65–68
Self-directed instructions, 279–280
Self-directed speech, 50–51, 60–62, 69
Self-esteem, 29–31
Self-help skills, 117
Self-monitoring, 36, 68–69
Self-motivation, 63–64
Self-organization, 25
Self-regulation, 25–26, 36, 65–68
Self-reliant level of executive functioning, 67. *See also* Executive functions
Self-restraint, 41
Sense of humor, adolescents and, 244–245
Shortcuts, impulse control and, 43
Shortsightedness, impulse control and, 43–44
Siblings, 127–128
Side effects of medication. *See also* Medication
  Clonidine, 324–325
  stimulant treatment and, 304–309
  Strattera, 315, 316
  tricyclic antidepressants, 320–322
Sleeping problems
  other problems associated with ADHD and, 116–117
  as a side effect of medication, 306, 317, 324–325
Sluggish cognitive tempo (SCT), 36, 150–151. *See also* ADHD—predominantly inattentive type

Smoking, 81–82, 95–96, 177
Social conflict, 105–106
Social cooperative level of executive functioning, 68. *See also* Executive functions
Social development, 26. *See also* Developmental processes
Social isolation, 270. *See also* Isolation; Time-outs
Social reciprocity level of executive functioning, 67–68. *See also* Executive functions
Social skills
ADHD changes with development and, 105–106
executive functions and, 65–68
medication and, 303
other problems associated with ADHD and, 118–119
overview, 217
priorities and, 288
retaining children in their grade, 261–262
school functioning and, 246
working on, 217–219
Social skills training group, 224
Social support, self-care for parents and, 174–175. *See also* Support groups
Special education programs. *See also* School functioning
adolescents and, 280–281
peer relationships and, 223–224
placement considerations, 258–260
Speech. *See also* Self-directed speech
development of, 69
other problems associated with ADHD and, 115
self-directed mental play and, 64–65
Splenium, 74. *See also* Brain structure
Sports, 222–223
SSRIs (selective serotonin reuptake inhibitors), 320. *See also* Medication
Stimulant treatment. *See also* Medication; Treatment
brain chemistry and, 75–76
decisions regarding, 309–312
how stimulants are prescribed, 312–314
how stimulants work, 300–304
myths regarding, 294–300
overview, 293–294
side effects of, 304–309
treatment options and, 154–155
when to stop, 314
Strattera, 314–316. *See also* Medication
Stress, 127, 169–172
Striatum, 77, 80. *See also* Brain structure
Structure, classroom and curriculum considerations and, 256–258
Student–teacher relationship. *See* Teacher–student relationship
Study skills, 246
Sugar consumption, myths regarding causes of ADHD and, 87–88
Suicide, medication and, 323
Support groups
becoming a scientific parent and, 13
diagnosis of ADHD and, 21
educating yourself following a diagnosis, 156–157
overview, 327–328
school placement considerations and, 259
seeking out professionals for evaluation and, 133
self-care for parents and, 145
sources for, 327–328
Supporting your child, 9, 31–33. *See also* Relationship with your child
Suspension from school, 271
Sustaining attention, 36–38, 53–54, 56
Symptoms of ADHD. *See also* ADHD in general; Diagnosis
changes in based on the situation, 108–112, 109*t*, 110*t*
other problems associated with ADHD, 112–118
Synapse functioning, 76, 85. *See also* Brain structure
Synergy, 9–10

T

Taking a break, adolescents and, 244–245
Taking care of yourself. *See* Self-care for parents
Taking turns, impulse control and, 41
Teachers. *See also* Classroom environments; School environment; Teacher–student relationship
behavior management methods for the classroom and, 265–273
choosing, 253–256
managing academic problems of adolescents and, 280–283
school management and, 264–265
symptoms changing with the situation and, 111
what to expect from the evaluation, 146–147
Teacher–student relationship, 247, 262, 281–282. *See also* Relationships; School functioning; Teachers
Teasing, dealing with, 219–220
Teens. *See* Adolescents

Television watching, 93–94, 221, 287
Temperament, 97
The Seven Habits of Highly Effective People (Covey), 6–10
Therapists, 134, 236–237. *See also* Professionals, working with
Thoughts
  guiding principles for raising a child with ADHD and, 164
  impulsive thinking, 45
  school management and, 279–280
  self-care for parents and, 176–177
  self-directed instruction and, 279–280
  self-directed speech and, 50–51
Thyroid hormone levels, 89–90
Tics, 306–307, 322
Time management, 25, 162–163, 173–174
Time-outs. *See also* Consequences; Punishment
  behavior management methods for the classroom and, 270–271
  expanding your use of, 203–204
  managing your child in public and, 206–207
  overview, 200–203
Toddler years, 96. *See also* Developmental processes
Tofranil. *See* Medication
Token system
  behavior management methods for the classroom and, 265–273
  overview, 195–198, 197*t*
  school management and, 264
  social skills and, 218–219
Tourette syndrome, 306–307
Toxin exposure, 81–82. *See also* Causes of ADHD
Transitions, 213–214
Treatment. *See also* Evaluating for ADHD; Medication
  adolescents and, 228, 243
  adults with ADHD and, 108
  costs of professional help, 135
  decisions regarding, 309–312
  EEG biofeedback or neurofeedback, 78
  facts versus fiction regarding, 24–25
  in other countries, 100–101
  school environment and, 136–138
  sluggish cognitive tempo (SCT) and, 151
  understanding the options for, 154–155
  what to expect from the evaluation, 142–147
  when to stop, 314
Treatment providers, 10–12. *See also* Communicating with schools and service providers
Tricyclic antidepressants, 319–322. *See also* Medication
Trust, 9. *See also* Relationship with your child
Tutoring, 265, 282–283

V

Verbal signs of approval, 188–189. *See also* Positive feedback
Vestibular system, 90
Video games, 287
Vision, 115
Visualization, 56–60
Vitamins in treatment, myths regarding causes of ADHD and, 88–89
Vyvanse. *See* Medication

W

Waiting for things, impulse control and, 41
Warnings, preparing your child for transitions and, 213–214
WatchMinder wrist watch, 162
Websites, 13–14, 156, 328. *See also* Information regarding ADHD
Wellbutrin, 322–323. *See also* Medication
When/then strategies, 214–215
Work functioning. *See* Employment functioning
Working memory. *See also* Memory
  guiding principles for raising a child with ADHD and, 163
  other problems associated with ADHD and, 114
  overview, 36
Worst-case scenario, adolescent "attitudes" and, 232–233

Y

Yeasts, myths regarding causes of ADHD and, 90–91

About the Author

Russell A. Barkley, PhD, ABPP, ABCN, is Clinical Professor of Psychiatry at the Virginia Treatment Center for Children and Virginia Commonwealth University School of Medicine. Dr. Barkley has worked with children, adolescents, and families since the 1970s and is the author of numerous bestselling books for both professionals and the public, including *Taking Charge of Adult ADHD.* A frequent conference presenter and speaker who is widely cited in the national media, Dr. Barkley is a recipient of awards from the American Academy of Pediatrics and the American Psychological Association, among other honors. His website is *www.russellbarkley.org.*

About the Authors